IMMUNOCYTOCHEMISTRY IN TUMOR DIAGNOSIS

DEVELOPMENTS IN ONCOLOGY

F.J. Cleton and J.W.I.M. Simons, eds.: Genetic Origins of Tumour Cells. 90-247-2272-1.
J. Aisner and P. Chang, eds.: Cancer Treatment and Research. 90-247-2358-2.
B.W. Ongerboer de Visser, D.A. Bosch and W.M.H. van Woerkom-Eykenboom, eds.: Neuro-oncology: Clinical and Experimental Aspects. 90-247-2421-X.
K. Hellmann, P. Hilgard and S. Eccles, eds.: Metastasis: Clinical and Experimental Aspects. 90-247-2424-4.
H.F. Seigler, ed.: Clinical Management of Melanoma. 90-247-2584-4.
P. Correa and W. Haenszel, eds.: Epidemiology of Cancer of the Digestive Tract. 90-247-2601-8.
L.A. Liotta and I.R. Hart, eds.: Tumour Invasion and Metastasis. 90-247-2611-5.
J. Banoczy, ed.: Oral Leukoplakia. 90-247-2655-7.
C. Tijssen, M. Halprin and L. Endtz, eds.: Familial Brain Tumours. 90-247-2691-3.
F.M. Muggia, C.W. Young and S.K. Carter, eds.: Anthracycline Antibiotics in Cancer. 90-247-2711-1.
B.W. Hancock, ed.: Assessment of Tumour Response. 90-247-2712-X.
D.E. Peterson, ed.: Oral Complications of Cancer Chemotherapy. 0-89838-563-6.
R. Mastrangelo, D.G. Poplack and R. Riccardi, eds.: Central Nervous System Leukemia. Prevention and Treatment. 0-89838-570-9.
A. Polliack, ed.: Human Leukemias. Cytochemical and Ultrastructural Techniques in Diagnosis and Research. 0-89838-585-7.
W. Davis, C. Maltoni and S. Tanneberger, eds.: The Control of Tumor Growth and its Biological Bases. 0-89838-603-9.
A.P.M. Heintz, C. Th. Griffiths and J.B. Trimbos, eds.: Surgery in Gynecological Oncology. 0-89838-604-7.
M.P. Hacker, E.B. Double and I. Krakoff, eds.: Platinum Coordination Complexes in Cancer Chemotherapy. 0-89838-619-5.
M.J. van Zwieten. The Rat as Animal Model in Breast Cancer Research: A Histopathological Study of Radiation- and Hormone-Induced Rat Mammary Tumors. 0-89838-624-1.
B. Löwenberg and A. Hogenbeck, eds.: Minimal Residual Disease in Acute Leukemia. 0-89838-630-6.
I. van der Waal and G.B. Snow, eds.: Oral Oncology. 0-89838-631-4.
B.W. Hancock and A.M. Ward, eds.: Immunological Aspects of Cancer. 0-89838-664-0.
K.V. Honn and B.F. Sloane, eds.: Hemostatic Mechanisms and Metastasis. 0-89838-667-5.
K.R. Harrap, W. Davis and A.N. Calvert, eds.: Cancer Chemotherapy and Selective Drug Development. 0-89838-673-X.
V.D. Velde, J.H. Cornelis and P.H. Sugarbaker, eds.: Liver Metastasis. 0-89838-648-5.
D.J. Ruiter, K. Welvaart and S. Ferrone, eds.: Cutaneous Melanoma and Precursor Lesions. 0-89838-689-6.
S.B. Howell, ed.: Intra-Arterial and Intracavitary Cancer Chemotherapy. 0-89838-691-8.
D.L. Kisner and J.F. Smyth, eds.: Interferon Alpha-2: Pre-Clinical and Clinical Evaluation. 0-89838-701-9.
P. Furmanski, J.C. Hager and M.A. Rich, eds.: RNA Tumor Viruses, Oncogenes, Human Cancer and Aids: On the Frontiers of Understanding. 0-89838-703-5.
J.E. Talmadge, I.J. Fidler and R.K. Oldham: Screening for Biological Response Modifiers: Methods and Rationale. 0-89838-712-4.
J.C. Bottino, R.W. Opfell and F.M. Muggia, eds.: Liver Cancer. 0-89838-713-2.
P.K. Pattengale, R.J. Lukes and C.R. Taylor, eds.: Lymphoproliferative Diseases: Pathogenesis, Diagnosis, Therapy. 0-89838-725-6.
F. Cavalli, G. Bonadonna and M. Rozencweig, eds.: Malignant Lymphomas and Hodgkin's Disease. 0-89838-727-2.
L. Baker, F. Valeriote and V. Ratanatharathorn, eds.: Biology and Therapy of Acute Leukemia. 0-89838-728-0.

IMMUNOCYTOCHEMISTRY IN TUMOR DIAGNOSIS

Proceedings of the Workshop on
Immunocytochemistry in Tumor Diagnosis
Detroit, Michigan—October 3-5, 1984

edited by

Jose Russo
Michigan Cancer Foundation

Springer-Science+Business Media, B.V.

Library of Congress Cataloging in Publication Data

Workshop on Immunocytochemistry in Tumor Diagnosis
(1984 : Detroit, Mich.)
Immunocytochemistry in tumor diagnosis.

(Developments in oncology)
Includes bibliographies.
1. Immunocytochemistry—Congresses. 2. Tumor markers—Analysis—Congresses. 3. Cancer cells—Identification—Congresses. 4. Cancer—Diagnosis—Congresses. I. Russo, Jose. II. Title. III. Series. [DNLM: 1. Diagnosis, Differential—congresses. 2. Histocytochemistry—congresses. 3. Immunochemistry—congresses. 4. Neoplasms—diagnosis—congresses.
W1 DE998N / QZ 241 W9258i 1984]
RC270.3.I44W67 1984 616.99'20756 85-10523

ISBN 978-1-4612-9636-2 ISBN 978-1-4613-2615-1 (eBook)
DOI 10.1007/978-1-4613-2615-1

Originally published by Martinus Nijhoff Publishing in 1985
Softcover reprint of the hardcover 1st edition 1985

Dedicated to:
MY PARENTS

CONTENTS

CONTRIBUTORS x

PREFACE xiii

ACKNOWLEDGEMENTS xv

Chapter 1
Organization of an Immunocytochemistry Laboratory 1
I. H. Russo

Chapter 2
Principles of Immunocytochemistry 12
L. A. Sternberger and N. H. Sternberger

Chapter 3
Use of Diagnostic Algorithms in Immunocytochemistry 21
A. E. Sherrod and C. R. Taylor

Chapter 4
Monoclonal Antibodies in Immunocytochemistry 31
H. Battifora

Chapter 5
Markers of Keratinocyte Differentiation in Preneoplastic and Neoplastic Lesions 59
C. J. Conti, G. I. Fernandez Alonso and A. J. P. Klein-Szanto

Chapter 6
Intermediate Filaments 72
R. J. Cote, T. M. Thomson and C. Cordon-Cardo

Chapter 7
Immunodiagnosis of Lymphoid and Mononuclear Phagocytic Neoplasms 83
E. S. Jaffe and J. Cossman

Chapter 8
Immunohistochemistry of Lymphomas in Frozen Tissue Sections 116
R. R. Tubbs

Chapter 9
The Use of Immunocytochemical Techniques in the Diagnosis of Lymphoreticular Proliferations 141
A. A. Giraldo and J. M. Meis

Chapter 10
Immunohistochemistry of Neuroendocrine Neoplasms of the Bronchopulmonary Tract and Skin 174
I. Lee, W. W. Franke, and V. E. Gould

Chapter 11
Immunocytology of Endocrine Tumors 183
K. Kovacs

Chapter 12
Immunocytochemical Demonstration of Cardionatrins in Human Atrial Myocardium 202
M. L. de Bold and A. J. de Bold

Chapter 13
Immunocytochemical Markers in Breast Cancer 207
J. Russo

Chapter 14
Immunocytochemical Studies in Breast Cancer Using Monoclonal Antibodies Against Breast Epithelial Cell Components and with Lectins 233
R. L. Ceriani, D. L. Hill, L. Osvaldo, C. Kandell and E. W. Blank

Chapter 15
Immunocytochemical Localization of Estrogen Receptors with Monoclonal Antibodies 264
G. L. Greene, W. J. King and M. F. Press

Chapter 16
Immunocytochemistry of an Estrogen-Regulated Protein (28K) in Estrogen Target Cells and Tissues 268
D. R. Ciocca

Chapter 17
Monoclonal Antibodies in the Diagnosis of Solid Tumors: Studies on Renal Carcinomas, Transitional Cell Carcinomas, and Melanoma 281
C. Cordon-Cardo

Chapter 18
Immunohistochemistry of Ovarian Tumors 293
R. E. Scully

Chapter 19
Immunopathology of Testicular Tumors 321
F. K. Mostofi, I. A. Sesterhenn and C. J. Davis, Jr.

Chapter 20
Immunopathology in Prostate and Bladder Tumors 337
I. Sesterhenn, F. K. Mostofi and C. J. Davis, Jr.

Chapter 21
Immunochemistry of Soft Tissue Tumors 362
A. R. Morales, E. W. Gould and M. Nadji

Chapter 22
A Review of DNA Flow Cytometric Preparatory and Analytical Methods 380
J. T. Thornthwaite, R. A. Thomas, J. Russo, H. Ownby, G. I. Malinin, F. J. Hornicek, T. W. Woolley, J. Frederick, T. I. Malinin, D. A. Vazquez and D. Seckinger

INDEX 399

CONTRIBUTORS:

H. BATTIFORA, M.D., Division Pathology, City of Hope National Medical Center, Duarte, CA 91010.

E.W. BLANK, Ph.D., Department of Pathology, John Muir Memorial Hospital, 2055 North Broadway, Walnut Creek, CA 94596.

R.L. CERIANI, M.D., Ph.D., John Muir Cancer and Aging Research Institute, 2055 North Broadway, Walnut Creek, CA 94596.

D.R. CIOCCA, M.D., Laboratorio de Reproduccion y Lactancia (LARLAC), Casilla de Correo 855, Mendoza 5500, Argentina.

C.J. CONTI, Ph.D, The University of Texas Science Park, Research Division, P.O. Box 389, Smithville, Texas 78957.

R. COTE, Ph.D., Department of Pathology, Memorial Sloan-Kettering Cancer Center, New York, NY 10021.

C. CORDON-CARDO, M.D., Ph.D., Department of Pathology Memorial Sloan-Kettering Cancer Center, New York, NY 10021

J. COSSMAN, M.D., Hematopathology Section, Laboratory of Pathology, National Cancer Institute, National institute of Health, Bethesda, MD 20205.

C.J. DAVIS, M.D., Department of Genitourinary Pathology, Armed Forces Institute of Pathology, Washington, DC 20306.

A. J. de BOLD, Ph.D., Department of Pathology, Queen's University Hotel-Dieu Hospital, Kington, Ontario, Canada K7L3H6.

M.L. de BOLD, Ph.D., Department of Pathology, Queen's University, Hotel-Dieu Hospital, Kington, Ontario, Canada K7L3H6

G.I. FERNANDEZ ALONSO, Ph.D., Centro de Estudio Oncologicos, Academia Nacional de Medicina, Buenos Aires, Argentina.

W.W. FRANKE, M.D., Department of Pathology, Rush Medical College, Rush-Presbyterian-St Luke's Medical Center, 1753 West Congress Parkway, Chicago, IL 60612.

J. FREDERICK, Ph.D., Department of Epidemiology, Michigan Cancer Foundation, 110 E. Warren Ave., Detroit, MI. 48201.

A.A. GIRALDO, M.D., Department of Pathology, St. John Hospital, Detroit, MI 48236.

E.W. GOULD, M.D., Department of Pathology, University of Miami, Jackson Memorial Medical Center, Miami, FL 33101.

V.E. GOULD, M.D., Department of Pathology, Rush Medical College, Rush-Presbyterian - St. Luke's Medical Center, 1753 West Congress Parkway, Chicago, IL. 60612.

G.L. GREENE, Ph.D., The University of Chicago, The Ben May Laboratory for Cancer Research, 5841 S. Maryland Ave., Chicago IL 60637.

D.L. HILL, Ph.D., John Muir Cancer and Aging Research Institute, 2055 North Broadway Walnut Creek, CA 94596.

F.J. HORNICEK, Ph.D., Surgical Research Laboratories, Department of Surgery, University of Miami, School of Medicine, Miami, FL 33101.

E.S. JAFFE, M.D., Hematopathology Section, Laboratory of Pathology, National Cancer Institute, National Institute of Health, Besthesda, MD 20205.

C.KANDELL, Ph.D., John Muir Cancer and Aging Research Institute, 2055 North Broadway, Walnut Creek, CA 94596.

W. J. KING, Ph.D., The University of Chicago, The Ben May Laboratory for Cancer Research, 5841 S. Maryland Avenue, Chicago, IL 60637.

A.J.P. KLEIN-SZANTO, M.D., The University of Texas Science Park, Research Division, P.O. Box 389, Smithville, TX 78957.

K. KOVACS, M.D., Ph.D., Department of Pathology, St Michael's Hospital, 30 Bond Street, Toronto, Ontario M5B1W8.

I. LEE, M.D., Department of Pathology, Rush Medical College, Rush-Presbyterian St. Luke's Medical Center, 1753 West Congress Parkway, Chicago, IL 60612.

G.I. MALININ, Ph.D., Department of Physics, Georgetown University, Washington, DC 20057.

T.I. MALININ, M.D., Department of Surgery, University of Miami, School of Medicine, Miami, FL 33101.

J.M. MEIS, M.D., Department of Pathology, The University of Texas, System Cancer Center, M.D. Anderson Hospital and Tumor Institute, 6723 Bertner Avenue, Houston, TX 77030.

A.R. MORALES, M.D., Department of Pathology, University of Miami, Jackson Memorial Medical Center, Miami, FL 33101.

F.K. MOSTOFI, M.D., Department of Genitourinary Pathology, Armed Forces Institute of Pathology, Washington, DC 20306.

N. NADJI, M.D., Department of Pathology, University of Miami, Jackson Memorial Medical Center, Miami, FL 33101.

L.OSVALDO, M.D., Department of Pathology, John Muir Memorial Hospital, 2055 North Broadway, Walnut Creek, CA 94546.

M.F. PRESS, Ph.D., The University of Chicago, The Ben May Laboratory for Cancer Research, 5841 S. Maryland Avenue, Chicago, IL 60637.

H. OWNBY, Ph.D., Biological Resources Unit, Research Division, Michigan Cancer Foundation, 110 E. Warren Ave, Detroit, MI 48201.

I.H. RUSSO, M.D., Department of Pathology, Michigan Cancer Foundation, 110 E. Warren Ave., Detroit, MI 48201.

J. RUSSO, M.D., Department of Pathology, Michigan Cancer Foundation, 110 E. Warren Ave., Detroit, MI 48201

R.E. SCULLY, M.D., James Homer Wright Pathology Laboratories, Massachusetts General Hospital, Boston, MA 02101.

D. SECKINGER, M.D., Department of Pathology, Cedars Medical Center, 1400 N.W. 12th Avenue, Miami, FL 33136.

I. SESTERHENN, M.D., Department of Genitourinary Pathology, Armed Forces Institute of Pathology, Washington, DC 20306.

A.E. SHERROD, M.D., Department of Pathology, University of Southern California, School of Medicine, 2025 Zonal Avenue, Los Angeles, CA 90033.

L. A. STERNBERGER, M.D., Center for Brain Research, University of Rochester, Medical Center, Rochester, NY 14642.

N.H. STERNBERGER, M.D., Center for Brain Research, University of Rochester, Medical Center, Rochester, NY 14642.

C.R. TAYLOR, M.D., Ph.D., Department of Pathology, University of Southern California, School of Medicine, 2025 Zonal Ave., Los Angeles, CA 90033.

R.A. THOMAS, M.S., Ratsom Inc., 7620 S.W. 147 Court, Miami, FL 33193.

T.M. THOMSON, Ph.D., Memorial Sloan-Kettering Cancer Center, New York, NY 10021.

J.T. THORNTHWAITE, Ph.D., Department of Pathology, Cedars Medical Center 1400 N.W. 12th Avenue, Miami, FL 33136.

R.R. TUBBS, D.O., Department of Pathology, The Cleveland Clinic Foundation, 9500 Euclid Ave., Cleveland, OH 44106.

D.A. VAZQUEZ, M.S., ASCP, Department of Pathology, Cedars Medical Center, 1400 N.W. 12th Ave., Miami, FL 33136.

T. WOOLLEY, Ph.D., College of Medicine, East Tennessee State University, Johnson City, TN 37614.

PREFACE

There is no doubt that the advent of immunocytochemical techniques, by enhancing our ability to detect specific cell products or markers, has opened new avenues in the understanding of human diseases, and in our ability to perform better diagnosis in surgical pathology.

The rapid development of this field has resulted in thousands of publications in the literature regarding immunocytochemistry in diagnostic pathology. This explosion of knowledge makes necessary publications summarizing what are the main markers available and how they can be used in the diagnosis of tumors. The need of a more organized and structured knowledge was evident during the workshop in Immunocytochemistry of Tumor Diagnosis that took place in the City of Detroit on October 1984. This book is the result of that workshop in which 22 chapters are focusing on the main subject of differential diagnosis of tumors.

Jose Russo, M.D.
Editor

ACKNOWLEDGEMENTS

I wish to thank my many associates at the Michigan Cancer Foundation for their help in the preparation of this manuscript. I give thanks to Dr. Irma H. Russo for her continual support and encouragement; to Mr. Kalem Amin Hasan for his meticulous and conscientious work in typing a great part of the manuscript. I want to acknowledge the pecuniary support of the Ida Faigle Charitable Foundation and an Institutional Grant from the United Foundation of Greater Detroit, that made possible Chapters 1 and 13 of this book. Finally, I wish to thank Ortho Diagnostic Systems, Inc., for their sponsorship of the Immunocytochemistry Workshop in Tumor Diagnosis, that was held in Detroit, Michigan October 3-5, 1984, which was the base of this book.

IMMUNOCYTOCHEMISTRY IN TUMOR DIAGNOSIS

1

ORGANIZATION OF AN IMMUNOCYTOCHEMISTRY LABORATORY

IRMA H. RUSSO, M.D.

I. INTRODUCTION

Modern day histopathology laboratories are becoming increasingly complex due to the rapid and constant development of new techniques leading to a more precise and accurate identification of tissue or cell type, secretory activity, extra cellular substances or specific cell type markers.

The need for precise cell type identification is more acute when the pathologist has to diagnose and classify neoplasms since the extent and mode of a patient's treatment, patient's prognosis and clinicopathologic correlations are all dependent upon the exact identification of the cell or origin of a given tumor.

The arsenal of surgical pathologists has traditionally counted with the use of histochemical techniques that could be applied to formalin-fixed, paraffin-embedded tissues, whereas the detection of sophisticated markers, such as secretory products, were relegated to the clinical laboratory for their identification and quantitation in serum.

In the past several decades, though, a remarkable array of methodological advances has emerged allowing the extension and expansion of morphologic observations to include physiologic and biochemical parameters; these are the immunocytochemical methods. These methods have been extensively employed in the classification of renal glomerular and interstitial diseases, as well as in other immunologically mediated diseases (1). However, their use in the diagnosis and classification of neoplastic conditions are more recent, and are based upon the presence or absence of specific tumor markers. These markers represent a heterogeneous group of substances that are either specifically synthesized or secreted by a given cell type and whose presence is detected on the cell surface, in its cytoplasm, in tissue extracts or in circulating plasma of the patient bearing a tumor. They are represented by a broad array of substances, such as hormones, enzymes and immunoglobulins.

The identification of a cell according to its antigenic constitution had an enormous success with the introduction of immunofluorescence methods by Coons and associates in 1941. However, the obvious disadvantages of immunofluorescence, such as the need for frozen sections, the use of a fluorescence microscope, the lack of morphologic detail and the transient nature of the reaction, did inhibit the widespread application of this method, which remained circumscribed to very specialized laboratories.

The development of methods utilizing enzyme - conjugated antibodies, and later the introduction of the immunoglobulin - enzyme bridge method of Mason et al (2) and the peroxidase - antiperoxidase method of Sternberger et al (3), provided the tools to expand this technology beyond the highly specialized laboratory. These methodologies have shown to be highly sensitive, and can be applied to fixed and paraffin or plastic embedded materials, thus permitting the localization of most antigens that are of interest to the surgical pathologist. The availability of this technology has revolutionized the present day practice of Pathology and is changing the way classical anatomic pathology is practiced. Besides, it is rapidly building a bridge between the pure morphologist and the clinical laboratory by allowing precise cell, organ or function identification. As a consequence, no present day laboratory of pathology can face the diagnosis of tumors without the assurance of one or more immunohistochemical techniques.

2. LABORATORY ORGANIZATION

The same goals and objectives outlined for the general histopathology laboratory would apply to the immunocytochemistry section. However, the more specialized nature of the techniques employed and the need to use specific antibodies require a careful evaluation of the laboratory's needs. Therefore, the following points must be assessed before committing personnel and budget to immunocytochemistry.

a. Daily workload
b. Number of "problem" cases that could be solved by the use of tumor markers
c. Type of pathology more frequently submitted for diagnosis.
d. Availability of skilled personnel.
e. Availability of adequate controls.
f. Availability of adequate equipment.

If the laboratory director concludes that immunocytochemistry performed in house is justified, or the laboratory has a teaching or research orientation, and counts with the adequate number of skilled personnel, then the most critical point becomes the type of equipment required.

3. LABORATORY EQUIPMENT

The type of equipment needed will depend exclusively of the type of immunocytochemical techniques chosen. At the present time the following are the most commonly used techniques:

3.1 Immunofluorescent staining methods (4).

3.1.1 Direct immunofluorescence - Fluorochrome conjugated directly to the primary antibody.

3.1.2 Indirect immunofluorescence.

Two stage procedure - Primary unconjugated antibody - Fluorochrome conjugated secondary antibody.

Specimen condition: Frozen sections.

Equipment requirement: Cryostat - Fluorescence microscope - Photographic camera attachment.

Draw backs:

a. Requirement of frozen tissue.
b. Low sensitivity in fixed tissue.
c. Background fluorescence.
d. Lack of morphological detail
e. Requires rigorous controls
f. Transient reaction. Requires photographic record.

3.2 Enzyme conjugated antibodies

3.2.1 Immunoperoxidase staining method (5).

A. Direct - Horseradish peroxidase conjugated to primary antibody.
B. Indirect - Two stage procedure - Primary unconjugated antiserum peroxidase - conjugated secondary antiserum.
C. Unlabeled - antibody bridge method (2)
D. Peroxidase - antiperoxidase method (3)
E. Double bridge peroxidase - antiperoxidase (6)

Specimen condition: Frozen section, or fixed (formalin, B5, Bouin's, Zenker's) paraffin-embedded tissues.

Equipment requirement: Routine histopathology equipment.

Advantages: a. High sensitivity
b. Absence of background - high signal to noise ratio.
c. Permits retrospective studies.
d. Excellent preservation of morphological detail.
e. Stains are permanent.
f. Does not require special equipment.

Draw backs a. Requires rigorous controls.
b. Nonspecific background staining.

3.2.2 Biotin - Avidin Immunoenzymatic procedures (7)

A. Bridged biotin - avidin technique. Biotin labeled antibody - avidin - biotin labeled enzyme.

B. Labeled avidin - biotin technique. Biotin labeled antibody - enzyme labeled avidin.

Specimen conditions: Frozen sections or fixed (formalin, B5, Bouin's Zenker's) - paraffin embedded tissues.

Equipment requirement: Routine histopathology equipment.

Advantages: a. High sensitivity
b. Permits retrospective studies.
c. Excellent preservation of morphological detail
d. Stains are permanent
e. Does not require special equipment

Drawbacks: a. Requires rigorous controls
b. Non-specific background

3.3 Ultrastructural immunocytochemistry (8).

A. Peroxidase conjugated method
B. Peroxidase-antiperoxidase method.
C. Immunoferritin method.
D. Protein A - gold method

Specimen condition: Electron microscopy fixation - Pre-embedding or post-embedding treatment.

Equipment requirement: Plastic embedding facilities, Ultramicrotome, electron microscope, dark room facilities.

Advantages: a. High sensitivity
b. Excellent correlation with morphology

Draw backs: a. Requires specialized equipment
b. Requires special fixation
c. Does not allow retrospective studies.

4. SCREENING PANELS

Definitive tumor identification by immunocytochemical techniques requires absolute and specific tumor markers. Although certain markers provide a high degree of confidence, such as breast MC5 antigen (9) or prostate specific antigen, a great percentage of antigens, however, is present in related or unrelated tumors or tissues, what makes are necessary to screen any given tumor with a series of antibodies, in order to narrow down the diagnostic possibilities or to reach a definitive diagnosis. Thus, the need to develop screening panels to categorize tumors within a given tissue or cell type.

TUMOR SUSPECTED TO BE DERIVED FROM:	SCREENING PANEL: ANTIGENS DETECTED
Adenocarcinoma of the colon, cervix, breast; differentiation of mesotheliomas from metastatic carcinomas	Carcinoembryonic antigen (CEA).
Breast carcinoma, extramammary Paget's disease	Casein Alpha-Lactalbumin Pregnancy Specific Glycoprotein (SP1) Placental Protein 5(PP5). Placental Lactogen MC5 monoclonal Ab against fat globule membrane
Carcinomas - Differentiation from sarcomas	Keratin
Carcinomas from bladder, cervix, colon, other tumors.	Blood group isoantigens
Gastrointestinal tumors and carcinoids	Pancreatic islet cell and gastrointestinal hormones (insulin, glucagon, somatostatin, gastrin, vasoactive intestinal peptide, pancreatic polypeptide, cholecystokinin.)
Gliomas from other tumors.	Glial fibrillary acidic protein (GFAP)
Hemangiomas, hemangiosarcomas.	Factor VIII-related antigen
Hepatocellular carcinomas	Alpha-1-antitrypsin Alpha-fetoprotein Hepatitis B antigen
Histiocytic lymphomas, monocytic leukemia.	Lysozyme
Mesotheliomas, differentiation from metastatic carcinomas and other tumors.	Mesothelioma antigen, keratin, CEA.

TUMOR SUSPECTED TO BE DERIVED FROM:	SCREENING PANEL: ANTIGENS DETECTED:
Mesenchymal and muscle cells	Vimentin
Muscle, smooth and skeletal; myoepithelial cell proliferation	Actin Desmin Myoblobin Myosin
Nervous tissue specific protein	S100
Neurons, diffuse neuroendocrine system	Neuron specific enolase
Oat cell carcinoma with neurosecretory granules	Oat cell carcinoma plasma membrane antigen Histaminase
Ovarian carcinoma	Alkaline phosphatase (Regan isoenzyme)
Ovarian granulosa and theca cell tumors	Estradiol
Pituitary tumor cell type	Pituitary hormones (adrenocorticotrophin, growth hormone, prolactin, thyroid stimulating hormone, luteinizing hormone, follicle stimulating hormone)
Prostatic carcinoma	Prostatic acid Phosphatase Prostate specific antigen
Testicular Sertoli and Leydig cell tumors	Testosterone
Testicular germ cell tumors	Alpha-fetoprotein
Thyroid adenomatous nodules, adenomas, carcinomas	Thyroglobulin
Medullary thyroid carcinoma and C-cell hyperplasia	Calcitonin Histaminase
Trophoblastic neoplasms, differentiation of ovarian and testicular germ cell tumors	Chorionic gonadotropin Placental Lactogen
Viral origin carcinomas	Herpes simplex-associated antigen

Screening Panels have to be also utilized in the diagnosis of lymphomas/ leukemias which can be characterized by a large number of polyclonal and monoclonal antibodies.

LYMPHOMAS/LEUKEMIAS SUSPECTED TO BE DERIVED FROM (10-12):	SCREENING PANEL:ANTIGEN DETECTED:
B cell lymphomas, differentiation of lymphomas from carcinomas, lymphoma from hyperplasia	Immunoglobulins: heavy chain, IgM, IgG, IgD, IgA; light chain Kappa, Lamba
Synthesized immunoglobulin	Immunoglobulin J-chain
Pan T cell	OKT1 (Anti-Leu 1)
Peripheral T lymphocytes	OKT3 (anti-Leu 4)
Inducer/helper T lymphocytes	OKT4 (anti-Leu 3a,b)
Thymocytes	OKT6 (anti-Leu 6)
Suppressor/cytotoxic T lymphocytes	OKT8 (anti-Leu-2a)
Monocytes, null cells, granulocytes	OKM1
B lymphocytes, activated T lymphocytes, some monocytes.	OKla1 (anti-HLA-DR)
Activated and/or proliferating cells	OKT9
Hematopoietic stem cells and activated lymphocytes	OKT10
Peripheral T lymphocytes	OKT11 (Anti-Leu-5)
B cells, granulocytes	OKB2
B cell	OKB7
Monocytes, platelets	OKM5

5. FUNCTIONAL CONSIDERATIONS

The determination as to the type of technique to be used and the number and type of antigens to be detected will depend on the orientation of the histopathology laboratory, whether it is service, education or research.

Once it is decided that the peroxidase-anti-peroxidase or the avidin - biotin method will be used, it is important to keep in mind that the basic needs of these methodologies are satisfied with the equipment usually available in a routine histopathology laboratory. Fixation, automatic tissue processing and embedding, sectioning, deparaffinization and observation at the light microscope can blend easily with the every day workload. However, the success of immunohistochemical techniques depends greatly of the skill of the histotechnologists performing the test and of developing adequate protocols for each given set of tissues and antibodies.

Pathology laboratories performing immunohistochemical stain have to be categorized based upon their workload, specialized area developed and degree of complexity of the testing performed in the following categories:

Level I - Small laboratory receiving small surgical specimens and having to decide only occasionally difficult diagnostic problems; has all basic instrumentation for histology. All tissue available is formalin-fixed, paraffin-embedded. No technical assistance for method development.

Should have availability of commercial kits for:

1) Adenocarcinoma screening: Carcinoembryonic antigen
Keratin
2) Prostatic carcinoma screening: Prostatic acid phosphatase.
Prostate specific antigen
3) Mesenchymal and muscle cell screening: Actin
Desmin
Vimentin

Level II - Medium size-hospital associated laboratory with active surgical service. Sufficient skilled personnel for frozen section and special fixation procedure. No research or method development.

Should have availability of most screening series of polyclonal antibodies and selected monoclonal antibodies.

Level III - Large Pathology Laboratory with active oncology service. Sufficient skilled personnel for frozen sections, special techniques, antibody titration, selection of adequate controls, immunoelectron microscopy.

Should have available the following polyclonal and monoclonal antibodies:

Neuropathology Section	- Brain screening series
Hematopathology	- Lymphoma/leukemia screening series.
Dermatopathology	- Immunoglobulins, complement antibodies.
Immunopathology	- method development. Special markers, testing of experimental antibodies.
Nephropathology	- Immunoglobulins, complement, fibrinogen antibodies.

Level IV - Specialized research oriented laboratory handling selected cases or referrals. It counts with highly skilled personnel with special training in method development, antibody titration, immunoelectron microscopy, use of monoclonal antibodies.

Should have a complete inventory of most polyclonal and monoclonal antibodies available, updated information on new antibodies developed and easy accessibility to new antibodies for titration and testing before its marketing.

6. INVENTORY CONTROL AND RECORDS

Inventory control is one of the most crucial problems in the immunocytochemistry laboratory due to the relative short shelf life of the antibodies, their different storage conditions, the small volume package in every kit, the difficulty in determining the volume (or number of drops) utilized per test and the number of tests performed with each reagent bottle.

An effective inventory control requires a well organized system with which all the persons involved in either purchasing reagents or performing the test are familiar, such as a stock record card system (13). The supervisor of the immunocytochemistry laboratory plays an essential role in setting the levels of on-hand supplies, which should be maintained to a minimum for those reagents with short shelf life, but to a medium or high level, although taking into consideration the rate of usage, when the reagent can be kept frozen for lengthy periods of time.

7. QUALITY CONTROL

Immunocytochemical techniques are qualitative, meaning that a reaction in a given specimen is either present or absent, and the results of these tests are yes or no, positive or negative. The reactions can be semiquantitated, and the degree of positivity or negativity is visually estimated and expressed as negative, weakly, moderately or strongly positive, or as 0, +, ++, +++ as a discrete variate with four possible values.

Quality control in immunocytochemistry relies heavily on the positive and negative tissue controls run simultaneously with the unknown specimen. The following conditions have to be carefully adjusted.

7.1 Specimen Collection:

Adhere, preferably to one fixative so controls and experimentals will be processed under the same conditions.

7.2 Always freeze a representative fragment of tissue and fix another in B5 if the primary fixative is formalin.

7.3 With every test run the following controls:

- One known positive control.
- One known negative control.
- One section incubated with pre-immune serum.

- One section incubated with the primary antiserum preabsorbed with the specific and related antigens.
- One section in which the bridge antiserum has been deleted.
- One section incubated with hydrogen peroxide to assess the presence of endogenous peroxidase.
- One section incubated with the peroxidase antiperoxidase complex alone to assess nonspecific affinity of the reagent to tissue structures.

8. TROUBLESHOOTING

Problem	Cause	Solution
Nonspecific background staining	Residual embedding medium	Heat slides to 60 degrees prior to deparaffinization
	Endogenous peroxidase activity	Pretreat sections with 0.3% H2O2 in methanol for 30 min.
	Nonspecific binding of various immunoglobulin reagents.	use blocking immunoglobulin as first step.
	Antibodies of unwanted specificity.	Absorption of antiserum with tissue extracts free of the specific antigen under study. Dilute primary antiserum.
	Diffusion of intra cellular antigens	Prompt fixation, choose more adequate fixative.
	Complement mediated binding	Use complement-free serum.
	Binding of antiserum via Fc fragment.	Use Fab fragment.
No reaction in formalin-fixed tissue	Masked immunoreactive sites	Incubate sections in 0.1% trypsin solution in 0.12% calcium chloride, pH 7.8 with 0.1M sodium hydroxide for 20-30 min. at 37°C (14).

REFERENCES

1. DeLellis RA: Diagnostic immunohistochemistry in tumor pathology: An Overview. In: DeLellis RA (ed), Diagnostic Immunohistochemistry. Masson Monographs in Diagnostic Pathology. Masson Publishing USA, Inc. 1981, pp 4-5.
2. Mason TE, Phifer RF, Spicer SS, Swallow RA and Dreskin RB: An immunoglobulin-enzyme bridge method for localizing tissue antigens. J Histochem Cytochem 17:563-569, 1969.
3. Sternberger LA and Joseph SA: The unlabeled antibody enzyme method of immunohistochemistry. J Histochem Cytochem 18:315-333, 1970.
4. Bhan AK: Application of monoclonal antibodies to tissue diagnosis. In DeLellis RA (ed) Advances in Immunohistochemistry. Masson Monographs in Diagnostic Pathology. Masson Publishing, USA, Inc. 1984, pp.1-29.
5. Nakane PK, and Pierce GB, Jr: Enzyme labeled antibodies. Preparation and application for localization of antigens. J Histochem Cytochem 14:929-938, 1966.
6. Vacca LL, Abrahams SJ and Naftchi NE: A modified peroxidase antiperoxidase procedure for improved localization of tissue antigens: Localization of substance P in rat spinal cord. J Histochem Cytochem 28:297-307, 1980.
7. Guesdon JL, Ternynch T and Avrameas S: The use of avidin biotin interaction in immunoenzymatic techniques. J. Histochem Cytochem 27:1131-1139, 1979.
8. Roth J: Light and electron microscopic localization of antigen with the protein A-gold (PAg) technique. In: Advances in immunohistochemistry, DeLellis RA. (ed) Masson Publishing, USA, 1984, pp. 43-66.
9. Russo J and Russo IH: Immunocytochemistry of human breast cancer and its prognostic implications (Abst). Breast Cancer Res. Conference. Intl Assoc. Breast Cancer Res., London, 1985.
10. Foon KA, Schroff, RW and Gale RP: Surface markers on leukemia and lymphoma cells: Recent advances. Blood 60:1-19, 1982.
11. Goding JW and Burns GF: Monoclonal antibody OKT-9 recognizes the receptor for transferrin on human acute lymphocytic leukemia. J Immunol 127: 1256-1258, 1981
12. Nadler LM, Ritz J, Griffin JD, Todd RF,III, Reinherz EL and Schlossman SF: Diagnosis and treatment of human leukemias and lymphomas utilizing monoclonal antibodies. Prog. Haematol 12:187-225, 1981.
13. McLendon WW and Henry JB: Administration of the clinical laboratory. In: Clinical Diagnosis and Management by Laboratory Methods. Henry JB (ed) WB Saunders Company, Philadelphia, London, Toronto. 16th ed. 1979, pp. 1977-1994.
14. Walker RA: Immunohistochemistry of biological markers of breast carcinoma In: Advances in Immunohistochemistry. DeLellis RA,(ed). Masson Publishing, USA, 1984, pp. 223-241.

2

PRINCIPLES OF IMMUNOCYTOCHEMISTRY*

L.A. STERNBERGER AND N.H. STERNBERGER

This outline will:

1. discuss the reasons for avoiding the covalent labeling of second antibodies in immunocytochemistry.
2. present a comparison between PAP and ABC methods.
3. discuss advantages and precautions in production and use of monoclonal antibodies for immunocytochemistry.
4. discuss advantages of using mouse or rat ClonoPAP made from monoclonal antiperoxidase.
5. show that immunocytochemistry with monoclonal antibodies permits dissection of biochemical processes in situ.
6. propose that the lesion in Alzheimer's disease and related disorders involves a disturbance in a specific neurofilament phosphorylation site.

All labels currently used in immunocytochemistry yield adequate staining intensity. The sensitivity of an immunocytochemical method does, therefore, not depend on the label itself, but rather on the manner in which a label is used (1). Second antibodies (for all indirect methods) have to be serum-derived, rather than monoclonal, in order to yield the broad applicability basic to the use of indirect methodology. Because of contaminants in

*This research was supported by grants from the Multiple Sclerosis Society, The National Science Foundation (BNS 8205643), and The National Institutes of Health {NS 17665, NS 21681 (Javits Award) and HD 12921}. The capable assistance of Francis Murant and Kristina Klingbiel is gratefully acknowledged.

immunoglobulin employed for production of second antibodies, the serum antibodies are likewise contaminated with nonspecific antibodies. These react directly with the tissue even in the absence of first antibody (2). The contaminating antibodies are present whether the second antibody is labeled, as in labeled antibody methods, or unlabeled, as in unlabeled antibody methods. The contaminants contribute to background if labeled. However the principle of the unlabeled antibody method (3) assures that only the specific anti-immunoglobulin is localized while nonspecifically reacting antibodies remain invisible. Basic to the unlabeled antibody method is the principle that, although second antibodies are heterogeneous, each individual antibody molecule possesses two identical idiotypic sites. Second antibodies in the unlabeled antibody method react twice, first with the first antibody (or with a tissue contaminant) and then again with the third layer reagent which is peroxidase-antiperoxidase (PAP) or another antigen-antibody complex (1). Since PAP is an affinity-purified reagent, it will react only with those components of second antibody which have reacted with immunoglobulin specifically and not with those components that have reacted with nonspecific tissue constituents. Furthermore, if it would have happened that PAP were contaminated with a constituent crossreactive with a tissue contaminant with which the nonspecific components of the second antibody would have reacted, again the reaction remains unvisualized. The reason is that any putative contaminant in PAP would, by definition, not be antiperoxidase and, therefore, even if reacting with a second antibody, it would not bind peroxidase and again not become visualized. Thus, the unlabeled antibody principle incorporates a dual specificity amplification.

Sensitivity of an immunocytochemical method is not evaluated by staining intensity. The true sensitivity is measured by the ratio of specific staining intensity to background staining intensity.

There is another factor which contributes to background in labeled antibody methods. This is due to nonspecific attachment of polymers that form as a result of the labeling process itself. For this reason, protocols for careful preparation of antibody conjugates include a final purification step in which polymers are separated from monomeric conjugates (4). An exception is the avidin-biotin complex method (ABC method) in which complexes are purposely produced during the staining procedure with the apparent aim of providing larger deposits (5). Since such large deposits are likely to increase staining intensity but at the same time to decrease sensitivity, we have compared staining by the PAP method with the ABC method. We found that at low dilutions of monoclonal antibodies (1:2,000) the PAP method was 12 times more sensitive than the ABC method. At high dilutions (1:512,000), the PAP method was twice as sensitive as the ABC method (Figure 1). When staining

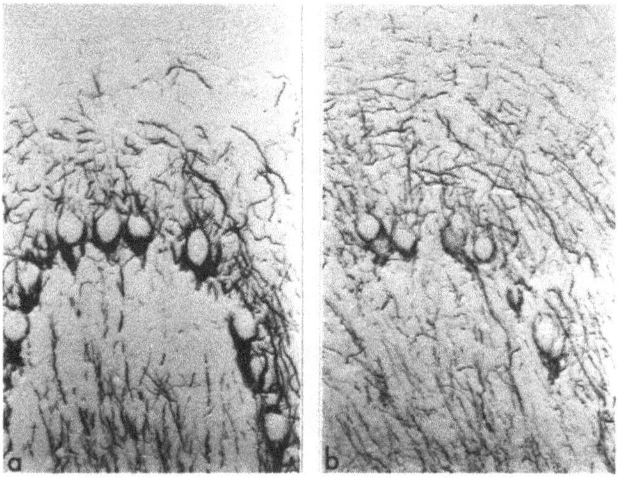

Figure 1. Rat cerebellum, serial paraffin sections, treated for 24 hr with monoclonal antiphosphorylated neurofilament antibody 07-5, diluted 1:512,000. a, PAP method. b, ABC method. X200.

intensity in the PAP method was plotted against antibody dilution, staining remained maximal to a dilution of 1:128,000, then decreased sharply with a 50% maximal intensity staining at a dilution of approximately 1:256,000. In this range, the method provided a steep curve that permitted differentiation between large and small concentrations of antibodies or tissue antigen. In contrast, the dilution curve with the ABC method was flat and permitted no distinction between high and low concentrations of antigen. Furthermore, the ABC method gave background and, indeed, provided a good stain for myelin even in the absence of any antibodies. Thus, the ABC method did not distinguish between significant and insignificant amounts of antigen or between small amounts of antigen and nonspecific material.

The behavior of the ABC method can be explained by the unpredictable and large size of the enzyme complex used. When the tissue epitope density is low, the large complex will amplify the signal obtained by the immunocytochemical reaction for the tissue antigen. As we increase the epitope density, the amount of detected complex deposited does not increase significantly because of steric hindrance of these large complexes. Although the complex itself possesses many peroxidase subunits, it is expected that the enzymatic activity of a good proportion of them is masked in the interior of the complex. Therefore, at high epitope density, the staining intensity conferred by the few reacting peroxidase complexes does not match that of the many reacting PAP complexes consisting of regular units of three peroxidases and two antiperoxidases.

In PAP, affinity-purified from antisera to peroxidase, the enzymatic activity of some of peroxidase is inhibited to varying extents. Usually about 30% of the original peroxidatic activity. The inhibition is due to antibodies in sera that react close to the enzymatic site of peroxidase. The advent of monoclonal antibodies gave us the opportunity to prepare rat and mouse PAP only with antiperoxidases that react with peroxidase away from the specific combining site. As a consequence, it turned out that ClonoPAP prepared from monoclonal antibodies provided much higher staining intensities and sensitivities than PAP affinity-purified from mouse and rat antisera to peroxidase.

There are three reasons for using monoclonal antibodies in immunocytochemistry:

1. They will only react with specific and crossreacting epitopes (serum derived or purified antibodies may react in addition with irrelevant antigens and there are no good controls to eliminate this possibility absolutely).
2. Monoclonal antibodies permit the detection of epitopes in individual antigens and properly selected antibodies can, therefore, be used for studying posttranslational changes in situ.
3. Monoclonal antibodies can be used to discover novel antigens.

It is important in the preparation of monoclonal antibodies to use an assay method which is identical to that employed in the intended use of the antibodies once prepared.

Using immunocytochemistry as a method of selection, we prepared 135 monoclonal antibodies reactive with brain tissue. Out of these antibodies (6), 37 were neuron-specific, 44 reacted with other interesting structures, and the remainder were discarded. Among the 44 antibodies, one was specific to the blood-brain barrier. With this antibody, deficiency in the blood-brain barrier has been visualized in lesions of chronic relapsing experimental allergic encephalitis prior to cellular infiltration or to deficiency in myelin basic protein or myelin-associated glycoprotein (7). Another antibody was specific to cilia of choroid plexus and respiratory epithelium (8).

The immunocytochemical staining patterns of 37 neuron-specific monoclonal antibodies previously described fell into four groups: I) "antisynapse-associated" (9), II) "antineurofibrillar", III) "antiperikaryonal-neurofibrillar", and IV) a single antibody reactive with a widely distributed epitope that covered the patterns of II as well as III. Antibodies of groups II, III and IV were shown to be specific to neurofilament triplet subunits, even though there was little overlap in staining patterns between groups II and III (10). We have examined nine of these antibodies as to their ability to distinguish functional states of neurofilaments dependent upon phosphorylation (11). Upon digestion with phosphatase, electroblot staining of neurofilament components was abolished with the five antibodies from group II, enhanced with the three antibodies from group III, and unaffected

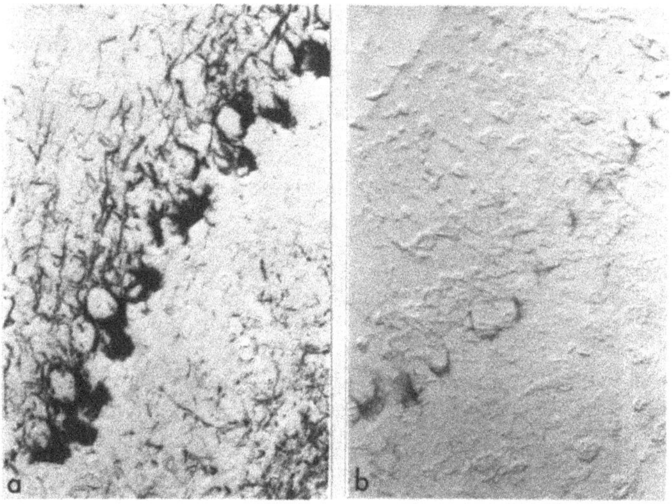

Figure 2. Rat cerebellum. 7 μm-thick paraffin sections. Antibody 06-17 from group II. A, section treated with buffer before immunocytochemistry. Staining of group II antibodies reveals axons and axon terminals, but no cell bodies or dendrites. B, upon treatment with trypsin and phosphatase before immunocytochemistry, staining is diminished. ClonoPAP technique. X200.

with antibody IV. Immunocytochemical staining of Bouin-fixed paraffin sections of rat brain was unaffected by phosphatase pretreatment. With antibodies of group II, predigestion with trypsin also left staining unaffected, but when followed by phosphatase, staining was diminished with three out of five antibodies (Figure 2). In contrast, predigestion with trypsin abolished all staining with each antibody from group III. If followed by phosphatase, staining reappeared but the group III pattern was replaced by a group II pattern. Staining of this pattern was again abolished upon a second treatment with trypsin (Figure 3). The antibody from group IV lost most of its group II and III staining patterns, when sections were digested with trypsin. The group II pattern reappeared and, indeed, was enhanced upon a subsequent phosphatase treatment, and reduced again upon a second trypsin treatment. Staining by four out of five antibodies from group II was inhibited by inorganic phosphate. The data indicate that certain nerve cell bodies, their dendrites and at least proximal axons possess non-phosphorylated neurofilaments and that long fibers, including terminal axons, possess phosphorylated neurofilaments. We proposed that phosphorylation may be a factor in stabilizing compacted forms of neurofilaments and that heterogeneity of the compacted structures may play a role in a possible multiplicity of function within individual nerve cells.

We found in collaborative studies with Drs. Don Price, Linda Cork and Jürg Ulrich that in Alzheimer's disease, Down's syndrome and related disorders, phosphorylation occurs already in the cell body. In normal tissues, phosphorylated neurofilaments are never seen in cell bodies. This premature phosphorylation is not merely a damming up of the phosphorylation process, but rather a specific disturbance of phosphorylation involving only selected neurofilament phosphorylation sites. We, therefore, propose that the pathogenesis of

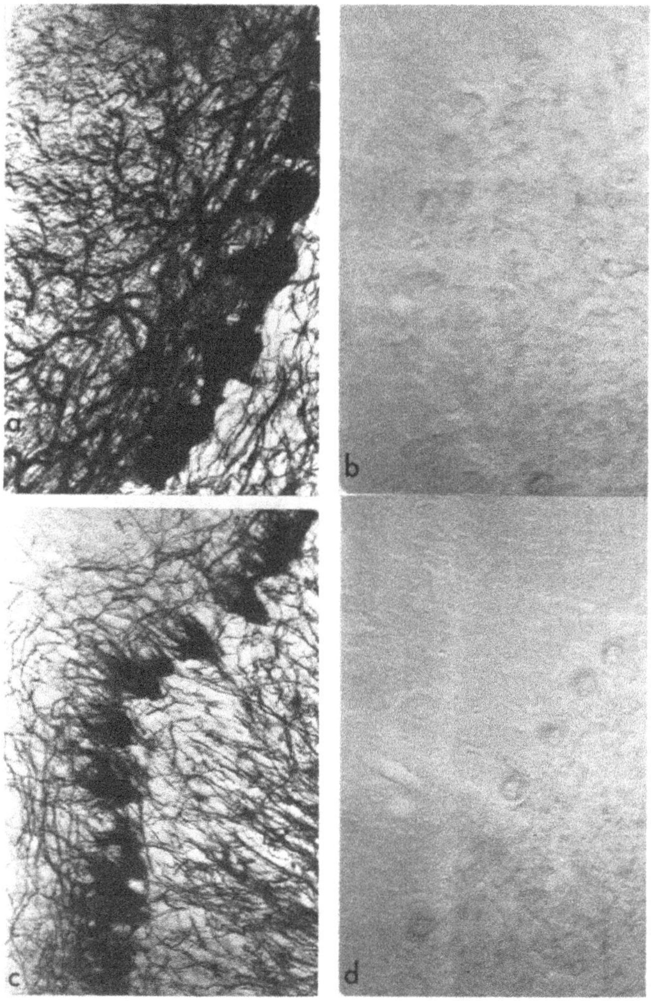

Figure 3. Rat cerebellum. 15 μm-thick Vibratome sections. Antibody 02-135 from group III. A, section treated with buffer before immunocytochemistry. Staining of group III antibodies reveals perikarya and dendrites, some axons, but not thin axons or axon terminals. B, treatment with trypsins before immunocytochemistry abolishes the staining. C, treatment with trypsin, followed by phosphatase causes reappearance of staining, but the group III pattern has been replaced by a group II pattern. D, treatment with trypsin, phosphatase and again trypsin, leads to a second disappearance of staining. ClonoPAP technique. X200.

Alzheimer's disease involves a metabolic disturbance that is restricted to a specific kinase among the possible heterogeneous pool of neurofilament or cytoskeleton-associated kinases.

REFERENCES

1. Sternberger LA: Immunocytochemistry, Third Edition. John Wiley, New York, in press.
2. Dougherty RM, Marucci AA, DiStefano HS: Application of immunohistochemistry to the study of avian leukosis virus. J Viral Biol (15):149-157, 1972.
3. Sternberger LA, Hardy PH Jr, Cuculis JJ, Meyer HG: The unlabeled antibody-enzyme method of immunohistochemistry. Preparation and properties of soluble antigen-antibody complex (horseradish peroxidase-anti-horseradish peroxidase) and its use in identification of spirochetes. J Histochem Cytochem (18):315-333, 1970.
4. Boorsma BM, Steefkerk JG: Periodate or glutaraldehyde for preparing peroxidase conjugates. J Immunol Meth (30):245-256, 1979.
5. Hsu SM, Raine L, Fanger H: Use of avidin-biotin-peroxidase complex (ABC) in immunoperoxidase techniques. A comparison between ABC and unlabeled antibody (PAP) procedures. J Histochem Cytochem (59):777-785, 1981.
6. Sternberger LA, Harwell LW, Sternberger NH: Neurotypy: regional individuality in rat brain detected by immunocytochemistry with monoclonal antibodies. Proc Natl Acad Sci USA (79):1326-1330, 1982.
7. Sternberger NH, Murant FG, Parkison JA, Kies MW: EAE in the Lewis rat: An immunocytochemical study. Transact Am Soc Neurochem (15):143, 1984.
8. Ostermann E, Sternberger NH, Sternberger LA: Immunocytochemistry of brain-reactive monoclonal antibodies in peripheral tissues. Cell Tiss Res (228):459-473, 1983.
9. Sternberger NH: Monoclonal antibodies to synapse-associated antigens. Transact Am Soc Neurochem (15):199, 1984.
10. Goldstein MA, Sternberger LA, Sternberger NH: Microheterogeneity of neurofilament proteins. Proc Natl Acad Sci USA 80:3101-3105, 1983.
11. Sternberger LA, Sternberger NH: Monoclonal antibodies distinguish phosphorylated and nonphosphorylated forms of neurofilaments in situ. Proc Natl Acad Sci USA 80:6126-6130, 1983.

3

USE OF DIAGNOSTIC ALGORITHMS IN IMMUNOCYTOCHEMISTRY

A.E. Sherrod, M.D. and Clive R. Taylor, M.D., D. Phil.

> "The adventurous physician goes on, and substitutes presumption for knowledge. From the scanty field of what is known, he launches into the boundless region of what is unknown."
>
> Thomas Jefferson (1763-1826)

One of the most challenging aspects of diagnostic histology is to determine the site of origin of poorly differentiated metastatic deposits. While many factors contribute to the reliability and validity of this diagnosis, the most critical factor is the standing and credibility (1) of the pathologist performing the examination. A histologic diagnosis is an opinion based upon experience and attained with a varying degree of confidence. In instances of uncertainty, a wise pathologist will consult one or more colleagues and a diagnosis may be reached by consensus; an exercise in the democratic process that is equally as fallible in pathology as in the political arena. A wise pathologist may also resort to one or more of several ancillary techniques designed to provide additional information upon which a rational diagnosis may be founded.

Circumstantial evidence is admissible, such as the known presence of tumor elsewhere, or a social or family history, or even the reported statistical incidence of different tumor types at the site in question; but such evidence should be considered last, rather than first, in reaching a diagnosis. If orthodox light microscopy alone does not permit a confident diagnosis, then the pathologist may search for microstructural clues, such as the presence of "prickles or intracellular bridges" (presumptive squamous carcinoma) or intracellular striations or fibrils (presumptive rhabdomyosarcoma), recognizing that faith and imagination, fired by circumstantial evidence, play large parts in determining whether or not these features are perceived in a particular tumor. Electron microscopy may also be of value in providing ultrastructural evidence of squamous differentiation, muscle cell differentiation, or glandular differentiation, but often the pathologist does not have material available for electron microscopic studies; even if material is available the time for processing and examination in most institutions produces an inordinate delay in reaching the final diagnosis. Furthermore, relatively few surgical pathologists are versed in the art of electron microscopic interpretation, and only major centers have electron microscopists with experience of using the technique for tumor diagnosis.

Histochemical stains (2,3) have proven of value in some instances, such as in the demonstration of PAS-positive material or mucins in suspected adenocarcinomas, or in the use of "melanin" (silver) stains in suspected melanoma. However, these types of histochemical stains lack true specificity in terms of defining particular cell or tumor types, and can do no more than sway the pathologist in one direction or another. More specific histochemical techniques, dependent upon the reaction of substrate to reveal the presence of a particular enzyme within a cell series, are notoriously susceptible to the adverse effects of fixation or paraffin embedding and thus are not applicable to routinely processed tissues.

The advent of immunocytochemistry promises tangible advantages in the precise definition of cell types that escape morphological recognition. It must be admitted that the range of antibodies currently available, although extensive (e.g. from Ortho Diagnostics, Carpinteria, California), is inadequate for the purpose in hand, and that in the use of immunohistochemical methods for classification of tumors we stand at the beginning, but it is a beginning full of promise.

Table 1 lists one approach to the use of immunohistochemical methods in facilitating diagnosis of unknown tumors. The antigens listed are those for which there is reasonable evidence in the literature concerning their general utility and the reproducibility of staining. A number of other antibodies of equal or greater potential value have been described (e.g. anti-pancreatic cancer antigen, anti-lung cancer antigen) (4-11), but data relating to their usefulness are either nonexistent, or limited, or subject to such controversy that no recommendation can at present be given. Even with the antibodies/antigens described, it must be remembered that not all antibodies of a named specificity (e.g. anti-keratin) in fact have identical specificity [many antibodies (antisera) will show overlapping specificities--only monoclonal antibodies may be said to have identical specificity and then only if demonstrated experimentally or if derived from the same clone.]

An initial approach in our laboratory is to screen tumors of unknown origin with monoclonal (or conventional) antibodies against carcinoembryonic antigen (CEA), keratin and vimentin (Lab Systems, Inc., Chicago, Illinois). The great majority of carcinomas will show positivity of at least a proportion of the carcinoma cells for CEA or keratin or both (Table 1). Squamous carcinomas show a propensity for more extensive positivity with anti-keratin antibody. Adenocarcinomas more frequently are positive with anti-CEA, but may show positivity for cytoskeletal keratin filaments if suitably processed (especially if trypsinized). The observation of this "overlap" precludes the formulation of a dogmatic approach to diagnosis. Vimentin positivity is seen in sarcomas, carcinomas being uniformly negative (12). One residual problem concerns the antibodies themselves; clearly not all anti-CEA antibodies

Table 1. Undifferentiated Tumors — Screening with Anti-CEA, Anti-PAN Keratin,[1] Anti-Vimentin

Results of Preliminary Screening	Preliminary Conclusion
CEA+ Keratin+ Vimentin-	Adenocarcinoma;[2] some squamous carcinomas (not sarcomas)
CEA- Keratin+ Vimentin-	Probable squamous carcinoma; transitional cell carcinoma; some adenocarcinomas;[2] mesothelioma
CEA+ Keratin- Vimentin-	Probable adenocarcinoma[2]
CEA- Keratin- Vimentin+	Probable sarcoma; astrocytic and ependymal tumors (not carcinoma)
CEA- Keratin- Vimentin-	Some neuronal/neuroendocrine tumors; possibly some myosarcomas; otherwise no useful conclusion
CEA+ Keratin+ Vimentin+	Probable technical artefact—no useful conclusion

[1] Anti-PAN Keratin — antiserum reactive with range of different molecular weight keratins; some monoclonals versus cytokeratin also are claimed to show very broad reactivity for epithelial cells (12) with occasional adenocarcinomas giving little or no reactivity.

[2] Results represent most frequently reported findings; exceptions are not uncommon reflecting either differences in antibody, variations in technique or "rogue" tumors.

(antisera) are identical, many containing activity against NCA (nonspecific cancer antigen) in addition to CEA (13). Antisera with significant NCA activity, in addition to CEA specificity, show a wider spectrum of positivity in tumors than highly purified CEA antibodies or monoclonal antibodies against CEA. Even with the use of monoclonal antibodies to CEA (Hybritech Inc., La Jolla, California), we are still learning new information concerning the range of reactivity of different anti-CEA monoclonal antibodies and the patterns of staining of various neoplasms. Colonic carcinoma almost always shows some degree of positivity for CEA using the most sensitive techniques (14,15), but significant reactivity may be found, indeed may be expected, in many other adenocarcinomas of endodermal derivation, including carcinomas of pancreas, stomach and lung. Breast carcinoma also may show significant positivity in 30%-50% of the cases (16,17). Tumors with definite squamous differentiation less often are CEA positive, but a proportion of CEA-positive cells may be observed in squamous carcinomas derived from cervix or lung.

Similarly, antibodies against keratin derived from different sources may not show a uniform pattern of positivity (18,19). Some antibodies seem mainly to detect cross-linked keratin, the type of keratin found in keratinizing squamous epithelium, while other antibodies more readily detect the non-linked keratin that exists as part of the cytoskeleton of diverse epithelial cell types, including those not of squamous epithelial origin; thus mesothelial tumors and many adenocarcinomas show varying degrees of positivity with such antibodies (19). Trypsinization adds another variable, but to obtain reproducible results in tissues fixed in formalin the general opinion is that trypsin digestion is required (20).

The initial screening with antibodies to CEA, keratin and vimentin gives information that is relative rather than absolute, and serves to point the pathologist towards one differential diagnosis rather than another. It may lead to a choice of a battery of second-stage immunostains (Table 2) in an attempt to define more precisely the tumor under investigation. Again the range of antibodies available for seeking more precise definition of tumors is limited, but it grows rapidly.

If the lesion is thought to be an adenocarcinoma, then several antibodies may be utilized in an attempt to identify the organ of origin; which one of these antibodies is selected for staining in any particular case depends upon circumstantial evidence and overall clinicopathologic correlations. For example, in a female with a tumor of unknown origin, it would be logical to stain with antibody against secretory epithelial membrane antigen and lactalbumin (or other breast related antigens), which, following absorption, may be made relatively specific for breast tissue (21-24); whereas staining with antibody against prostate-specific acid phosphatase would make little sense. In the male, of course, the situation is reversed; the probability of breast cancer is very small and the primary choice would be antibody against prostate-specific acid phosphatase (PSAP) or prostate-specific epithelial antigen (PSA) (25-27). With these antibodies positivity provides strong

Table 2. Secondary Screening for Specific Tumor Groups

A. PRESUMPTIVE CARCINOMA (Vimentin-, CEA±, PAN Keratin±[1])

CEA+	High MW Keratin+ Low MW Keratin(±)	→ Squamous carcinoma	
	High MW Keratin- Low MW Keratin+	→ Many adenocarcinomas (esp. endodermally derived tissues)	→ Stain as in B (below)
CEA-	High MW Keratin+ Low MW Keratin(±)	→ Squamous carcinoma	
	High MW Keratin- Low MW Keratin+	→ Some adenocarcinomas; mesothelioma, transitional cell carcinoma	→ Stain as in B (below)

B. PRESUMPTIVE ADENOCARCINOMA (CEA±, Low MW Keratin+)

Stain for possible product according to clinico-pathologic indications: e.g.,

Prostatic acid phosphatase Prostate specific epithelial antigen	+	Prostate
Milk fat globule antigen Lactalbumin	+	Breast
Thyroglobulin/T3/T4	+	Thyroid
Calcitonin	+	Medullary carcinoma of thyroid
Parathormone	+	Parathyroid
Alpha-fetoprotein	+	Hepatoma, germ gell (yolk sac) tumor
Human chorionic gonadotropin	+	Choriocarcinoma, germ cell tumor, some lung and breast carcinomas

C. PRESUMPTIVE CARCINOMA (non-carcinoma) (Vimentin+)

Stain according to clinico-pathologic indications: e.g.,

Desmin (±) actin, myosin	+	Myosarcomas
Factor VIII antigen	+	Angiosarcomas (including Kaposi)
Glial fibrillary antigen	+	Astrocytomas, ependymomas (in CNS)
Common leucocyte antigen	+	Lymphoma (or less probable granulocytic or histiocytic tumors)
Lysozyme	+	Granulocytic sarcoma; some histiocytic proliferations
LN-1	+	Follicular center cell tumor
LN-2	+	Probable B cell lymphoma; less likely histiocytic tumor
Kappa/lambda light chain	+	B cell lymphoma, myeloma (monoclonal)
S-100	+	Melanoma; some Schwannomas, neurilemomas and liposarcomas
Melanoma antigens	+	Melanoma

[1] High MW (molecular weight) keratin characterizes squamous carcinoma; low MW keratin typical of other epithelial tumors. Again results represent a consensus where it exists; conflicting data not uncommon in individual cases.

evidence for the site of origin of the primary tumor; PSAP and PSA are essentially confined to prostatic tissue or prostatic carcinomas, and the great majority of prostatic carcinomas, even if poorly differentiated, show at least some positivity with one or both of these antibodies.

Likewise, the presence of thyroglobulin or thyroxin within an undifferentiated tumor is strong evidence for a thyroid origin of that neoplasm (28), and the presence of calcitonin is considered almost diagnostic of medullary C cell carcinoma, the only exception being the possibility of ectopic production of these hormones by tumors of thyroid origin (29), and this is a relatively rare event. Similar considerations apply to the demonstration of positivity with antibody to parathormone (30).

The use of antibodies against alpha-fetoprotein or HCG provides less definitive information, for these antigens are not restricted to single tumor types. Alpha-fetoprotein characteristically is found in liver cell carcinomas, but not in all cases, and may also be found in embryonal carcinoma and yolk sac tumors. Human chorionic gonadotropin has an even wider range of distribution. Characteristically, of course, it is present in choriocarcinomas; however, significant HCG positivity has been observed in carcinomas of breast and lung and in seminomas and other germ cell tumors (1,31,32).

There are, in addition, reports of a number of other antibodies of potential value in the definition of the site of origin of adenocarcinomas. These include reports of other breast-specific antigens (23,24), antigens specific to pancreatic (5) and lung carcinomas (7-11), colon carcinoma antigens (4) and antigens found only in melanoma (33-37). Some of these antibodies have given positive results in paraffin sections; some appear to give positivity only in frozen sections (e.g. most of the anti-melanoma monoclonal antibodies currently available). Results are at this time preliminary; any investigator seeking to use these reagents for diagnostic purposes should be sure to develop a direct experience of the pattern of reactivity of these antibodies against representative examples of known tumor types. Finally, most of the hormones are demonstrable in paraffin sections by use of immunohistologic techniques with conventional or monoclonal antibodies (1,31,32); these utilized in conjunction with more recently available antibodies, such as neuron-specific enolase (38), permit accurate definition of endocrine and neuroendocrine tumors.

In the complete absence of detectable staining for keratin and CEA, assuming of course that controls have given the anticipated pattern of results attesting to the validity of the stain, it is probable that the tumor in question is not a carcinoma; positivity for vimentin filaments confirms this impression, whereas lack of reactivity for all these antibodies (CEA, keratin and vimentin) would be unhelpful, suggesting a tumor with little functional differentiation. Positivity for vimentin leads the pathologist to follow a different pattern of responses in attempting to more precisely define the type of tumor (Table 2).

A stain for common leukocyte antigen will serve to distinguish lymphomas and other leucocyte-derived tumors from all other sarcomas. At present, most of the available antibodies (e.g. from Hybritech Inc., La Jolla, California) against common leucocyte antigen work well only on fresh cells or frozen sections; however, antibodies that will give positive results on paraffin sections recently have become available (39) (Dako, Santa Barbara, California). If lymphoma is suspected, then as described above, common leucocyte antigen will be positive, and staining for kappa and lambda light chains and for heavy chain classes may define a monoclonal population of B cells giving a diagnosis of B cell lymphoma, the precise type being decided on morphologic considerations. The LN series of monoclonal antibodies (Techniclone, Costa Mesa, California) (40-42) also is particularly valuable in this context. LN-1 reacts with normal follicular center cells and follicular center cell lymphomas; LN-2 reacts with the majority of B-cells and many histiocytes, and with most B-cell lymphomas (little data is available regarding reactivity with histiocytic tumors); LN-3 is an anti-Ia-like antibody that reacts with many B-cells, histiocytes and some T-cells; it reacts positively with many lymphomas. All three antibodies give excellent results on B-5 fixed paraffin sections; reactivity is less intense and more variable following formalin fixation. Lysozyme (muramidase) will be positive in granulocytic sarcomas and in most, but not all, histiocytic proliferations including malignant histiocytosis (43). It is important to realize that lysozyme is not specific for these cell types, but may be found in some adenocarcinomas, particularly adenocarcinomas derived from the salivary glands, lacrimal glands and stomach.

Positive staining for factor VIII antigen, according to our present understanding, appears to be confined to tumors of endothelial cell origin, and has particularly been utilized in the recognition of Kaposi's sarcoma (44), including the gay-related immunodeficiency variant of this disorder. Actin, myosin and myoglobulin are widely distributed in many cells, but intense positivity is most often observed in rhabdomyosarcomas and to a lesser degree in leiomyosarcomas (32). Astrocytic neoplasms may be encountered extending directly from central nervous tissues, or one may occasionally find embryonic nests or extensions or neural elements into the soft tissues of the head and neck. Tumors of astrocytic derivation, or embryonic nests containing astrocytes, will show positivity when stained with antibody against glial fibrillary acidic protein (45). Many additional monoclonals versus glial cells and neurones have recently been reported (46), but data is not yet available concerning their patterns of reactivity in CNS neoplasms.

The antibodies described here are predominantly those giving reproducible results on paraffin sections. A huge range of antibodies reacting only with antigens in frozen sections has been described; the utility of these antibodies remains debatable within the current modus operandi of the surgical pathologist, who continues to rely primarily upon the formalin-paraffin section for diagnosis. With currently available antibodies it already is clear that wisdom dictates that a frozen block of tissue be set aside (and stored either in liquid nitrogen or at -70C) on all suspected tumors, as insurance against the eventuality that immunohistochemical stains will be required beyond what is possible in routinely processed tissue. In the longer term, the necessity for being able to perform a range of immunohistologic stains may force the surgical pathologist to seriously revise the current approach to fixation and processing, with the development of fixatives and embedding procedures that are more compatible with immunohistochemical techniques.

Conclusions

Clearly, immunohistology offers a potential means of precise cellular recognition that will become more extensively utilized as new antibodies are developed and characterized. It seems certain that such stains will become an essential part of the practice of diagnostic histopathology in the next decade.

REFERENCES

1. Taylor CR, Kledzik G: Immunohistologic techniques in surgical pathology—a spectrum of "new" special stains. Human Pathol 12:590-596, 1981.
2. Culling CFA: Histopathological and Histochemical Techniques: Butterworths, London, pp 1, 151, 1974.
3. Lillie RD: Histopathologic Technic and Practical Histochemistry. McGraw Hill, London, p 107, 1965.
4. Herlyn M, Steplewski Z, Herlyn D, et al: Colorectal carcinoma-specific antigen: detection by means of monoclonal antibodies. Proc Natl Acad Sci USA 76:1438-1452, 1979.
5. Metzgar RS, Gaillard MT, Levine SJ, et al: Antigens of human pancreatic adenocarcinoma cells defined by murine monoclonal antibodies. Cancer Res 42:654-659, 1982.
6. Cuttitta F, Rosen S, Gazdar AF, et al: Monoclonal antibodies that demonstrate specificity for several types of human lung cancer. Proc Natl Acad Sci USA 78:4591-4595, 1978.
7. Minna JD, Cuttitta R, Rosen S, et al: Methods for production of monoclonal antibodies with specificity for human lung cancer cells. In Vitro 17:1058-1070, 1981.
8. Kasai M, Saxton RE, Holmes EC, et al: Membrane antigens detected on human lung carcinoma cells by hybridoma monoclonal antibody. J Surg Res 30:403-408, 1981.
9. Sikora K, Wright R: Human monoclonal antibodies to lung cancer antigens. Br J Cancer 43:696-700, 1981.
10. Mulshine JL, Cuttitta F, Bibro M, et al: Monoclonal antibodies that distinguish non-small cell from small cell lung cancer. J Immunol 131:497-502, 1983.
11. DeSchryver-Kecskemeti K, Kyriakos M, Bell CE Jr, et al: Pulmonary oat cell carcinomas. Expression of plasma membrane antigen correlated with presence of cytoplasmic neurosecretory granules. Lab Invest 41:432-436, 1979.
12. Osborn M, Weber K: Biology of disease: tumor diagnosis by intermediate filament typing: a novel tool for surgical pathology. Lab Invest 48:372-394, 1983.
13. Pattengale PK, Taylor CR, Engvall E, et al: Direct visualization of normal cross-reacting antigen (NCA) in neoplastic granulocytes. Am J Clin Pathol 73:351-355, 1980.

14. Ahnen DJ, Nakane PK, Brown WR: Ultrastructural localization of carcinoembryonic antigen in normal intestine and colon cancer: abnormal distribution of CEA on the surfaces of colon cancer cells. Cancer 49:2077-2090, 1982.
15. Wiley EL, Mendelsohn G, Eggleston JC: Distribution of carcinoembryonic antigens and blood group substances in adenocarcinoma of the colon. J Lab Invest 44:507-513, 1981.
16. Whittekind C, von Kleist S, Sandritter W: (Comparative immunohistological studies on the localization of the carcinoembryonic antigen in benign and malignant breast tissue.) Acta Histochem (Suppl) 25:83-87, 1982.
17. Walker RA: Demonstration of carcinoembryonic antigen in human breast carcinomas by the immunoperoxidase technique. J Clin Pathol 33:356-360, 1980.
18. van Muijen GNP, Ruiter DJ, Ponec M, et al: Monoclonal antibodies with different specificities against cytokeratins. Am J Pathol 114:9-17, 1984.
19. Debus E, Moll R, Franke WW, et al: Immunohistochemical distinction of human carcinomas by cytokeratin typing with monoclonal antibodies. Am J Pathol 114:121-130, 1984.
20. Hautzer NW, Wittkuhn JF, McCaughey WRE: Trypsin digestion in immunoperoxidase staining. J Histochem Cytochem 28:52-53, 1980.
21. Imam A, Taylor CR, Tokes ZA: Immunohistochemical study of the expression of human milk-fat-globule membrane glycoprotein-70. Cancer Res (in press).
22. Lee AK, DeLellis RA, Rosen PP, et al: Alpha-lactalbumin as an immnohistochemical marker for metastatic breast carcinoma. Am J Surg Pathol 8:93-100, 1984.
23. Cardiff J, Taylor R, Wellings JR, et al: Monoclonal antibodies in immunoenzyme studies of breast cancer. Ann NY Acad Sci 420:115-126, 1983.
24. Teramoto YA, Meriani R, Wunderlich D, et al: The immunohistochemical reactivity of a human monoclonal antibody with tissue sections of human mammary tumors. Cancer 50:241-249, 1982.
25. Naritoku WY, Taylor CR: A comparative study of the use of monoclonal antibodies using three different immunohistochemical methods: an evaluation of monoclonal and polyclonal antibodies against human prostatic acid phosphatase. J Histochem Cytochem 30:253-260, 1982.
26. Nadji M, Tabei SZ, Castro A, et al: Prostatic origin of tumors. An immunohistochemical study. Am J Clin Pathol 73:735-739, 1980.
27. Kuriyama M, Loor R, Wang MC, et al: Prostatic acid phosphatase and prostate-specific antigen in prostate cancer. Int Adv Surg Oncol 5:29-49, 1982.
28. Kawaoi A, Okano T, Nemoto N, et al: Simultaneous detection of thyroglobulin (Tg), thyroxine (T4), and triiodothyronine (T3) in nontoxic thyroid tymors by the immunoperoxidase method. Am J Pathol 108:39-49, 1982.
29. Kameda Y, Harada T, Ito K, Ikeda A: Immunohistochemical study of the medullary thyroid carcinoma with reference to C-thyroglobulin reaction of tumor cells. Cancer 44:2071-2082, 1979.
30. Ordo~nez NG, Iba~nez ML, Samaan NA, Hickey RC: Immunoperoxidase study of uncommon parathyroid tumors. Report of two cases of nonfunctioning parathyroid carcinoma and one intrathyroid parathyroid tumor-producing amyloid. Am J Surg Pathol 7:535-542, 1983.
31. DeLellis RA: Diagnostic Immunohistochemistry. New York, Masson, 1981.
32. Mukai K, Rosai J: Applications of immunoperoxidase techniques in surgical pathology, In: Progress in Surgical Pathology. Edited by CM Fenoglio, M Wolff, New York, Masson, 1980.

33. Reisfeld RA: Monoclonal antibody to human malignant melanoma. Nature 298:325-326, 1982.
34. Brown JP, Woodbury RG, Head CE, et al: Quantitative analysis of melanoma-associated antigen P97 in normal and neoplastic tissues. Proc Natl Acad Sci USA 78:539-543, 1981.
35. Stuhlmiller GM, Borowitz MJ, Croker BP, et al: Multiple assay characterization of murine monoclonal antimelanoma antibodies. Hybridoma 1:447-460, 1982.
36. Carrel S, Accolla RS, Carmagno AL, et al: Common human melanoma-associated antigens detected by monoclonal antibodies. Cancer Res 40:2523, 1980.
37. Thompson JJ, Herlyn MF, Elder DE, et al: Use of monoclonal antibodies in detection of melanoma associated antigen in intact human tumors. Am J Pathol 107:357-361, 1982.
38. Tapia FJ, Polak JM, Barbosa AJA, et al: Neuron-specific enolase is produced by neuroendocrine tumors. Lancet 1:808-811, 1981.
39. Gatter KC, Alcock C, Heryet A, et al: The differential diagnosis of routinely processed anaplastic tumors using monoclonal antibodies. Am J Clin Pathol 82:33-43, 1984.
40. Epstein AL, Marder RJ, Winter J, et al: Two new monoclonal antibodies (LN-1, LN-2) reactive in B5 fixed paraffin embedded tissues with follicular center and mantle zone human B lymphocytes and derived tumors. J Immunol (in press).
41. Okon E, Felder B, Epstein A, et al: Monoclonal antibodies reactive with B lymphocytes and histiocytes in paraffin sections. Cancer (in press).
42. Marder RJ, Variakojis D, Silver J, Epstein AL: Immunohistochemical analysis of human lymphomas with monoclonal antibodies to B cell and Ig antigens reactive in paraffin sections. Lab Invest (in press).
43. Robb-Smith AHT, Taylor CR: Lymph Node Biopsy. London, Miller Heyden Ltd, and New York, Oxford University Press, 1981.
44. Mukai K, Rosai J, Burgdorf WH: Localization of factor VIII-related antigen in vascular endothelial cells using an immunoperoxidase method. Am J Surg Pathol 4:273-276, 1980.
45. Pasquier B, Pasquier D, Tanous AM, et al: Detection of glial fibrillary acidic protein in central nervous tumors using an immunohistochemical method. Preliminary study of 33 cases. Sem Hop Paris 56:1720-1721, 1980.
46. Miller CA, Benzer S: Monoclonal antibody cross-reactions between Drosophila and human brain. Pros Natl Acad Sci USA 80:7641-7645, 1983.

4

MONOCLONAL ANTIBODIES IN IMMUNOCYTOCHEMISTRY

HECTOR BATTIFORA, M.D.

1. INTRODUCTION

The application of immunohistochemical methods to the solution of diagnostic problems in the surgical pathology of neoplasms has progressed considerably in recent years. In large measure, this welcome development stems from the advent of the technique of somatic cell hybridization for the manufacturing of monoclonal antibodies (mabs) (1). This technological breakthrough permits the production of chemically uniform, monospecific antibodies, and has the added advantage that purification of the antigens is no longer obligatory. Thus, it has been possible to prepare antibodies that have varying degrees of tissue or cell-differentiation specificity, using intact cells (and therefore a complex mixture of antigens) used as immunogens.

A large number of mabs with important investigational applications have been developed in recent years. Some of these mabs have been found to be useful tools in surgical pathology. I will review our experience with the antibodies we most frequently use to solve common problems in tumor diagnosis. These are antibodies to keratins, leukocyte common antigen, protein S100, milk fat globule-derived antigen and antibodies to basal lamina antigens. All of these, with the exception of antiserum to protein S100, are recently developed monoclonal antibodies.

2. KERATINS

In recent years much attention has been devoted to the study of the intermediate filaments (IFs) which are a family of fibrous proteins with a diameter of 8-10 nanometers and are a part of the cytoskeleton of higher eukaryotic cells. Members of this family are differentially expressed by various tissues and can be identified using specific antibodies. The family of IFs was initially subdivided according to the tissue from which they were initially isolated: neurofilaments and glial filaments from the central nervous system, vimentin from mesenchymal cells, desmin from muscle and keratins from epithelial cells, (for review see reference 2). Keratins are a family of water insoluble, intracellular fibrous proteins present in abundance in cells of the epidermis and its appendages, where they are, for the most part, responsible for cytoarchitectural support (2,24-26).

Recent studies have shown that keratin filaments are present in almost all epithelia, both in vivo and in culture (2,7,9,24-26). Keratin filaments may be identified ultrastructurally when they are laterally aggregated and form the familiar tonofilaments of squamous and other epithelial cells. Often, however only dispersed keratin filaments exist within epithelial cells and cannot be distinguished from other IFs by electron microscopy but may be readily identified by immunochemical and immunohistological means (21). Thus, antibodies to keratins are more sensitive than electron microscopy for the purpose of identifying epithelial lineage.

About 19 subclasses of keratins have been identified by two dimensional gel electrophoresis (7). Low molecular weight keratins predominate during early embryogenesis and in the dividing cells of the skin (12,13). Maturation of epidermal cells is accompanied by increases in the high molecular weight keratins (14,28). There is now clear evidence that different keratin classes are expressed by various epithelia and their derived neoplasms and that the type of keratin subclass expressed may vary depending on the cell origin, maturation stage, and growth conditions (7,10,11).

Monoclonal antibodies with limited specificity to keratins of various molecular weights have been prepared by several laboratories (6,11,129). Utilizing these antibodies it has been possible to correlate the expression of specific keratin classes with various types of epithelial differentiation (6,7,8,10,11). Thus, monoclonal antibodies with limited range of keratin specificity may prove valuable for the subclassification of epithelial tumors. We have done extensive clinical testing of two monoclonal antibodies prepared against human epidermal callus keratins. These antibodies, which are designated as AE1 and AE3, react with keratins of different molecular weights. Antibody AE1 recognizes predominantly low molecular weight, acidic keratins in the range of 40Kd to 56Kd. Antibody AE3 recognizes higher molecular weight, primarily basic, keratins in the range of 46Kd to 67Kd. Using these antibodies it was established that the 40,46 and 52 Kd keratin classes are expressed by virtually all epithelial. The high molecular weight keratins 65-67Kd, on the other hand are unique to keratinized epidermis (28,29).

We have examined a large number of human neoplasms and normal tissues with these antibodies using several immunohistochemical methods and various modalities of specimen preparation. Antibody AE1 has shown great sensitivity and broad specificity for keratins under a variety of fixation and staining methods and because of its broad specificity it is a sensitive detector of the epithelial lineage. We compared the immunoreactivity of antibody AE1 with various "homemade" rabbit anti-whole human callus keratin antisera against a panel of several hundred human neoplasms. The immunostains obtained with the monoclonal antibody were easier to interpret because of their cleaner background and greater intensity. We obtained similar results when AE1 was compared with two commercially available antisera to keratins (21).

2.1 <u>Staining of normal tissues with antibodies AE1 and AE3:</u>

Epithelial cells such as those of the skin, mucosae, ducts of secretory glands and gastrointestinal lining normally stain intensely with both AE1 and AE3 (Fig.1). However, in the epidermis the reaction above the basal layer is weak with AE1, but strong with AE3. This is due to the abundance of high-molecular-weight keratins in the upper layers of the skin. The epithelial-reticular cells of the thymus as well as Hassal's corpuscles give a strong positive staining (Fig.2). Tissues of mesenchymal, hematopoietic and neural origin do not exhibit detectable keratin with AE1.

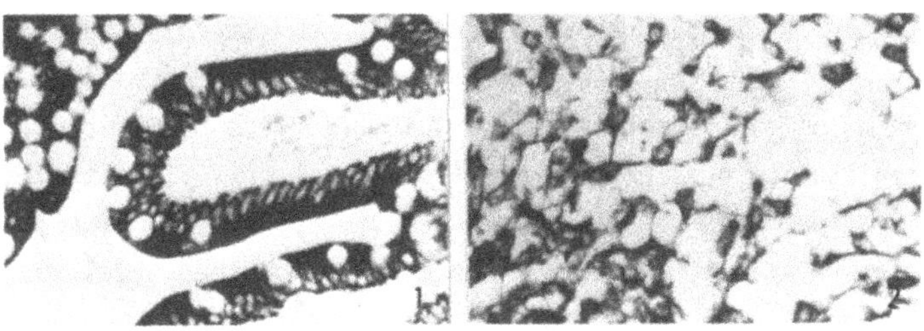

FIGURE 1. Normal jejunal mucosa stained with mab to keratins AE1. Note strong staining only of the epithelial cells Formalin fixed, paraffin embedded, ABC method. FIGURE 2. Sections of infant thymus, stained with mab AE1. Note strong expression of keratins by the epithelial reticular cells and the Hassal's corpuscle. Formalin fixed, paraffin embedded, ABC method.

2.2 Immunohistochemistry of Tumors with Antibody AE1:

Our results to date with AE1 are summarized in Tables I and III. There is good correlation between the AE1-detectable keratin in neoplastic cells and their cell or origin. There are, however, some departures from this rule. Hepatocellular and renal cell carcinoma give positive staining whereas normal hepatocytes and renal tubular cells do not. It is now well established that hepatocytes and tubular cells of the kidney contain keratins but of a class not usually detectable with ordinary antisera or AE1 (30,31). During the process of neoplastic transformation and diseases such as hepatitis, different classes of keratins, detectable by AE1, may be expressed by hepatocytes (32-34). Mallory alcoholic hyaline, for example, is strongly stained with antibody AE1.

Table 1. Neoplasm which are always positive with monoclonal antibody AE1.

	No. of Cases Studied
- Squamous carcinoma, irrespective of degree differentiation	- 200
- Adenocarcinoma even if poorly differentiated	- 500
- Oat cell carcinoma (intermediate type)	- 15
- Epithelial and mixed mesothelioma	- 16
- True thymoma	- 50
- Germ cell tumors (except seminomas)	- 50
- Synovial sarcoma	- 24
- Epithelioid sarcoma	- 8
- Chordoma	- 4

Tumors of mesenchymal, neural or hematopoietic origin fail to express keratins. However, epithelioid sarcoma and synovial sarcoma, which are classified as soft tissue neoplasms, consistently express keratins detectable with AE1. These neoplasms may share a common histogenesis, but their cell of origin is not known and both, (perhaps significantly) resemble epithelium by light and electron microscopy. Similarly, normal mesothelium, (believed to be mesoderm-derived epithelium) is strongly positive for keratins. Expectedly, mesotheliomas of epithelial and mixed type (and some of pure spindle cell type) are also keratin positive. It can be stated that the type of intermediate filament expressed by these tumors, parallels their epithelial phenotype, histogenetic considerations notwithstanding.

Table 2. Neoplasms which are negative with monoclonal antibody AE1.

	No. of Cases
- Soft tissue tumors (except synovial and and epithelioid sarcoma)	- 90
- Hematopoietic tumors (mostly lymphomas)	- 180
- Malignant melanoma	- 70
- Neuroblastoma	- 12
- Meningioma	- 10
- Glioma	- 10
- Paraganglioma	- 12
- Seminoma	- 24

Table 3. Neoplasms which are sometimes positive with antibody AE1.

	No. of Cases
- Oat cell carcinoma, classical (lymphocyte like)	- 12 (50% focal)
- "Carcinoids"	- 16 (+ 70% Uniform)
- Neuroendocrine carcinoma of skin	- 17 (75% Uniform)

2.3 Diagnostic Applications AE1:

Because of its sensitivity and broad specificity as a nearly universal detector of the epithelial phenotype AE1 has rapidly become one of our most useful diagnostic mabs. We use it frequently in our laboratory to solve problems which heretofore were the domain of the electron microscope. For example, it is often difficult, to distinguish undifferentiated or poorly differentiated carcinoma from malignant lymphomas and amelanotic melanoma. The demonstration of keratins in the neoplastic cells effectively rules out lymphomas and melanoma (Fig.3). To avoid basing a diagnosis on a negative result, it is best to approach this problem with a multi-antibody panel, as shown in the illustrative cases (see below). As shown in Table I, we found keratins in all cases of squamous cell carcinoma which we studied, including the poorly differentiated types. Similarly, every case of breast carcinoma (more than 200 studied) showed strong staining of virtually every tumor cell with AE1 (Fig.4). Metastatic tumors were as strongly stained as were their respective primaries (Fig.5). The presence of readily demonstrable keratins within metastatic breast cancer cells suggests that AE1 could be used to detect micrometastases in lymph nodes and bone marrow; tissues not normally harboring keratin-containing cells. Thus, single neoplastic cells can readily be identified with this antibody (Fig. 6).

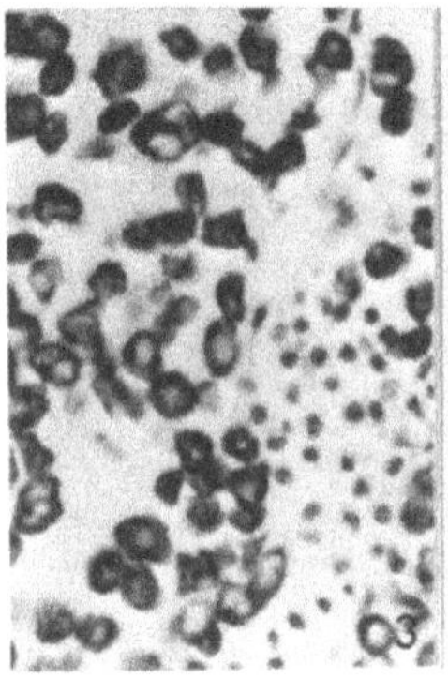

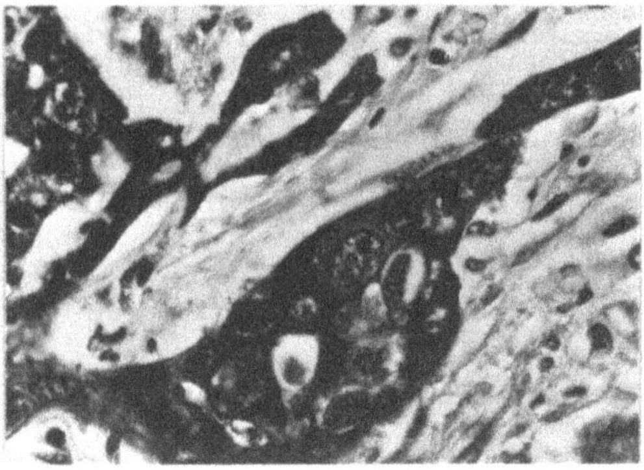

FIGURE 3. Ductal carcinoma of the breast, metastatic to the liver. Alcohol Fixation, paraffin embedded. Stained with AE1. FIGURE 4. Lobular carcinoma of the breast, metastatic to a lymph node. The subcapsular sinuses contain keratin-positive neoplastic cells. Formalin fixed, paraffin embedded, ABC stained with antibody AE1.

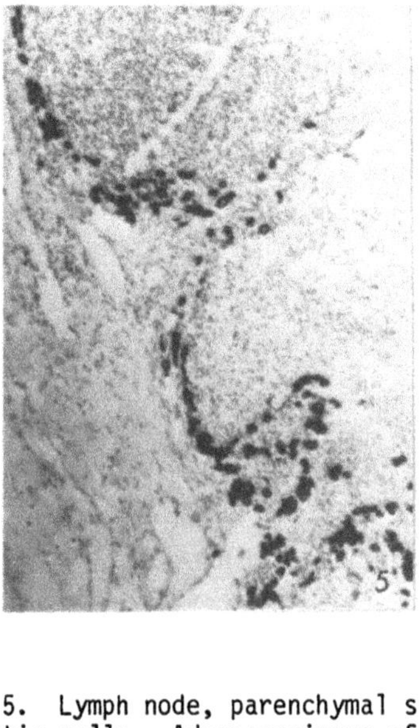

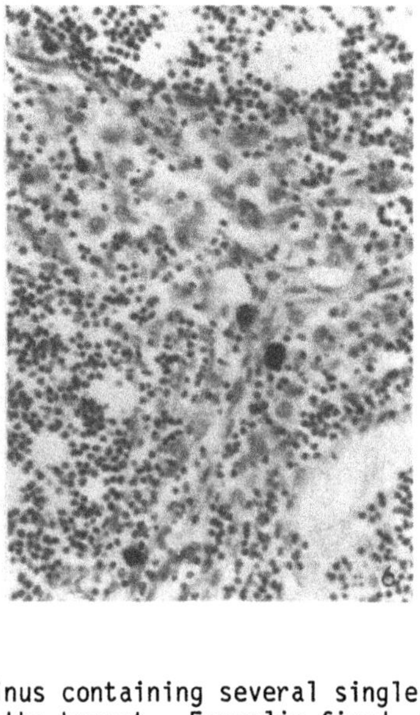

FIGURE 5. Lymph node, parenchymal sinus containing several single neoplastic cells. Adenocarcinoma of the breast. Formalin-fixed, AE1 stained with the ABC method. FIGURE 6. Predominantly lymphocytic thymoma. AE1 stained. Notice strong staining of the body of the neoplastic epithelial cells. The lightly counterstained lymphocytes are negative for keratin.

2.4 Thymoma:

The distinction between thymoma and lymphoma involving the anterior mediastinum can often be problematic. In such cases immunohistochemistry with antisera against keratins or with monoclonal antibody AE1 will readily reveal the epithelial nature of the neoplastic cells (15). In thymomas, even in those with an apparent predominance of non neoplastic lymphocytes, immunohistochemistry will reveal a surprisingly large number of epithelial cells (the neoplastic cells of true thymomas) which are regularly distributed among the unreactive lymphocytes (Fig.7). This sharply constrasts with the picture seen in lymphoma involving the thymus, where no keratin-containing cells are detected or, if present, they appear as discrete aggregates ascribable to residual thymic tissue. When the electron microscope is used in these cases, the foci of residual thymus may lead to sampling error. Such errors are easily avoided with immunohistochemistry because of the larger amount of tissue examined.

2.5 Germ Cell Tumors:

As noted in Table I, all germ cell tumors except seminoma express keratins. Primitive germ cells of the testes do not express detectable keratin; seminoma, a neoplasm of primitive germ cells believed to be incapable of somatic differentiation fails to express keratins (Fig.8).

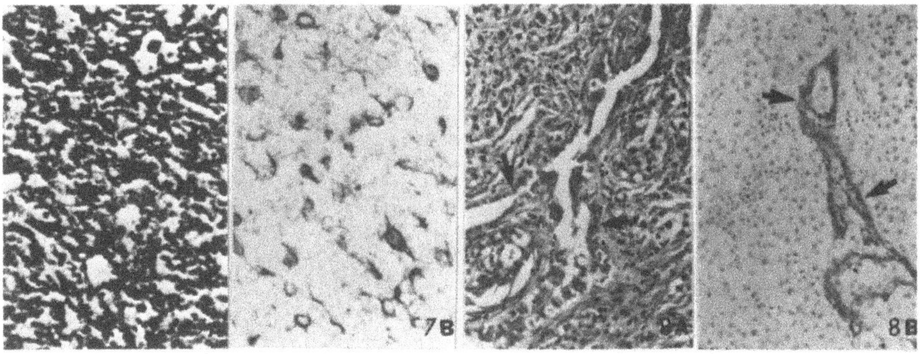

FIGURE 7. Large cell lymphoma of the anterior mediastinum (proven with lymphocyte marker study) A and B keratin stained with mab AE1. Note absence of keratin in the neoplastic cells (A) and a focus of residual thymic tissue and mature lymphocytes (B). The entrapped epithelial cells are strongly positive for keratins. FIGURE 8. Testicular seminoma surrounding portion of the rete testis. A: Hematoxylin and eosin, B:AE1, stained. Note that only the epithelium of the rete testis stains for keratins, the neoplastic cells are entirely negative.

On the other hand keratins are the first IFs to appear in the embryo and accordingly, are expressed (albeit often focally) by embryonal carcinoma, a neoplasm characterized by a variable degree of somatic differentiation (Fig.9). These findings may have practical application in the distinction between anaplastic seminoma and embryonal carcinoma (16).

2.6 Spindle Cell Carcinoma:

Spindle cell carcinoma is often misdiagnosed as sarcoma. In cases arising in the epidermis the differential diagnosis should include spindle cell melanoma and fibrous histiocytoma. Keratins may be demonstrated with mab AE1 within the cytoplasm of the spindle cells in most cases of spindle cell carcinoma but neither melanomas nor fibrous histiocytomas contain keratins (Fig.10).

2.7 Mesenchymal Neoplasms:

The diagnosis of monophasic synovial sarcoma is difficult and often controversial. The discovery of expression of keratins by synovial sarcoma, in particular by the spindle cell component (albeit, focally in most instances) paved the way for the separation of monophasic synovial sarcoma from other spindle cell sarcomas (36). In every example of biphasic synovial sarcoma that we have studied with mab AE1, there was strong immunostaining of the epithelial component (Fig.11A). In these

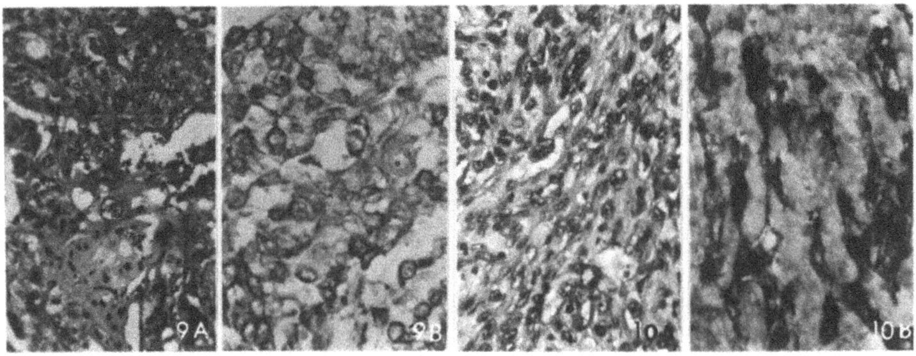

FIGURE 9. Embryonal cell carcinoma of testes. A: Hematoxylin and eosin, B:AE1 stained section. Notice that most tumor cells contain keratin although in variable proportions. FIGURE 10. Large skin neoplasm diagnosed by previous biopsies as malignant fibrous histiocytoma. A: Hematoxylin and eosin, predominantly spindle cell growth closely mimicking a sarcoma. B: Frozen section of same tumor stained with antibody AE1. Notice heavy staining of the cytoplasm of the spindle cells.

cases, however, focal staining of the spindle cell component was also observed. We carried out the same study in seven samples of monophasic or predominantly monophasic synovial sarcomas, focal staining of the spindle shaped neoplastic cells was detected (Fig. 11B). Epithelioid sarcoma, a neoplasm believed to be histogenetically related to synovial sarcoma, is occasionally mistaken for other sarcomas, in particular rhabdomyosarcoma. We have two cases in our consultation files in which this error was made by the referring pathologist. The tumor cells in both cases contained abundant and uniformly distributed keratins, as shown with antibody AE1 (which rules out rhabdomyosarcoma) (Fig.12). Seventy percent of epitheliod sarcomas have demonstrated keratin with conventional antikeratin antisera (37). Conceivably, a larger percentage, perhaps nearly 100% could be positive if monoclonal antibodies to low molecular weight keratins were used since everyone of eight cases that we have studied with AE1 was strongly positive. Chondromas, chondrosarcomas and chordoid sarcomas have, in our experience failed to show evidence of expression of keratins with antibody AE1. Chordoma, a tumor of the epithelial notochord, produced uniform and strong staining for the presence of keratins. These findings could be useful in cases of diagnostic difficulty between chordoma, chordoid sarcoma and chondrosarcoma.

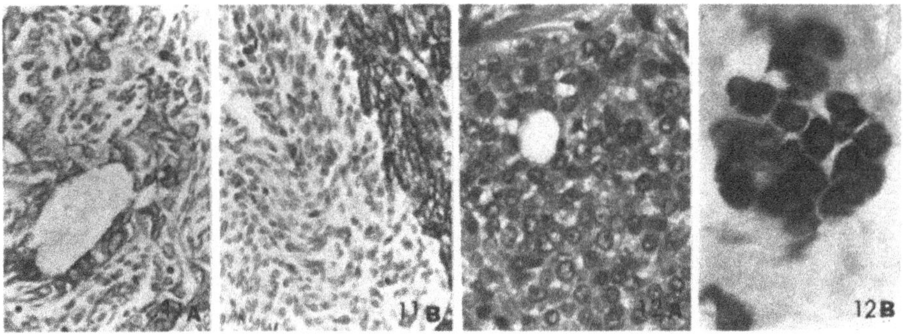

FIGURE 11. Synovial sarcoma, AE1 stained. A: Classifical biphasic pattern. Notice predominant staining of the epithelial component. B: Predominantly monophasic synovial sarcoma. Notice strong but focal staining of the spindle cells. FIGURE 12. Epithelioid sarcoma which had been previously diagnosed as rhabdomyosarcoma. A: Hematoxylin and eosin, B: AE1 stained section, formalin fixation, paraffin embedded, no counterstain. Notice strong cytoplasmic staining indicating the presence of keratins.

2.8 Neuroendocrine Carcinoma:

Not every sample of neuroendocrine carcinoma contained keratins demonstrable with antibody AE1, but the majority did. This adds to the growing body of evidence against the neural-crest origin of these neoplasms, since true neural crest-derived neoplasms such as melanoma and neuroblastoma consistently fail to express keratins. Further, these findings could be diagnostically useful. For example, small cell carcinoma of the skin (Merkel cell tumor) is often misdiagnosed as cutaneous lymphoma. We have studied fourteen cases of Merkel cell tumor, and eleven of these contained readily demonstrable, uniformly distributed keratins as detected by AE1 (unpublished data). Therefore, a positive stain for keratins, given this differential diagnosis, would effectively rule out lymphoma.

3. ANTIBODIES TO LEUKOCYTE COMMON ANTIGEN:

A larger number of mabs prepared against leukocyte antigen have become available in recent years. The majority of these antibodies are however specific for lymphocyte subsets. Antibodies to antigens such as Ia (Dr) react with a broad spectrum of white blood cells but are not specific for hematopoietic cells (30-40) Several mabs that have restricted specificity for leukocytes, but that are widely expressed by leukocytes and hematopoietic neoplasms, have recently been described (41-45).

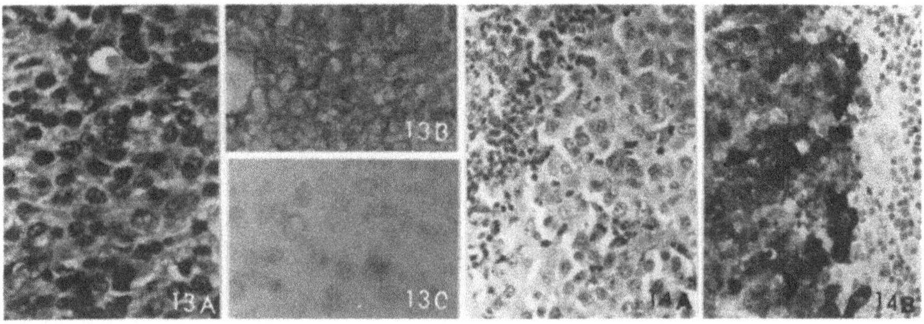

FIGURE 13. Biopsy of axillary lymph node originally diagnosed as metastatic melanoma. A: Hematoxylin and eosin, B: Frozen section stained with antibody T29/33 by indirect immunofluorescence, C: Control. Additional work-up revealed presence of several B cell markers. The diagnosis was changed to large cell lymphoma. FIGURE 14. Typical malignant melanoma metastatic to a lymph node. A: Hematoxylin and eosin. B: S100 stained, formalin fixed, paraffin embedded. ABC method. Notice strong immunoreactivity of the neoplastic cells and occasional nuclear staining.

Such antibodies can play a major role in the solution of the familiar problem of distinguishing undifferentiated carcinoma, amelanotic melanoma, or sarcoma from lymphoma (Fig.13). It appears that most (if not all) of these antibodies recognize members of a family of high-molecular weight glycoproteins designated as T200 or leukocyte common antigen (LCA) (41). The antigen is partially or completely destroyed or masked by fixation. Some anti LCA antibodies react with leukocytes fixed in various fixatives (44-46). However, in our experience, reliable and reproducible results are only obtained with frozen sections. Furthermore most other surface markers employed in the phenotyping of hematopoietic neoplasms are sensitive to fixation. Snap-freezing of suspected lymphomas is thus always desirable. It should be stressed that anti LCA antibodies are tissue but not tumor-specific and that, by themselves cannot help in the distinction between benign and malignant lymphoid lesions. Nevertheless, in the case of neoplasms of uncertain origin but with definite malignant histologic appearance the antibodies can be very useful in the identification of hematopoietic lineage.

3.1 Antibody T29/33:

For more than four years, we have been using an antibody to LCA prepared by Dr. Ian Trowbridge, Department of Cancer Biology, Salk Institute, La Jolla, Ca. The antibody, designated as T29/33 was made against a human T-cell leukemic line. Chemical characterization of the antigen recognized by T29/33 has shown it to be a high (200kd) molecular weight glycoprotein (41).

The antigen recognized by T29/33 (also referred to as T200) does not survive ordinary fixation. With short term incubation in formalin or alcohol, some preservation of the antigen may be observed and occasionally positive results in paraffin embedded tissue may be obtained (46). The results are unreliable, however, fixation is therefore not recommended with this mab. We have studied a wide spectrum of hematopoietic neoplasms with antibody T29/33. Negative results are unusual but we, as well as and others, have found them in rare plasmacytomas, in two or four true histiocytic lymphomas and rarely in acute lymphoblastic leukemia. It is important, from a practical standpoint that we have not yet come across a bona fide large cell lymphoma (other than the true histiocytic type) that failed to react with T29/33 (43,47,48). However, it is theorectically possible that some lymphomas do not express detectable quantities of antigen. False positive results are rare. In our initial work with T29/33 we used immunofluorescence to study frozen sections of more than 100 human neoplasms over a wide histogenetic spectrum. Many poorly differentiated carcinomas, (well characterized by electron microscopy and antikeratin antisera) were included in this series. In more recent years we have used the sensitive ABC method on frozen sections almost exclusively and have not yet found a convincing case of false positivity with this antibody. Borowitz and Stein have reported an example of rhabdomyosarcoma which reacted positively with T29/33 (48). We observed one spindle cell sarcoma having relatively intense cytoplasmic staining with this antibody. Because antigen T200 is located only in the cell membrane in hematopoietic cells, this was not considered a false positive result. However, because monoclonal antibodies recognize a narrow portion of the antigen (epitope), a true cross reaction, that is that recognition of a similar epitope in an unrelated molecule is a possibility. However, this is a rare occurrence (49). Antibodies directed against LCA are particularly useful in the distinction between undifferentiated carcinoma, amelanotic melanoma, and large cell lymphoma (see below).

4. ANTIBODIES TO S100 PROTEIN:

S100 protein is an acidic protein, originally isolated from brain tissue, its designation derives from its solubility in 100% ammonium sulfate. Early work suggested that the protein was brain specific and could be used as a marker of glial cell differentiation (50). More recent studies have shown that it may be found in a variety of cells of non neural origin such as chondrocytes, myoepithelium, interdigitating reticulum cells of lymph nodes and Langerhans cell of the skin (51,52), S100 protein has been detected in a number of human tumors including melanoma, schwannoma, granular cell tumor, adenoma of salivary gland and chordoma (51-58). Despite this apparent lack of specificity, antisera to S100 protein, if properly applied, especially together with antibodies to other markers, may be very useful diagnostic aids. Antisera to S100 protein are particularly useful for the diagnosis of amelanotic malignant melanoma since positive results are found in the majority of cases, (52,54). The staining pattern characteristically involves the cytoplasm and occasionally the nuclei (Fig.14). The antisera are also helpful in the diagnosis of soft tissue tumors. Virtually all benign nerve sheath tumors give positive results with antisera to S100 protein, whereas only 59% of malignant schwannomas have positive immunoreactivity, and often only focally (55). Benign and malignant fibrous histiocytic tumors fail to show presence of S100 protein, thus the antisera may be helpful in the distinction between these tumors and nerve sheath tumors. Sporadic positive results are obtained in a variety of mesenchymal tumors such as lipoma, liposarcoma, chondrosarcoma and fibromatosis (55). Because negative results are very rare with amelanotic melanoma, antisera against S100 protein have, as their principal diagnostic role to distinguish amelanotic and spindle cell melanoma from unrelated, but histologically similar neoplasms.

5. ANTIBODIES AGAINS MILK FAT GLOBULE DERIVED ANTIGEN (MFGDA) AND THEIR USE IN THE DIAGNOSIS OF MESOTHELIOMA.

Because the milk fat globules are enveloped by portions of the apical cell membrane of the breast epithelium, they are a convenient source of plasma membrane for use as immunogen (59-61). Numerous conventional and monoclonal antibodies have been raised with cell membranes obtained from human milk. The resulting antibodies have often shown relative tissue specificity for breast epithelium and its tumors. In most cases, however, they have shown broad specificity, reacting with several epithelia and neoplasms of non-breast origin (62). Because mab AE1 is superior as detector of epithelial lineage, these antibodies to MFGDA are less useful for this purpose. However, some of the MFGDA, by virtue of their more restricted specificity have practical uses. For example, some of these antibodies distinguish epithelial from mesothelial cells. We have explored the application of a monoclonal antibody against MFGDA which was originally designated as 1.10F3 (83) but is currently designated as HMFG-2, (Seward Labs, London). The antibody recognizes determinants present in high molecular weight components (400Kd) in normal and neoplastic mammary cells (64). By immunohistochemistry, the antibody stains the apical membranes reactivity with HFMG-2. In well-differentiated carcinomas, apical staining may be intense. The antigen recognized by this mab is also expressed by a variety of adenocarcinomas of diverse origin. We obtained reliable and reproducible results in formalin fixed tissue, with no need for protease digestion of the sections. The important feature of this antibody and which is responsible for its clinical usefulness is its lack of reactivity with normal, irritated, or neoplastic mesothelial cells (Fig. 15). We have compared several antisera as well as monoclonal antibodies to keratin, antisera to CEA and antibody HFMG-2 against 12 mesotheliomas and 100 adenocarcinomas (65). Our results showed 100% staining of mesotheliomas and adenocarcinomas with the antikeratin antisera and with monoclonal antikeratin antibody AE1. On the other hand, none of the mesotheliomas and 85% of the adenocarcinomas stained with antibody HFMG-2 (Figs. 16,17). As shown in Table IV all breast, lung, and ovarian adenocarcinomas stained with HFMG-2. This is of particular significance since these are the most common adenocarcinomas involving pleura or peritoneum and the last two mentioned are the most likely to have a clinical and histopathologic picture simulating mesothelioma. Carcinoembryonic antigen was expressed by fewer adenocarcinomas. Moreover, two mesotheliomas reacted, although weakly, with the commercial CEA antiserum used in this study (Dako). The tendency for CEA antiserum to stain leukocytes and histiocytes strongly may be an obstacle in the interpretation of CEA immunostains of keukocyte-rich neoplasms. Although we conclude that antibody HMFG-2 is superior to CEA antiserum for the differential diagnosis between mesothelioma and adenocarcinoma we recommend that both be used, because occasional adenocarcinomas which were negative with HMFG-2 antibody were CEA positive (66).

In a parallel study, we compared the diagnostic value of the same antibodies when applied to cytologic preparations from pleural fluids. We studied paraffin-embedded cell blocks which had been fixed in formalin, but we obtained comparable results from smears or cytospin preparations. The results are shown in Table V. Strong cytoplasmic staining with HFMG-2 was noted in most adenocarcinoma cells but reactive mesothelial cells failed to stain (Figs.18,19). The antibody permitted the recognition of neoplastic cells in low-power examination of the immunostains. That this may be a more sensitive means of identifying adenocarcinoma cells in effusive fluids has been suggested by the results of others who used similar antibodies (66,67).

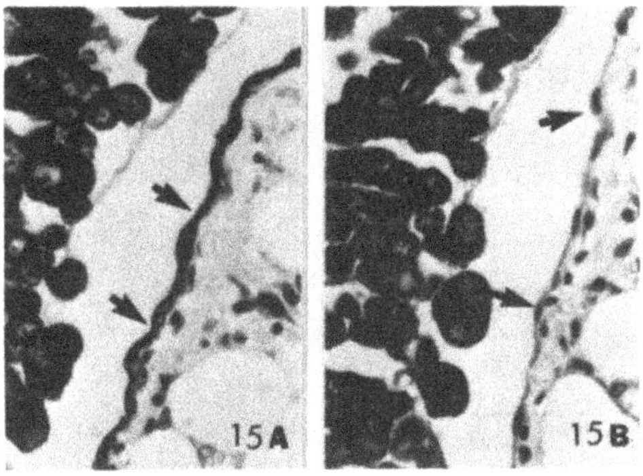

FIGURE 15. Poorly differentiated adenocarcinoma of ovarian origin, metastatic to omentum. The upper portion of both photographs shows part of an uninvolved lobule of omental fat covered by mesothelial cells (arrows). A: Keratin stained with antibody AE1, notice strong staining of neoplastic and mesothelial cells. B: Stained with antibody HFMG-2, notice that only the neoplastic cells but not the mesothelium stains. Formalin fixed, paraffin embedded, ABC method.

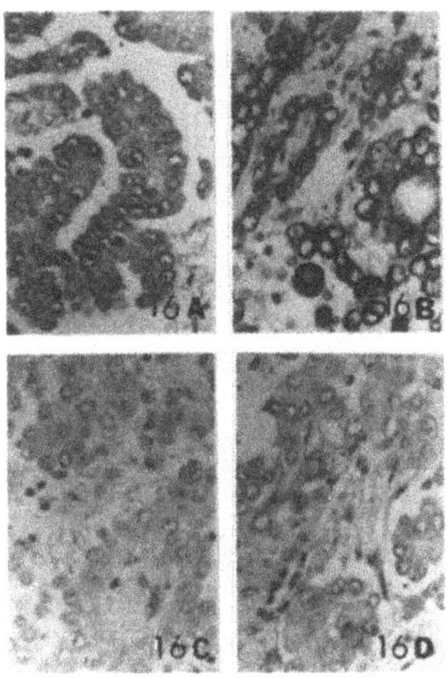

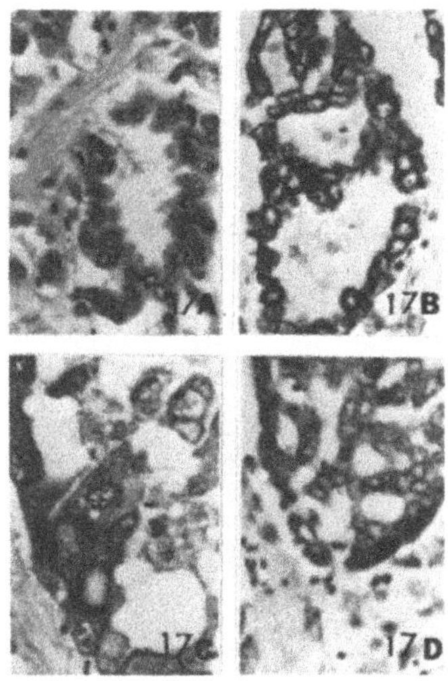

FIGURE 16. Typical epithelial mesothelioma from the pleura of an asbestos worker A. Hematoxylin and Eosin, B: AE1 antikeratin stain, C: Stained with HFMG-2, D: Stained with Antiserum to CEA. Notice strong expression of keratins by the malignant mesothelial cells, negativity with the antibody to HFMG-2 and weak positivity with CEA antiserum.

FIGURE 17. Adenocarcinoma of the lung involving the pleural surface. A: Hematoxylin and eosin, B: AE1 stained, C: HFMG-2, D: Anti CEA. Notice strong positivity for keratins, HFMG-2 and CEA.

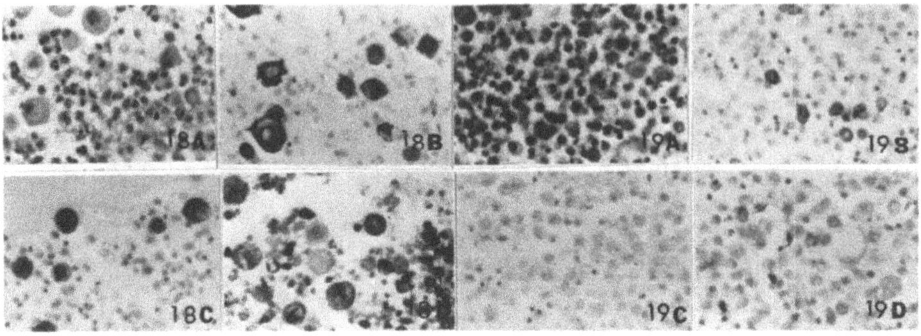

FIGURE 18. Cell block of a poorly differentiated adenocarcinoma of gastric origin in pleural effusion. A Hematoxylin and eosin, B: AE1, C: HFMG-2, D: CEA. Notice strong immunoreaction with all the antibodies and staining of leukocytes with CEA. FIGURE 19. Cell block of serous effusion from a patient in cardiac failure containing irritated mesothelial cells. A: Hematoxylin and eosin, B: AE1, C: HFMG-2, D: CEA. Notice keratin expression by the mesothelial cells, negative staining with HFMG-2 and staining of macrophages and leukocytes with CEA antiserum.

Table 4. IMMUNOSTAINING OF TISSUES WITH MESOTHELIOMA PANEL

	ANTIBODY		
DIAGNOSIS	AE1	MFG-2	CEA
MESOTHELIOMA	13/13	0/13	2/13
ADENOCARCINOMA:			
Breast*	22/22	22/22	18/22
Lung*	24/24	24/24	24/24
Ovary*	14/14	14/14	10/14
Stomach	8/8	6/8	5/8
Colon	6/6	4/6	3/6
Kidney	5/5	4/5	1/5
Prostate	5/5	0/5	0/5
Miscellaneous	13/13	9/13	4/13
% of Adenoca stained	100%	86%	69%
% of * marked	100%	100%	86%

Table 5 IMMUNOSTAINING OF SEROUS FLUIDS WITH MESOTHELIOMAS PANEL

CYTOLOGIC DIAGNOSIS	ANTIBODY AE1	MFG-2	CEA
REACTIVE MESOTHELIUM	12/12	0/12	0/12
MESOTHELIOMA	1/1	0/1	0/1
ADNOCARCINOMA			
Breast	6/6	6/6	4/6
Lung	2/2	2/2	2/2
Ovary	2/2	2/2/	2/2
Miscellaneous	12/12	10/12	9/12
% of Adenoca stained	100%	91%	77%

6. ANTIBODIES TO BASAL MEMBRANE ANTIGENS:

In recent years, antisera and monoclonal antibodies have been prepared against collagen type IV and laminin, the two major components of the basement membrane (68-70). These antibodies provide us with the most specific stains of the basement membrane to date and are useful in several aspects of histological diagnosis. We have used a monoclonal antibody to collagen type IV, a generous gift to Drs. D.W. Hollister and R.E. Burgeson (68). The antibody is specific for human collagen type IV and does not cross react with any other type of collagen. The best results are obtained on frozen sections or on alcohol-fixed tissues. Formalin fixation is often responsible for negative results. Mesenchymal as well as epithelial basement membranes are outlined with minimal or no background staining.

We have studied more than 100 adenocarcinomas of the breast with this antibody (unpublished observations). An intact basement membrane is consistently visible around ductal carcinoma in situ (Fig.20). In contrast, no such basement membrane can be seen around invasive carcinoma (Fig.21). It has been suggested that invasive carcinoma cells are capable of production of new basal lamina. This may be the case in squamous carcinoma of the cervix, but this is a controversial subject (71-73). Our findings, in the case of breast carcinoma, nevertheless, indicate that the antibody may be useful in distinguishing stromal infiltration from intralobular extension. Similarly, the antibody may help in separating tubular carcinoma from microglandular adenosis. In the latter, a well-defined basal lamina can be demonstrated with the immunoperoxidase technique around the glandular structures.

The antibody may allow the distinction between benign tumors of schwannian origin and non-neural tumors of similar histology. In the former, a large amount of basal membrane material is made by the tumor cells and can be identified readily with electron microscopy or with ntibodies to collagen type IV or laminin (Fig.23) (74). These antibodies can also be applied to the distinction between capillaries, (which have a basal lamina) and lymphatics, (which do not) (75). Antibodies to laminin, the second most abundant component of the basement membrane, have been used with results comparable to those obtainable with antibody to collagen type IV. We have studied, in parallel with antibodies to collagen type IV, a monoclonal antibody to laminin, a generous gift of Dr. E. Ruoslahti (70). The results are similar to those obtained with the monoclonal anti collagen IV antibody but the combined use of the two antibasement membrane antibodies as a "cocktail" result, in most instances, in stronger staining of the basal lamina because they have an additive effect.

7. REPRESENTATIVE CLINICAL EXAMPLES

The following clinical cases have been chosen to illustrate the clinical applications of the antibodies discussed in preceding pages. It is noteworthy that in many instances an unambiguous diagnosis be obtained by the combined use of two or more of these antibodies as panels to avoid basing a diagnosis on a negative result. It should also be emphasized that the problems cases illustrated here are frequent ones. Another point worth re-emphasizing is that successful application of immunodiagnostic methods - as is the case with transmission electron microscopy - depends in great part on narrowing of the diagnosis to a small number of possibilities by conventional histologic examination.

7.1. CASE #1: A 59-year-old woman was seen at a referring hospital because of a mass located in the axillary tail of the right breast. A biopsy revealed a poorly differentiated neoplasm (Fig.22A) The biopsy was examined by several pathologists and their opinions were divided between large cell lymphomas and medullary carcinoma. The controversy persisted even after electron microscopy and several histochemical stains were done. The case was then referred in consultation to our laboratory. Immunohistochemical study was done on frozen sections using antibody T29/33 and AE1. Strong membrane positivity with T29/33 and negative staining with AE1 were shown by these cells (Figs.22B,C). These results indicated that the correct diagnosis was lymphoma. The patient was then placed on a therapeutic lymphoma protocol which resulted in rapid resolution of the tumor.

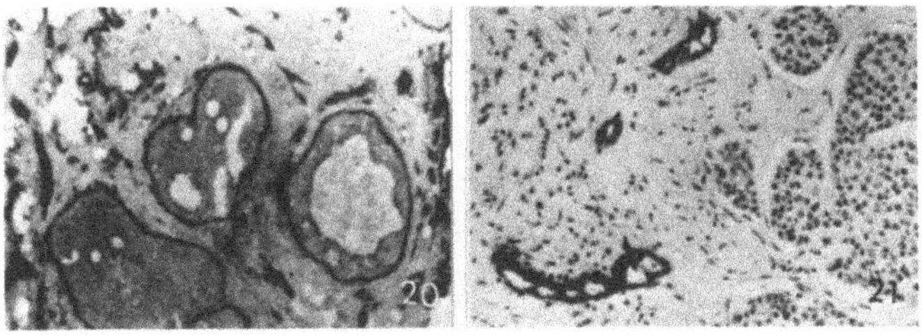

FIGURE 20. Duct carcinoma in situ of the breast (two cases) stained with antibody to collagen type IV. Notice staining of epithelial basal lamina as well as mesenchymal vascular basal lamina. Both frozen sections. ABC method. FIGURE 21. Infiltrating carcinoma of the breast stained with monoclonal antibody to collagen type IV. Duct carcinoma, usual type, notice no basal lamina material around the neoplastic nests but ample immunoreactivity on the basal lamina of the blood vessels.

Comment: The distinction between large cell lymphoma and undifferentiated carcinoma is often difficult. We know, for example four cases of extranodal lymphoma involving the breast which were misdiagnosed as medullary carcinoma and underwent mastectomy.

The antigens recognized by the mabs comprising the antibody panel we used in this case are mutually exclusive. That is to say, lymphomas never express keratins and carcinoma does not have antigen T200. Conversely, all large cell lymphomas are T200 positive, and will react with antibody T29/33 and all carcinomas will (at least focally) be positive for the presence of keratins with mab AE1.

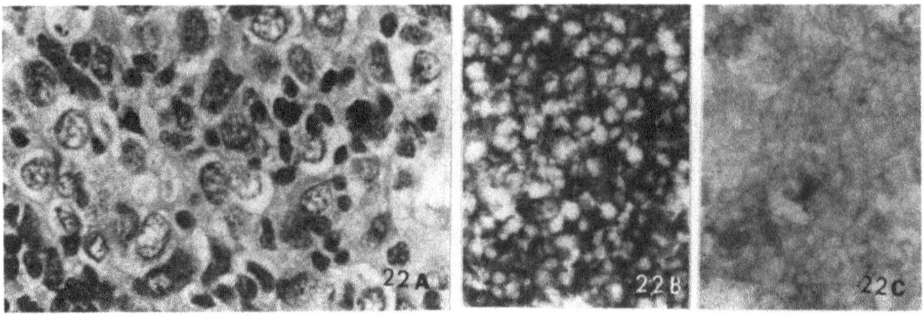

FIGURE 22. Lesion of microglandular adenosis of the breast. A: Hematoxylin and eosin. B: Stained with mab to collagen type IV. C: Stained with mab T 29/33.

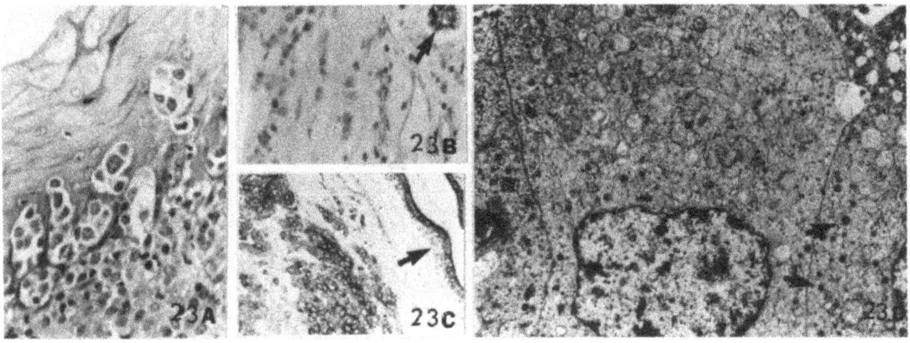

FIGURE 23. Epithelioid schwannoma, A: Electron micrograph depicting the typical enveloping cell processes and multilayered basal lamina-like material. B: Section stained with mab to collagen type IV. Notice immunoreactive haloes around the tumor cells corresponding to the basal lamina shown by the electron microscope. C:S100 stained section showing strong immunostaining of nuclei and cytoplasm. D. Electron microscopy revealing the presence of neuroendocrine granules.

7.2. CASE #2: The patient, a 61-year-old man presented to another hospital with symptoms of upper airway obstruction. A large tumor involving the endolarynx was found and biopsied. The specimen was initially interpreted as malignant amelanotic melanoma, probably primary in the larynx. The paraffin embedded material was submitted in consultation to our laboratory. As a diagnostic panel in this case, we used antiserum to S100 protein and mab AE1. The results are depicted in Fig.23A. The light microscopic features of the tumor are indeed consistent with amelanotic melanoma. Clusters of neoplastic cells are seen invading the mucosa. However, the neoplastic cells intensely stained with mab AE1 and not with antiserum to S100 protein (Figs.23B,C,D). This is opposite to the results expected from melanoma which expresses S100 protein in virtually every case and is always keratin negative. The tumor was therefore classified as epithelial in origin. Electron microscopy revealed the presence of numerous dense-core granules within the cytoplasm of the neoplastic cells and led to a diagnosis of neuroendocrine carcinoma (Fig.23D).

Comment: In cases where the diagnosis has been narrowed to carcinoma vs melanoma the antibody panel chosen in case 2 is usually adequate to obtain a firm diagnosis. If lymphoma cannot be excluded and frozen tissue is available antibody T29/33 is added to the panel.

7.3. CASE #3: The patient, a 68-year-old man developed a slowly growing subdermal mass in his left nostril. The skin over the lesion did not appear particularly abnormal. A wedge biopsy revealed a neoplasm made up exclusively of spindle cells forming short bundles. The differential diagnosis was between atypical fibrous xanthoma, spindle cell carcinoma and spindle cell melanoma. Immunohistochemical study was done using the same antibody panel as the preceding case. The results, shown in Fig.24, were the reverse of those in case 2 in that the neoplastic cells were strongly stained with antiserum to S100 protein and not with antibody to keratin AE1. A diagnosis of spindle cell melanoma was rendered in view of these results. Eight months later the patient developed regional lymph node metastasis, and later disseminated metastases which were biopsied and had the appearance of typical non spindle melanoma and were still S100 protein immunoreactive.

Comment: Accurate dignosis, by conventional means, is often difficulty in cases of spindle cell tumors of the skin. The clinical features are usually of no help because the three most common entities which enter the differential diagnosis, AFX, melanoma and spindle cell carcinoma all present on sun-damaged skin in the elderly and have similar

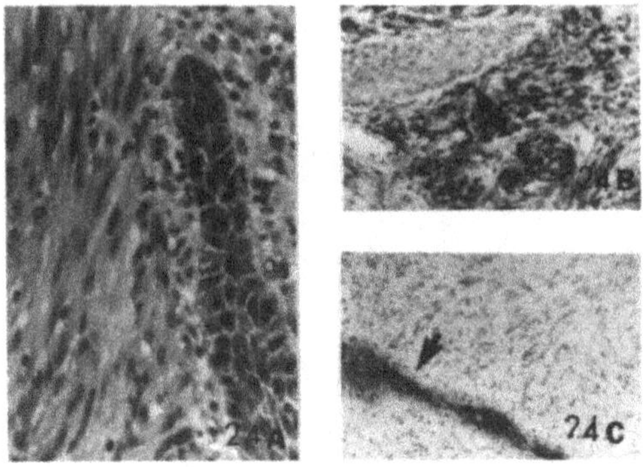

FIGURE 24. Sections from a patient with a squamous cell carcinoma of the tongue treated surgically who developed, 8 months later, neck lymphadenopathy. A: Hematoxylin and eosin, representative view of the tongue lesion. B: Frozen section of neck mass, stained with mab T29/33, notice intense membrane stain. C: Parallel frozen section stained with mab AE1. The diagnosis of large cell lymphoma was further supported by monoclonal light chain staining and other B cell markers.

gross and histologic appearance. Because AFX has a benign behavior, it is imperative to distinguish it from melanoma and carcinoma which are malignant neoplasms and need more aggressive treatment. We have found that AFX expressed neither keratins nor S100 protein, whereas spindle cell carcinoma can be readily recognized by its expression of keratins with antibody AE1. Spindle cell melanoma, as in this case, will not stain with AE1 but will give positive results with antiserum to S100 protein.

7.4. CASE #4: This patient, a 56-year-old man presented to another hospital with recurring left pleural effusion. Atypical cells were presented in cytological preparations of the pleural fluid. A pleural biopsy revealed a tumor with epithelial and glandular appearance which was interpreted as adenocarcinoma. Our studies with a panel of antibodies which included AE1, HMFG-2 and antiserum to CEA is shown in Fig.16, the neoplastic cells express keratins but are negative with antibodies HMFG-2 and anti CEA. Because the vast majority of adenocarcinomas involving the pleural surfaces are positive with all antibodies in this panel (see table IV) these results suggested that the patient had a mesothelioma. In addition electrophoresis of glycosaminoglycans of the pleural fluid demonstrated a preponderance of hyaluronic acid. Electron microscopy showed that the tumor cells had abundant long sinuous microvilli. These two results are strongly supportive of the diagnosis of mesothelioma. The patient was subjected to palliative pleural decortication. During the thoracotomy it was noted that both pleural surfaces were studded with tumor. Additional evidence favoring mesothelioma was later obtained when a history of occupational exposure to asbestos was elicited.

EPILOGUE:

Methodological advances in the field of immunohistochemistry coupled with the advent of the production of monoclonal antibodies are revolutionizing tissue diagnosis and promised greater diagnostic accuracy in surgical pathology. In this communication we have shown a small group of mabs which are frequently used in our laboratories to solve common problems of histopathologic diagnosis. Undoubtedly, many more antibodies with practical applications to surgical pathology will soon be developed. Libraries of antibodies to antigens expressed by the various tissues and their derived neoplasms are likely to be developed. The possibility is clearly at hand that monoclonal antibodies will be utilized for identification of increasing numbers of marker substances which have not only diagnostic, but also prognostic significance.

References

1. Kohler, G and Milstein, C: Continuous cultures of fused cells secreting antibody of predefined specificity. Nature (Lond) (256):495-497, 1975.
2. Lazarides E: Intermediate filaments as mechical integrators of cellular space. Nature (283):249-256, 1978.
3. Denk H, Krepler R, Artlieb U,: Proteins of intermediate filaments: An immunohistochemical and biochemical approach to the classification of soft tissue tumors. Am J Pathol (110):193-208, 1983.
4. Ramaekers FCS, Puts JJG, Kant A,: Use of antibodies to intermediate filaments in the characterization of human tumors. Cold Spring Harbor Symposia on Quantitative Biology, (46):331-339, 1982.
5. Osborne M and Weber K: Tumor diagnosis by intermediate filament typing. Lab Invest (48):372-394, 1983.
6. Gown AM and Vogel AM: Monoclonal antibodies to human intermediate filament proteins: II distribution of filament proteins in normal human tissues. Am J Pathol (114):309-321, 1984.
7. Moll R, Franke WW, Schiller DL,: The catalogue of human cytokeratin polypeptides: Patterns of expression of cytokeratins in normal epithelia, tumors and cultured cells. Cell (31):11-24, 1982.
8. Scheffer C, Tseng G, Jarvinen MJ,: Correlation of specific keratins with different types of epithelial differentiation: Monoclonal antibody studies. Cell (30):361-372, 1982.
9. Franke WW, Applelhans B, Schmid E,: Identification and characterization of epithelial cells in mammalian tissues by immunofluorescence microscopy using antibodies to prekeratin. Differentiation (15):7-25, 1979.
10. Nelson WG, Battifora H, Santana H and Sun TT: Specific keratins as markers for neoplasms with a stratified epithelial origin: Monoclonal antibody analysis. Cancer Research (44): 1600-1603, 1984.
11. Debus E, Weber K, and Osborn M: Monoclonal cytokeratin antibodies that distinquish simple from stratified squamous epithelial: Characterization on human tissues. The Embo Journal (1):1641-1647, 1982.
12. Banks-Schlegel SP: Keratin alterations during embryonic epidermal differentiation: A Presage of Adult Epidermal Maturation. J. Cell Biol (93):551-559, 1982.
13. Moll R, Moll I, and Wiest W: Changes in the pattern of cytokeratin polypeptides in epidermis and hair follicles during skin development in human fetuses. Differentiation (23):170-178,1982.
14. Nelson WG and Sun TT: The 50-and-58-kdalton keratin classes as molecular markers for stratified squamous epithelial: Cell culture studies. J Cell Biol (97):244-251, 1983.
15. Battifora H, Sun TT, Rao S, and Bahu R: Antikeratin antibodies in tumor diagnosis: Thymomas. Human Pathol (11):635-641, 1980.
16. Battifora H, Sheibani K, Tubbs RR,: Antikeratin antibodies in tumor diagnosis: distinction between seminoma and embryonal carcinoma. Cancer (54):843-848, 1984.
17. Nagle RB, McDaniel KM, Clark VA,: The use of antikeratin antibodies in the diagnosis of human neoplasms. Am J Clin Pathol (79):458-466, 1983.

18. Gatter KC, Abdulaziz Z, Beverley P,: Use of monoclonal antibodies for the histopathological diagnosis of human malignancy. J Clin Pathol (35):1253-1267, 1982.
19. Madri JA and Barwick KW: An immunohistochemical study of nasopharyngeal neoplasms using keratin antibodies: epithelial versus nonepithelial versus nonepithelial neoplasms. Am J Surg Pathol (6):143-149, 1982.
20. Miettinen M. Lehto V and Virtanen I: Nasopharyngeal lymphoepithelioma: Histological diagnosis as aided by immunohistochemical demonstration of keratin. Virchows Arch (Cell Pathol) (40):163-169, 1982.
21. Taxy JB, Battifora H and Hidvegi D: Nasopharyngeal Carcinoma: Electron Microscopy and a comparison of three antikeratin antisera. Lab Invest (50):59a, 1984 (abstr).
22. Sieinski W, Dorsett B and Ioachim HL: Identification of prekeratin by immunofluorescence staining in the differential diagnosis of tumors. Human Pathol (12):452-457, 1981.
23. Fuchs E and Hanukoglu I: Unraveling the structure of the intermediate filaments. Cell (34):321-334, 1983.
24. Gown AM and Vogel AM: Monoclonal antibodies to intermediate filament proteins of human cells: Unique and cross reacting antibodies. J Cell Biol (95):414-424, 1982.
25. Sun TT and Green H: Keratin filaments of cultures human epidermal cells. J Biol Chem (253):2053-2060, 1978.
26. Sun TT and Green H: Immuonfluorescent staining of keratin fibers in cultured cells. Cell (14):469-476, 1978
27. Sun TT, Shih C and Green H: Keratin cytoskeletons in epithelial cells or internal organs. Proc Natl Acad Sci USA (76):2813-2817, 1979.
28. Sun TT, Eichner R, Nelson WG,: Keratin classes: Molecular markers for different types of epithelial differentiation. J Invest Dermatol (81):109s-115s, 1983.
29. Woodcock D, Mitchell J, Eichner R, Nelson WG, Sun TT: Immunolocalization of keratin polypeptides in human epidermis using monoclonal antibodies. J Cell Biol (95):580-588, 1982.
30. Franke WW, Denk H, Kalt R, Schmid E: Biochemical and immunological identification of cytokeratin proteins present in hepatocytes of mammalian liver tissue. Exp Cell Res (131):299-318, 1981.
31. Holthofer H, Miettinen A, Lehto V-P,: Expression of vimentin and cytokeratin types of intermediate filament proteins in developing and adult human kidneys. Lab Invest (50):552-559, 1984.
32. Franke WW, Mayer D, Schmid E: Differences of expression of cytoskeletal proteins in cultured rat hepatocytes and hepatoma cells. Exp Cell Res (134):345-365, 1981.
33. Denk H, Franke WW, Eckerstorfer R: Formation and involution of Mallory bodies ("alcoholic hyalin") in murine and human liver revealed by immunofluorescence microscopy with antibodies to prekeratin. Proc Natl Acad Sci USA (76):4112-4116, 1979.
34. Denk H, Franke WW, Dragosics B, Zeiler I: Pathology of cytoskeleton of liver cells: Demonstration of Mallory bodies (alcoholic hyalin) in murine and human hepatocytes by immunofluorescence microscopy using antibodies to cytokeratin polypeptides from hepatocytes by immunofluorescence microscopy using antibodies to cytokeratin polypeptides from hepatocytes. Hepatology (1):9-20, 1981.

35. Miettinen M. Lehto V-P, Virtanen I: Keratin in the epthelial-like cells of classical biphasic synovial sarcoma. Virchows Arch (Cell Pathol) (40):157-151, 1982.
36. Miettinen M, Lehto V-P, Virtanen I: Monophasic synovial sarcoma of spindle-cell type: epithelial differentiation as revealed by ultrastructureal features, content of prekeratin and binding of peanut agglutinin. Virchows Arch (Cell Pathol) (44):187-199, 1983.
37. Chase D. Enzinger F. Weiss SW, Langloss JM: Keratin in epithelioid sarcoma: An immunohistochemical study. Am J Surg Pathol (8):435-441, 1984.
38. Brodsky FM, Parham P, Barnstable CJ: Monclonal antibodies for analysis of the HLA system. Immuno Rev (47):3-61, 1979.
39. Rouse RV, Parham P, Grumet FC, Weissman IL: Expression of HLA antigens by human thymic epithelial cells. Human Immunol (5):21-34, 1982.
40. vanRood JJ, de Vries RRP, Bradley BA: Genetics and biology of the HLA system. IN: The role of the major histocompatibility complex in immunobiology. Edited by Dorf ME, New York, Garland, pp 59-113, 1981.
41. Omary MB, Trowbridge IS, Battifora HA: Human homologue of murine T200 glycoprotein. J Exp Med (152):842-852, 1980.
42. Pizzolo G, Sloane J, Beverley P: Differential diagnosis of malignant lymphoma and nonlymphoid tumors using monoclonal antileukocyte antibody. Cancer (46):2640-2647, 1980.
43. Battifora H and Trowbridge IS: A monoclonal antibody useful for the differential diagnosis between malignant lymphomas and nonhematopoietic neoplasms. Cancer (51):816-831, 1983.
44. Warnke RA, Gatter KC, Falini B: Diagnosis of human lymphoma with monoclonal antileukocyte antibodies. NEJM (309):1275-1281, 1983.
45. Wood GS, Link DM, Warnke R: Pan-leukocyte monoclonal antibody L3B12: Characterization and application to research and diagnostic problems. Am J Clin Pathol (80):415-420, 1983.
46. Hsu S-M, Shang H-Z, Jaffe ES: Utility of monoclonal antibodies directed against B and T lymphocytes and monocytes in paraffin-embedded sections. Am J Clin Pathol (80):415-420, 1983.
47. Andres TL, Kadin ME: Immunologic markers in the differetial diagnosis of small round cell tumors form lymphocytic lymphoma and leukemia. Am J Clin Pathol (79):546-551, 1983.
48. Borowitz MJ, Stein RB: Diagnostic applications of monoclonal antibodies to human cancer. Arch Pathol Lab Med (108):101-105, 1984.
49. Dulbecco R, Unger M. Bolongna M: Cross-reactivity between Thy-1 and a component of intermediate filaments demonstrated using a monoclonal antibody. Nature (292):772-774, 1981.
50. Moore BW: A soluble protein characteristic of the nervous system. Biochem Biophys Res Commun (19):793-744, 1965.
51. Kahn HJ, Marks A, Thomas H, Baumal R: Role of antibody to S100 protein in diagnostic pathology. Am J Clin Pathol (79):341-347, 1983.
52. Nakajima T, Watanabe S, Sato Y: An immunoperioxidase study of S100 protein distribution in normal and neoplastic tissues. Am J Surg Pathol (6):715-727, 1982.
53. Cochran AJ, Duan-Ren W, Hershman Hr, Gaynor RB: Dectection of S100 protein as an aid in the identification of melanocytic tumors. Int J Cancer (30):295-297, 1982.
54. Nakajima T, Watanabe S, Sato T: Immunohistochemical demonstration of S100 protein in malignant melanoma and pigmented nevus, and its diagnostic application. Cancer (50):912-918, 1982.

55. Weiss SW, Langloss JM, Enzinger FM: The value of S100 protein in the diagnosis of soft tissue tumors with particular reference to benign and malignant schwann cell tumors. Lab Invest (49):299-308.1983.
56. Stefansson K. Wollman RL: S100 protein in granular cell tumors (granular cell myoblastomas). Cancer (49):1834-1838, 1982.
57. Nakazato Y, Ischizeki J, Takahashi K: Localization of S100 protein and glial fibroaxillary acidic protin-related antigen in pleomorphic adenoma of the salivary glands. Lab Invest. (46):621-626, 1982.
58. Nakamura Y, Becker LE, Marks A: S100 protein in human chordoma and human and rabbit notochord. Arch Pathol Lab Invest (46):621-626, 1982.
59. Ceriani RL, Thompson K. Peterson JA, Abraham S: Surface differentiation antigens of human mammary epithelial cells carried on the human milk fat globule, Proc Natl Acad Sci (47):582-586, 1977.
60. Taylor-Papadimitriou J, Peterson JA, Arklie J: Monoclonal antibodies to epithelium-specific components of the human milk fat globule membrane: Production and reaction with cells in culture. Int J Cancer (28):17-21, 1981.
61. Sasaki M, Peterson JA, Wara WM, Ceriani RL: Human mammary epithelial antigens (HME-Ags) in the circulation of nude mice implant with a breast tumor and non breast tumors. Cancer (48):2204-2210, 1981.
62. Sloane JP, Ormerod MG: Distribution of epithelial membrane antigen in normal and neoplastic tissues and its value in diagnostic tumor pathology. Cancer (47):1786-1795, 1981.
63. Arklie J, Taylor-Papadimitriou J, Bodmer W: Differentiation antigens expressed by epithelial cells in the lactating breast are also detectable in breast cancers. Int J Cancer (28):23-29, 1981.
64. Burchell J, Durbin H, Taylor-Papadimitriou J: Complexity of expression of antigenic determinants recognized by monoclonal antibodies HFMG-1 and HFMG-2 in normal and malignant human mammary epithelial cells. J Immunol (131):508-513, 1983.
65. Battifora H, Kopinski MI: distinction of mesothelioma from adeoncarcinoma: An immunohistochemical approach. Cancer, in press.
66. Epenetos AA, Conti IG, Taylor-Papapdimitriou J: Use of two epithelium-specific monoclonal antibodies for diagnosis of malignancy in pleural effusions. Lancet II:1004-1006, Nov. 6, 1982.
67. Ghosh AK, Mason DY: Immunocytochemical staining with monoclonal antibodies in cytologically "Negative" serous effusions from patients with malignant diasease. J. Clin Pathol (36):1150-1153, 1983.
68. Sakai LY, Engvall E, Hollister DW, Burgeson RE: Production and characterization of a monoclonal antibody to human type IV collagen. Am J Pathol (108):310-318, 1982.
69. Foellmer HG, Madri, JA, Furthmayr H: Methods in Laboratory investigation: Monoclonal antibodies to type IV collagen: Probes for the study of structure and function of basement membranes. Lab Invest (48):639-649, 1983.
70. Wewer U, Albrechtsen R, MAnthorpe M: Human laminin isolated in a nearly intact, biologically active form from placenta by limited proteolysis. J Biol Chem. (258):12654-12660, 1983.
71. Pertschuk LP, Boyce JG, Urcuyo R: An immunofluorescent study of basement membranes in squamous cell carcinoma of the cervix, vagina and vulva. Obst. Gynecol (49):417-420, 1976.
72. Frappart L, Berger G, Grimaud JA: Basement membrane of the uterine cervix: Immunofluorescence characteristics of the collagen component in normal or atypical epithelium and invasive carcinoma. Gyn Oncol (13):58-66, 1982.

73. Rubio CA, Biberfeld P: The basement membrane of the uterine cervix in dysplasia and squamous carcinoma: An immunofluorescent study with antibodies to basement membrane antigen. Acta Patho Microbiol Scand Sect A (83):744-748, 1975.

74. Miettinen M, Foidart J-M, Ekblom P: Immunohistochemical demonstration of laminin, the major glycoprotein of basement membranes, as an aid in the diagnosis of soft tissue tumors. Am J Clin Pathol, (79):306-311, 1983.

75. Barsky SH, Baker A, Siegal GP: Use of antibasement membrane antibodies to distinguish blood vessel capillaries from lymphatic capillaries. Am J Surg Pathol (7):667-677, 1983.

5

MARKERS OF KERATINOCYTE DIFFERENTIATION IN PRENEOPLASTIC AND NEOPLASTIC LESIONS

C.J. CONTI, G.I. FERNANDEZ ALONSO, AND A.J.P. KLEIN-SZANTO

In the last few years several laboratories have studied extensively the molecular events leading to the terminal differentiation of squamous epithelia. These studies have shown that the maturation of those stratified epithelia, also known as epidermoid or malpighian, is the result of a coordinated sequence of events that begins with cellular proliferation in the basal or germinative layer (1). The new cells are dislodged from the basal layer and, as they lose contact with the basement membrane, start synthesizing high-molecular-weight keratins (2) and other proteins unrelated to keratins that, in a later step of maturation, are cross-linked, forming a chemical-resistant envelope under the cell membrane (3). Simultaneously the keratins become stabilized by S-S bonds (2) and are organized into bundles of fibers, apparently by a basic protein of the matrix called filaggrin (4). At the same time, modified lysosomal bodies (membrane-coating granules or Odland bodies) secrete their products into the intercellular space, forming an impermeable lipid seal in the superficial epithelial layers, where most of the cellular organelles are lost by an unknown mechanism (5). All these events lead to the formation of a corneocyte, which is located at the most superficial layer of the epithelium, formed mainly from bundles of tonofilaments (keratins) embedded in an amorphous matrix (mainly filaggrin), and surrounded by a cell membrane under which a resistant envelope has been formed (1).

Most of the molecules that play a role in these processes have been identified, and isolated, and antibodies have been obtained against them. Some of these antibodies have been made available to pathologists in recent years. Monoclonal and polyclonal antibodies against keratins, for example, have become important tools in surgical and experimental pathology as markers of epithelial progeny (6). Although several subspecies of keratins have been described and most epithelia seem to have typical biochemical patterns of keratins (7), it has still not been possible to raise antikeratin antibodies that are specific for different types of epithelia. This is because keratin subspecies are immunologically closely related (8).

Other antibodies against differentiation products of squamous stratified epithelium, such as precursors of the envelopes (9,10) and filaggrin (11,12), are being studied, since they have great potential as diagnostic aids in pathology. One of their possible applications is as markers for isolated cells or anaplastic tumors that originate in squamous stratified epithelium or have some degree of epidermoid differentiation. The other important application of these antibodies is related to the fact that the differentiation patterns of premalignant and malignant lesions can alter the differentiation patterns, and, therefore, quantitative or qualitative modifications of these markers and changes in their localization can be found in different lesions. Using a battery of antibodies against products of differentiation of these epithelia may lead to a more rational classification of dysplastic and neoplastic lesions, and eventually allow researchers to document the epithelial progeny and the organ of origin of poorly differentiated tumors.

Precursors of the corneal envelope. As stated above, mature cells from stratified squamous epithelia form a 10-nm thick marginal bond, or corneal envelope, immediately beneath the plasma membrane. This structure was described years ago by electron microscopy (13), but not until the last few years did we learn that the envelope is formed in the upper spinous and granular layers by cross-linked soluble precursors catalyzed by the calcium dependent enzyme transglutaminase (3).

Two soluble precursors of the envelope have been isolated. The two molecules seem to be different biochemically and do not seem to be related immunologically. One of them is a 36K protein that was isolated from human and from bovine snout epidermis and was called keratolinin (10). The other precursor, called involucrin is a 92K protein that was isolated from human keratinocyte cultures

(9,15). Antibodies have been obtained against both precursors and the antiserum against involucrin is now commercially available.

In our laboratory we have used a different approach to obtain an immunoserum against the envelope and its precurors (14). We injected envelopes isolated from rat foot -pad epidermis into rabbits; the serum obtained after several booster inoculations was adsorbed against liver and spleen powder and purified keratins.

These antibodies seem to be useful for immunohistochemical studies, not only in fresh-frozen tissues but also in routinely prepared formalin fixed and paraffin-embedded tissues (15,16). However, when immuno-fluorescence techniques are employed in unfixed frozen sections, the involucrin staining appears in not less than three or four layers above the basement membrane and in a characteristic pericellular pattern that is probably related to the localization of the envelope (15). In formalinfixed tissues, (Figure 1) the peripheral pattern is not always observed, and the reaction is more diffuse in the cytoplasm of cells located suprabasally (16-18). This reaction can be carried out in formalin-fixed, paraffin-embedded blocks, even without enzymatic pre-treatment. Tissues processed in fixatives other than formaldehyde are also suitable for involucrin staining, but in our experience, ethanol fixation, a very effective procedure for keratin immunostaining, provides poor results. We have found other antibodies against envelope to produce similar results (14). However, since anti-involucrin antiserum is the only one that has been used in pathology, we will confine most of our discussions to this marker.

Involucrin in normal and pathological tissues. The involucrin staining pattern for normal and pathologic human skin was studied by Murphy et al. (18). Their study showed that cells of the upper third of the epidermis exhibit a homogeneous cytoplasmic involucrin pattern. Positive reaction was also obtained in the cells of the distal portion of the eccrine ducts and acrosyringium, the cells forming the inner root sheath of the hair follicle, the lining cells of apocrine ducts, and the follicular infundibula and isthmi. Skin lesions in which the differentiation process is altered are characterized by changes in the normal expression of involucrin. Four different patterns have been identified. The first is a homogeneous intracellular staining of the upper areas of the epithelium, similar in pattern to that of normal skin, that was found in epidermal hyperplasia and benign lesions such as lichen planus and keratoacanthomas. A second pattern, found in lesions with hyperplasia of basaloid keratinocytes such as seborrheic keratosis, is characterized by large confluent areas devoid of staining. A third pattern, a strong pericellular staining with little or no cytoplasmic reaction, is found in some benign neoplasms. The fourth pattern, which is unique to squamous cell carcinoma, is a mosaic patchy pattern with alternating areas of positive and negative cells. It is present in both invasive and in situ squamous cell carcinomas. In the invasive form the strongest staining is in the center of squamous nests. When inflammatory areas are present beneath the tumor, involucrin staining is usually decreased (18).

Said et al. (17) have described the staining pattern of squamous cell carcinomas in situ. In these lesions an abnormal pattern with irregular staining either was focal and localized to the lesion or extended to contiguous "normal" basal-layer areas; probably it was an expression of early dysplastic or preneoplastic changes. Basal cell carcinomas apparently do not express involucrin except when squamous horn cysts are present. Occasionally isolated cells stained strongly, and the overlying skin showed an abnormal pattern with positive basal cells.

The involucrin pattern of chemically induced mouse skin tumors has been studied in our laboratory (19). The pattern of squamous cell carcinoma is very similar to that described for the human counterpart.

Results of involucrin staining in human and mouse skin correlate well with the alterations of the differentiation process that characterize the respective epidermal lesions. When histopathologic observation indicates an accumulation of basal kerationcytes, involucrin expression decreases. Conversely, when lesions undergo rapid or increased cornification, the expression of this biologic marker is stronger.

Involucrin was also studied in white lesions of the human oral mucosa (20). Homogeneous leukoplakias exhibited a marked increase in the involucrin content of the spinous and granular layers (Figure 2). This contrasted markedly with the absence of this marker in the non-keratinized normal epithelia. In comparison with homogeneous leukoplakias, speckled (dysplastic) leukoplakias showed a relative decrease in involucrin immunostain. In situ and invasive carcinomas showed small but variable amounts of involucrin, which correlated well with the degree of differentiation (Figure 3). Involucrin also proved to be potentially useful in cervicovaginal pathology (16). Application of the involucrin immunostaining technique has been directed towards the differential diagnosis of dysplastic and neoplastic lesions. Non-neoplastic lesions, including mature and immature metaplasias, are positive for involucrin and have the same distribution pattern as normal epithelium, i.e., similar to normal epidermis. This pattern was also present in nonneoplastic viral lesions. Malignant lesions, however,are mainly negative or, when positive, show an altered pattern.

The majority (81%) of cervical intraepithelial neoplasias (CIN) of all degrees were negative. Using this technique, researchers can detect early stages of CIN by the absence of involucrin expression in the epithelium. However, extreme caution should be observed when inflammation is present in areas adjacent to the tumor since as we have already stated (see skin lesions), the presence of inflammation in a nonneoplastic lesion can cause a decrease in the intensity of involucrin staining or an alteration in its normal pattern. Although this complication can limit the use of the technique, involucrin immunostaining seems to be a useful tool in diagnosing cervicovaginal lesions. The results on CIN differ from those on carcinoma in situ of skin reported by Said (17). Further studies are necessary to discover why, but differences in the histologic type and the tumors biologic behavior may be the reason. It is possible, although not likely, that other envelope precursors such as keratolinin will not be modified by inflammation. Further exploration is warranted.

Normal lung tissues do not express involucrin but several lung lesions undergo epidermoid differentiation and do express the marker (20). For this reason, involucrin can be useful in diagnosting pathologic conditions of the respiratory tract epithelium. According to the study of Said et al. (21) involucrin staining is strongly positive in squamous metaplastic lesions in formalin -fixed tissue,but is either negative or positive for lung cancer

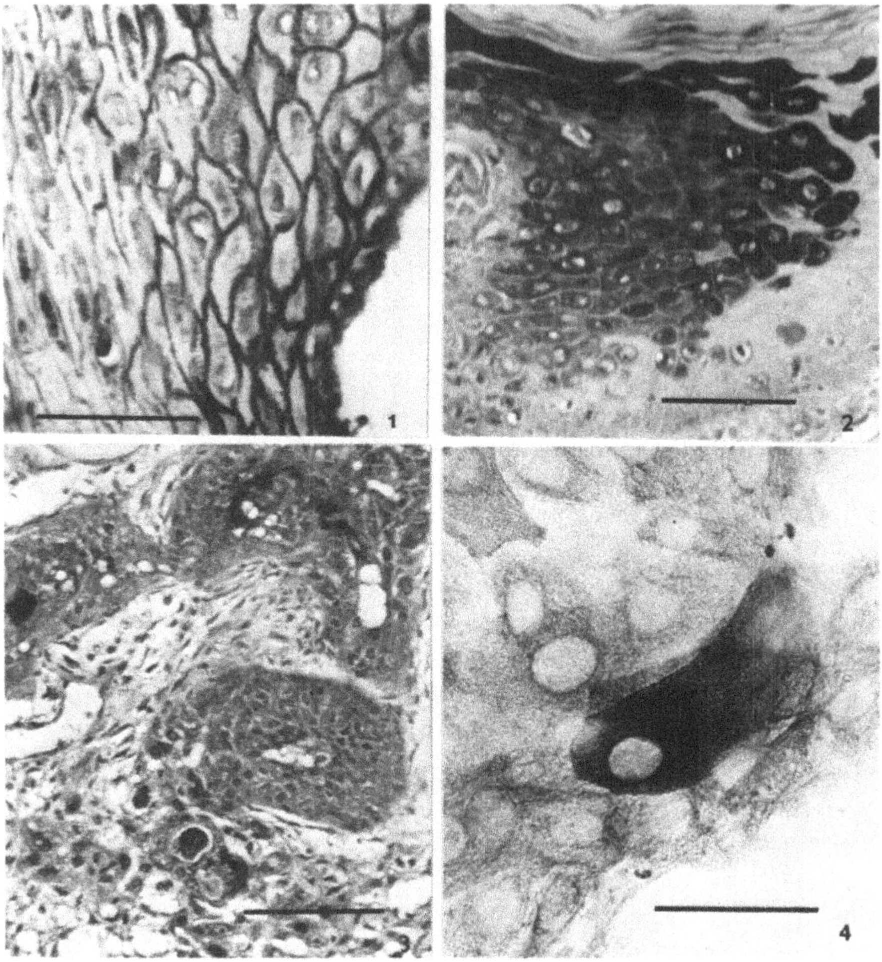

Figure 1. Human oral mucosa. Immunostaining for involucrin. Intense reaction beneath the plasma membrane (peripheral envelope-type pattern.) Immunoperoxidase (PAP) technique with rabbit anti-human involucrin. Formalin-fixed and paraffin embedded tissues. Hematoxylin counterstain. Bar = 100 μm. Figure 2. Leukoplakia of the human oral mucosa. Immunoperoxidase (PAP) staining for involucrin. Intense cytoplasmic difuse staining of granular and horny layers. No staining in basal cells. (Hematoxylin counterstain) Bar = 200 μm. Figure 3. Squamous cell carcinoma of the human oral mucosa stained for involucrin. Differentiated areas in centers of tumor nests show positive reaction. (Hematoxylin counterstain) Bar = 200 μm. Figure 4. Rat vaginal epithelial cell culture treated with 17 β-estradiol large differentiated cell showing intense reaction with rabbit antienvelope serum (14). Bar = 90 μm.

according to the histologic type and grade of differentiation. Small cell cancers are 100% positive; the staining is mostly focal and appears stronger in the larger cells of the tumor nests, showing a diffuse cytoplasmic pattern. Occasionally staining is peripheral, most often when immunofluorenscence techniques are used. Small cells adjacent to the tumor nests are always negative. Adenosquamous carcinomas are positive in squamouse cells lining squamous nests. The majority of adenocarcinomas are negative; the few positive cases showed staining in some large-cell foci that were probably undergoing some degree of squamous-cell differentiation. Approximately 50% of the large-cell undifferentiated carcinomas are positive for involucrin showing focal staining and a diffuse cytoplasmic pattern, sometimes stronger beneath the cell membrane. As a result of the studies, Said et al consider that involucrin may represent a specific marker for squamous differentiation in lung tumors.

Involucrin has also been used as a marker of squamous cell differentiation in tissue cultures and isolated cells. In keratinocyte cultures, large differentiated cells are strongly postive while the fast-replicating small undifferentiated cells are negative (22). In our laboratory, we have shown that large cells with positive staining for precursor of the envelope can be induced by ovarian hormones in vaginal keratinocyte cultures (23). (Figure 4) We have shown that this in vitro phenomenon correlates with our in vivo study, which revealed that involucrin and envelope are usually absent in the vaginal epithelium of ovariectomized rats and are induced by endogenous or exogeneous estrogenic hormones (24) (Figure 5).

Filament-aggregating protein (filaggrin). Filaggrin is a basic histidine-rich protein in keratohyalin granules and believed to be the electron-dense matrix that surrounds the bundles of keratin filaments in cornified cells (25,26). Filaggrin is synthesized in the upper spinous layers as a high-molecular weight phosphorylated precursor of approximately 350K (27). This precursor is apparently packed into the keratohyalin granules. When keratohyalin granules disappear in the transition between granular and horny layers, the high-molecular-weight precursor is dephosphorylated and partly degraded to form a lower-molecular-weight, highly basic, histidine-rich protein (25). The function of this protein is to aggregate keratin filaments, forming large, well-ordered macrofibrils, and to form the interfilamentous matrix seen in the lower stratum corneum (4).

Recently Harding and Scott have proposed a second function (26). They observed that filaggrin is further degraded, and that its complete proteolysis results in the formation of a concentrated pool of free amino acids and derivatives that allows the stratum corneum to retain water against the desiccating action of the environment. The two functions attributed to filaggrin are not mutually exclusive and probably represent sequential rather than alternative roles in the process of keratinization.

A polyclonal antibody against a 49K rat filaggrin, raised in goats by Dale and Ling, was used to study the localization of filaggrin in normal epidermis (11) and oral mucosa (28). A second antibody against a 28K mouse filaggrin was recently raised in rabbits (29). Both antibodies produce excellent immunohistochemical stainings with immunofluorescent techniques on frozen sections (29) or immunoperoxidase in paraffin-embedded tissues (11,30). In the latter instance, formalin-fixed tissue has been shown to be suitable without enzymatic pretreatment (30). However, tissues fixed in Zenker's fixative exhibit a stronger reaction (especially at lower serum concentrations). Zenker's fixative appears to be the first choice when preparing experimental tissues for filaggrin staining (11). The antimouse filaggrin serum prepared in our laboratory cross-reacts with other species and is suitable for pathologic studies in humans (12,30).

Filaggrin in normal and pathological epithe lia. The normal skin and epithelium of the oral mucosa of rat (11,28), mouse (29), and human (11,30) react strongly in the granular layer and no reaction has been detected in the basal and spinous layers. Staining of the stratum corneum was very variable, depending on the tissues. Dale and Ling (11) showed a positive reaction in the stratum corneum of the rat skin that was stronger in the two cell layers closest to the granular layer, but Dale et al. later found that the reaction in the oral epithelia was limited to the soft palate plus a weak, patchy area in the densely keratinized epithelium of the hard palate and tongue (28). A study carried out in our laboratory showed no immunostain in the stratum corneum of human oral mucosa (30).

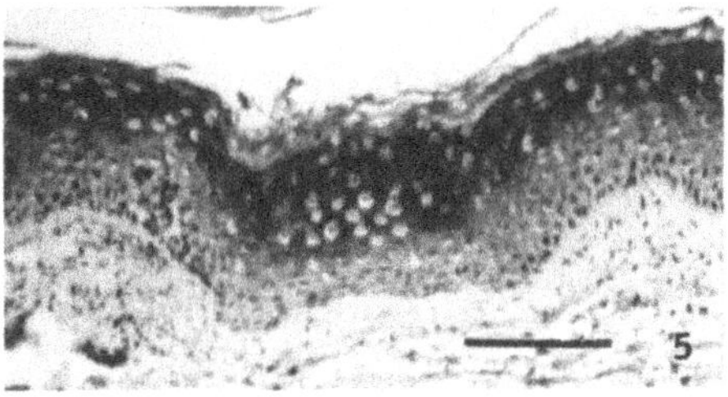

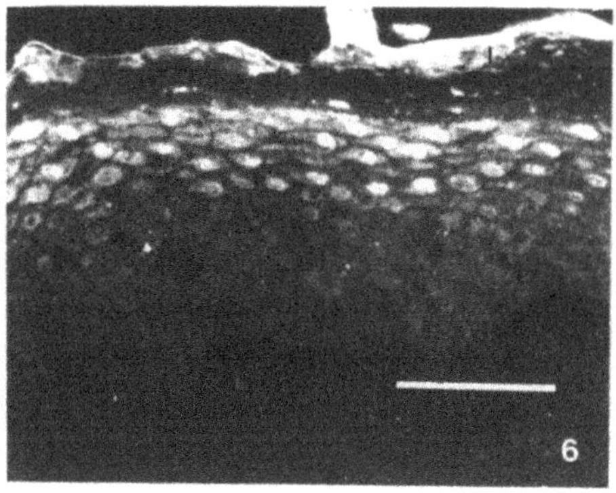

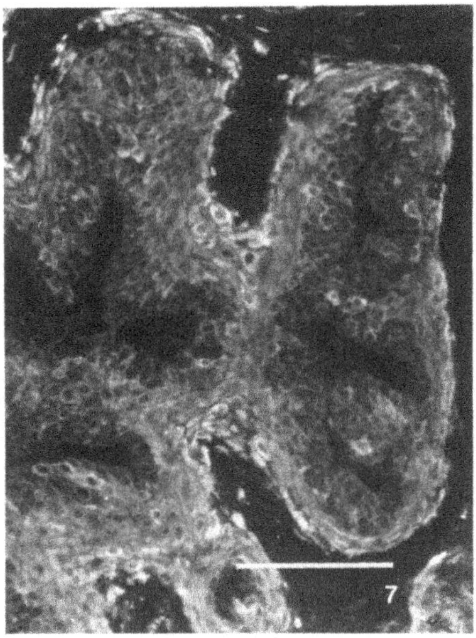

Figure 5. Rat vaginal squamous epithelium during estrous phase. Normal involucrin pattern: basal cells are negative while the upper layers show strong reaction (Hematoxylin counterstain) Bar = 200 μm. Figure 6. Hyperplastic mouse skin. Immunofluorescent staining with rabbit antifilaggrin. Intense reaction in the upper spinous and granular layers. Bar = 200 μm. Figure 7. Immunofluorescence pattern of filaggrin in a mouse skin papilloma. Heterogeneous reaction in the different layers, including staining of some basal cells. Bar = 200 μm.

The weak or absent reaction in areas of the stratum corneum has been postulated to be the result of either the loss of the protein at the time of terminal maturation or the physical or chemical masking of filaggrin in the dense areas of the stratum corneum. We have shown that pretreating the sections with trypsin, which has been very efficient in unmasking and producing immunoreaction in previously undetectable keratin filaments in the stratum corneum of human oral epithelium, is not effective in detecting filaggrin in the negative areas of the horny layer (30). This probably indicates that filaggrin is further degraded in the stratum corneum, as suggested by Harding and Scott (26).

Since filaggrin is a protein related to the process of maturation of the epithelium, lesions in which this process is altered show important changes in its expression and disbribution. In our experience, lesions of the human oral mucosa (30) present a different pattern according to the degree of alteration of the maturation process. Parakeratinized and hyperkeratotic lesions, such as leukoplakias and verrocous carcinoma, showed an intense staining of the horny layer with a patchy distribution, whereas the granular layer had a strong but less uniform reaction. These findings suggest that, in hyperkeratotic lesions, a less-mature horny layer is produced, in which situation the normal degradation of the filaggrin does not take place.

Using immunofluorescent techniques we also studied filaggrin in chemically induced papillomas and carcinoma of the mouse (20). Normal mouse skin shows positive staining restricted to the granular layer, as described for other epithelia. However, in skin that becomes hyperplastic as a result of treatment with a tumor promoter, fluorescence can be observed in both spinous and granular layers.

After continuous treatment with tumor promoters, the antifilaggrin fluorescence in the adult epidermis develops a pattern very similar to that described for newborn skin, i.e., stains the granular and horny layers. The papillomas induced with the same initiation-promotion protocol show an increase of filaggrin staining in all layers, whereas the most exuberant papillomas (preneoplastic) show a pleomorphic distribution of filaggrin with alternating positive and negative areas (Figure 7). The antifilaggrin reaction of squamous cell carcinoma is negative or, in some instances, slightly positive. We have found similar results in keratocacanthomas of the human skin (12) where we have detected a strong positive reaction in the spinous, granular, and horny layers.

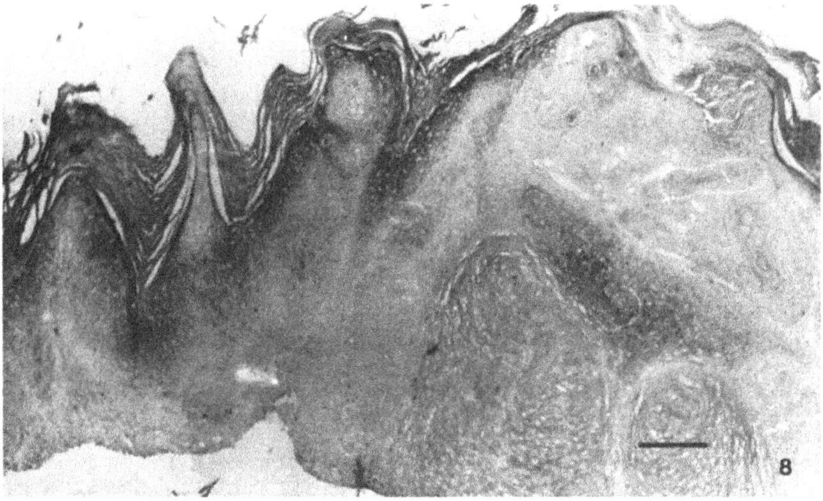

Figure 8. Immunoperoxidase (PAP) staining for filaggrin in a human skin keratoacanthoma. Positive reaction in upper spinous, granular, and horny layers. Bar = 500 μm.

From this study we conclude that filaggrin is a good marker of maturation and differentiation and its presence correlates with the absence of invasive growth.

References:

1. Matoltsy AG: Keratinization. J Invest Dermatol (67):20-25, 1976.
2. Green H: The keratinocyte as differentiated cell types. Harvey Lect (74):101-139, 1980.
3. Rice RH, Green H: The cornified envelope of terminally diff erentially human epidermal keratinocytes consists of cross-linked protein. Cell (11):417-411, 1977.
4. Dale BA, Holbrook KA, Steinert PM: Assembly of stratum corneum basic protein and keratin filaments in macrofibrils. Nature (276): 729-731, 1978.
5. Elias M: Lipids and the epidermis permability barrier. Arch Dermatol Res. (270):95-117, 1981.
6. Schlegel R, Banks-Schlegel S, MacLeod SA, Pinkus GS: Immuno-peroxidase localization of keratins in human neoplasm. Am J Pathol (101):41-50, 1980.
7. Moll R, Franke W, Schiller DL: The catalog of human cytokeratins: patterns of expression in normal epithelia, tumors, and cultured
8. Gigo O, Geiger B, Eshhar Z, Moll R, Schmid E, Winter S, Schiller DL, Franke WW: Detection of a cytokeratin determinant common to diverse epithelial cells by a broadly cross-reacting monoclonal antibody.
9. Rice H, Green H: Presence in human epidermal cells of a soluble protein precursor of the cross-linked envelope: activation of the cross-linking by calcium ions. Cell (18):681-684, 1979.
10. Zettergen JG, Peterson L, Wuepper KD: Keratolinin: The soluble substrate of epidermal transglutaminase from human and bovine tissue. Proc Natl Acad Sci USA (81):238-242, 1984
11. Dale BA, Ling SY: Immunologic cross-reaction of stratum corneum basic protein and a keratohyalin granule protein. J Invest Dermatol (72):257-261,1979.
12. Klein-Szanto AJP, Barr RF, Reiners JJ, Jr, and Mamrack MD: Filaggrin distribution in kerathoacanthomas and squamous cell carcinomas. Arch Pathol Lab Med (108):888-890, 1984.
13. Hashimoto K: Cellular envelopes of keratinized cells of the human epidermis. Arch Klin Exptl Dermatol (253):374-385, 1969.
14. Fernandez Alonso GI, Gimenez-Conti IB, Tasat DR, Larcher FM, Aldaz CM, Conti CJ: Unpublished data.
15. Banks-Schlegel S, Green H: Involucrin synthesis and tissue assemble by keratinocyte natural and cultural human epithelia. J Cell Biol (90):732-737, 1981.
16. Warhol MJ, Antonial DA, Pinkus S, Burke L, Rice RH: Immuno-peroxidase staining for involucrin: a potential diagnostic aid in cervicovaginal pathology. Hum Pathol (13):1095-1099,1982.
17. Said S. Sasson AF, Shintaku PL, Banks-Schlegel S: Involucrin in squamous and basal cell carcinomas of the skin: an immuno-histochemical study. J Invest Dermatol (82):449-452, 1984.
18. Murphy GF, Flynn TC, Rice R, Pinkus G: Ivolucrin expression in normal and neoplastic human skin: a marker for keratinocyte differentiation. J Invest Dermatol (82):453-457, 1984.
19. Conti CJ, Fernandez Alonso EI, Klein-Szanto AJP, Slaga TJ: Unpublished data.
20. Gimenez-Conti IB, Itoiz ME, Fernandez Alonso GI, Conti CJ, Klein-Szanto AJP: Manuscript in preparation.

21. Said, W., Nash, G., Sassoon, F., Shintaku, P.J., and Banks-Schlegel, S: Involucrin in lung tumors. A specific marker for squamous differentiation. Lab Invest (49):563-568, 1983.
22. Watt FM, Green H: Involucrin synthesis is correlated with cell size in human epidermal cultures. J Cell Biol (90):738-742, 1981.
23. Tasat D.R., Fernandez Alonso GI, Conti CJ: Marcadores biologicos de celulas epiteliales en cultivo. Medicina (43):725, 1983.
24. Tasat DR, DeLasHeras M, Meiss RP, Fernandez Alonso GI: Manuscript in preparation.
25. Scott TR, Harding AR: Studies on the synthesis and degradation of a high molecular weight histidine-rich phosphoprotein from mammalian epidermis. Biochim Biophys Acta (669):65-78, 1981.
26. Harding CR, Scott IR: Histidine-rich proteins (filaggrins): structural and functional heterogeneity during epidermal differentiation. J Mol Biol (170):651-673, 1983.
27. Meek RL, Londsdale-Eccles JD, Dale BA: Epidermal filaggrin is synthesized on a large messenger ribronucleic acid as a high-molecular-weight precursor. Biochemistry (22):4867-4871, 1983.
28. Dale BA, Thompson WB, Stern JB: Distribution of histidine-rich basic protein, a possible kertin matrix protein in rat oral epithelium. Arch Oral Biol (27):535-545, 1982.
29. Mamrack MD, Klein-Szanto AJP, Reiners JJ, Slaga TJ: Alteration in the distribution of the epidermal protein filaggrin during two-stage chemical carcinogenesis in the SENCAR mouse skin. Cancer Res (44):2634-2641, 1984.
30. Itoiz ME, Conti CJ, Lanfranchi HE, Mamrack MR, Klein-Szanto AJP: Immunohistochemical detection of filaggrin in preneoplastic and neoplastic lesions of the human oral mucosa (submitted for publication).

Acknowledgements:

This work was partially supported by DHHS, grant CA 34690 from the National Cancer Institute, NIH. G. I. Fernandez Alonso was supported by an ICRETT fellowship from the UICC Geneva-Switzerland. We thank Ms. P. Mutschink, Ms. J. Mayhugh, Ms. Karen Engel for expert secretarial help and Ms. J. Ing for excellent photographic support.

6

INTERMEDIATE FILAMENTS

RICHARD J. COTE, TIMOTHY M. THOMSON AND CARLOS CORDON-CARDO

I. INTRODUCTION

The intermediate filaments are a family of cytoskeletal differentiation-related proteins present in virtually all eukaryotic cells. First described during early electron microscopic studies of cellular structure, they were found to be intermediate in diameter between microtubules and microfilaments. They have only recently been recognized as a family of dynamic intracellular elements.

There are five classes of chemically and antigenically distinct intermediate filament proteins whose expression is related to the embryogenesis of cells. Cytokeratin filaments are expressed by epithelial cells, vimentin is in cells of mesodermal and neuroectodermal origin, desmin is found in myogenic cells, and glial fibrillary acidic protein and neurofilaments are expressed by cells of neuroectodermal origin.

Although the expression of intermediate filaments appears to be developmentally regulated, their function is not known. They are thought to be possibly involved in maintenance of cellular support, cell motility, intracellular organization, cell-cell and cell-matrix interactions and regulation of cellular events such as mitogenesis (1).

The expression of intermediate filaments is relatively well conserved during malignant transformation. Because of their distinct cellular distribution, they are becoming increasingly important in the identification and classification of normal and malignant tissues.

For more in-depth information on the analysis of intermediate filament proteins, the reader is referred to excellent reviews by Lazarides (1), Sun et al, (2), Moll, Franke, et al.(3), Osborn and Weber (4) and Steinert et al.(5).

2. BIOCHEMICAL AND IMMUNOCHEMICAL CHARACTERIZATION OF INTERMEDIATE FILAMENTS

Intermediate filaments account for up to 30% of the cellular protein. Like other cytoskeletal proteins they are generally insoluble in high and low salt detergents, but are extractable by denaturing solvents, either as whole molecules or as polypeptide constituents (1). As a result of recent advances in biochemical separation techniques and the development of specific antibodies, these proteins have been further subclassified and defined (Table 1).

2.1 Cytokeratins: Unlike most other intermediate filaments, which consist of only one type of protein, cytokeratins are a complex family of peptides ranging in molecular weight from 40,000 to 68,000 Daltons (D), with isoelectric points (PI) ranging from pH 5 to 8. There have been at least 19 different cytokeratins described (2,3). They are expressed in various combinations by epithelial cells. Recent work has indicated that different types of epithelia (e.g., simple vs. stratified) can be distinguished by their cytokeratin composition (2). Franke and co-workers have biochemically defined and catalogued the cytokeratins identified to date (3), while Sun and colleagues have suggested a unifying model for the differential expression of cytokeratin filaments (4).

TABLE 1. The Cytoskeleton Proteins

FILAMENTS	PROTEINS	DIAMETER	MOLECULAR WEIGHT
Microfilaments	Actin	7nm	42KD
	Myosin	15nm	460KD
Intermediate	Keratins	8nm	40-68KD
Filaments	Vimentin	10nm	52KD
	Desmin	10nm	53KD
	GFAP	8nm	51KD
	Neurofilaments	10nm	210/160/68KD
Microtubles	Tubulin	25nm	55/55KD

2.2 Vimentin: Vimentin appears to be the most evolutionary conserved intermediate filament protein (Cote and Thomson, unpublished data). It is thought to consist of a single peptide with a molecular weight of 52,000 to 57,000 D, depending on the species and extraction procedure, with a PI of 5.3. Vimentin filaments have been found to form perinuclear aggregates after exposure of live cells to Colcemid (6), a property they share with desmin filaments (7). Antibodies raised against vimentin from one species generally cross-react with vimentin from other species.

2.3 Desmin: The molecular weight and PI of desmin are 50-55,000 D and 5.4. Biochemically and immunologically distinct desmin proteins have been identified in different species. As previously mentioned, desmin forms perinuclear aggregates on exposure to Colcemid.

2.3 Glial Fibrillary Acidic Protin (GFAP): GFAP appears to consist predominantly on one major subunit with a molecular weight of 51,000 D and PI of 5.6. Originally thought to be related to neurofilaments, GFAP is a biochemically, immunologically and histogenically distinct intermediate filament protein.

2.5 Neurofilaments: Neurofilaments are composed of three subunits with molecular weights of approximately 210,000, 160,000 and 68,000 D with a PI of 5.65, 5.28, and 5.25, respectively. These subunits are antigenically related, however, each possess unique epitopes (8).

3. TISSUE DISTRIBUTION OF INTERMEDIATE FILAMENT PROTEINS (Table 2 and Table 3)

Cells derived from a particular histogenic pathway demonstrate a particular pattern of intermediate filament expression. This pattern is generally conserved during malignant transformation. Therefore, intermediate filament expression can provide information about the cellular origin of normal and malignant tissue, a feature which has contributed to the proliferation of studies concerning the detection and distribution of these proteins. Intermediate filaments can be detected in a variety of ways, ranging from biochemical and physical methods, electron microscopic studies and, most recently, through the development of specific antibodies. Heterologous antisera raised against intermediate filaments have been useful in the biochemical definition of this family of proteins. However, most of these types of reagents have been found to cross-react with multiple polypeptides of the intermediate filament family, as well as other non-intermediate filament antigents. The application of the hybridoma technology has resulted in the development of antibodies specific for the different subclasses of intermediate filament proteins. Using these reagents, the tissue distribution of these proteins has been studied using immunofluorescence, immunoperoxidase and immunoblotting techniques.

TABLE 2. Intermediate Filament Distribution of Normal Tissues

	CYTOKERATINS	VIMENTIN	DESMIN	GFAP[1]	NF[2]
1. ECTODERM					
A. Surface Ectoderm					
Epidermis	+	-	-	-	-
Glands	+	-	-	-	-
Breast	+	-	-	-	-
B. Neuroectoderm					
Neurons	-	-	-	-	+
Glial Cells	-	+ or -	-	+	-
Melanocytes	-	+	-	-	-
2. MESODERM					
Skeleton Muscles	-	+	+	-	-
Smooth Muscle	-	+	+ or -	-	-
Fibroblast	-	+	+ or -	-	-
Endothelium	-	+	-	-	-
Chondroblast	-	+	-	-	-
Osteoblast	-	+	-	-	-
Mesothelium	+	+	-	-	-
Leukocytes	-	+	-	-	-
Kidney Epithelium	+	+ or -	-	-	-
Prostate Epithelium	+	-	-	-	-
3. ENDODERM					
Bronchi	+	-	-	-	-
Lung	+	-	-	-	-
Thyroid	+	-	-	-	-
Gastrointestinal Tract	+	-	-	-	-
Pancreas	+	-	-	-	-
Liver	+	-	-	-	-
Ureter	+	-	-	-	-
Urinary Bladder	+	-	-	-	-

[1]GFAP: Glial Fibrillary Acidic Protein
[2]NF: Neurofilaments

TABLE 3. Intermediate Filament Patterns In Human Neoplasias

	CYTOKERATINS	VIMENTIN	DESMIN	GFAP[1]	NF[2]
CARCINOMAS	+	-	-	-	-
MUSCLE SARCOMAS:					
A) Rhabdomyosarcoma	-	+ or -	+	-	-
B) Leiomyosarcoma	-	+	+ or -	-	-
NONMUSCLE SARCOMAS:					
A) Liposarcoma	-	+	-	-	-
B) Angiosarcoma	-	+	-	-	-
C) Fibrosarcoma	-	+	+ or -	-	-
D) MFH[3]	-	+	+ or -	-	-
E) Schwannoma	-	+	-	-	-
MELANOMA	-	+	-	-	-
GLIOMAS	-	+ or -	-	+	-
NEUROBLASTOMA	-	-	-	-	+

[1]GFAP: Glial fibrillary acidic protein

[2]NF: Neurofilaments

[3]MFH: Malignant fibrous histiocytoma

3.1 Cytokeratins (Figure 1A ᑦytokeratin expression is restricted to cells of epithelial origin. Different cell types express characteristic sets of between 2 and 10 of the 19 distinct subspecies of cytokeratins that have been described (3). Sun and co-workers have shown that cytokeratins can be divided into two mutually exclusive subgroups, and that the expression of members of these subgroups can be related to epithelial morphology and different stages of epithelial cell differentiation (2). This analysis has been facilitated by the development of monoclonal antibodies which identify and distinguish these subgroups and can be used in immunochemical and·immunohistological analysis (9). Although epithelial cells generally only express cytokeratins, it has been found that metastatic malignant epithelial cells (particularly those found in ascitic or pleural fluid) and early embryonal cells can exhibit co-expression of cytokeratin and vimentin (10,11). Epithelial cells in culture often co-express vimentin and cytokeratins as well (12).

Human monoclonal antibodies recognizing both high and low molecular weight cytokeratins have been generated by our laboratory (13). Many of these antibodies have been derived from patients with epithelial tumors and may have developed in response to tumor cell breakdown with subsequent release of cytoplasmic contents.

3.2 Vimentin (Figure 1B): Vimentin is the most ubiquitous of the intermediate filaments. It is expressed by cells of mesodermal and neuroectodermal origin, and occasionally by cells of epithelial and myogenic origin. When present, it is co-expressed with other intermediate filament types, except in cells of mesodermal origin, where (in general) only vimentin is found. Vimentin is often expressed in non-mesodermal cultured cells, and can be the predominant intermediate filament protein expressed by cultured cells of neuroectodermal and myogenic origin.

3.3 Desmin (Figure 1C): Cells of myogenic origin express desmin, including skeletal, cardiac and smooth muscle and Purkinje fibers of the heart, vascular and aortic smooth muscle. In adult striated muscle, desmin is not expressed in filamentous form, but is concentrated at the Z-disk. Vascular smooth muscle can express both vimentin and desmin, and some types of aortic vascular smooth muscle apparently express only vimentin (14). Non-myogenic cells have been found to express desmin, including mesangial cells and arterioles of the kidney (15), and embryonal fibroblasts.

3.4 Glial Fibrillary Acidic Protein (Figure 1D): GFAP is expressed by cells of glial origin, including astrocytes, ependymal cells, oligodendrocytes and microglia. In most of these cells, GFAP is co-expressed with vimentin, however, gray matter astrocytes and oligodendrocytes only express GFAP. Malignant glial cells express GFAP and vimentin. When these malignant cells are cultured, there is decreased GFAP and increased vimentin expression with increasing passage, so that in many cultured gliomas only vimentin can be detected.

3.5 Neurofilaments (Figure 1E): Cells of neuronal origin express neurofilaments. This family of proteins appears to function as a 3-dimensional framework that provides support to axons. Neurofilaments have not been found to be co-expressed with vimentin in normal neuronal cells. However, cultured neuroblastomas express vimentin, and these cells are in fact poor expressors of neurofilaments.

4. IMMUNOHISTOCHEMICAL METHODS FOR THE DETECTION OF INTERMEDIATE FILAMENTS

The immunostaining methods have been previously described (16,17) and are generally well known. Fresh tissues are either fixed in 10% formaldehyde in phosphate buffer (PBS) or 95% ethanol and embedded in paraffin. Frozen tissue blocks are prepared by immersion of fresh tissue in isopentane pre-cooled in liquid nitrogen, embedded in OCT compound in cryomolds (Miles Laboratories, Inc., Naperville, IL) and stored at -70°C.

4.1 Immunofluorescence: Frozen tissue sections 4 to 8 microns thick are cut using a cryostat. Cryostat-cut sections are used unfixed, or are fixed for 10 minutes with either 10% formaldehyde in PBS, cold acetone or 95% ethanol. Tissue sections are washed three times in PBS for five minutes each, once in bovine serum albumin in PBS (BSA-PBNS), and then incubated with the appropriate suppressor serum (e.g., 10% normal goat serum in BSA-PBS) for 20 minutes. The suppressor serum in drained off and the primary anti-intermediate filament antibody added and incubated for one hour, the titration and appropriate dilution having been previously established. Sections are washed with PBS and incubated for 45 minutes with the secondary fluoresceinated antibody, which has also been previously titrated for optimal dilution (usually 1:40 in BSA-PBS). The secondary antibodies are affinity purified immunoglobulins, and in some instances washed extensively in PBS with the creation of turbulence using a magnetic stirring plate, and wet mounted in 90% glycerol in PBS and/or semi-permanently mounted Gelvatol.

The immunofluorescence procedures are usually performed at room temperature with the incubations in wet chambers. The specimens are examined with a fluorescence microscope equipped with epifluorescence, using a 100 watt mercury lamp.

4.2 Immunoperoxidase Procedure: Formalin-fixed and paraffin-embedded sections are deparaffinized for these techniques. Frozen sections can also be used with these methods. The sections are quenched for 30 minutes in 0.03% hydrogen peroxide in PBS, or for 15 minutes in 1% periodic acid, in order to remove endogenous peroxidase activity. For intermediate filament analysis, deparaffinized sections are usually treated with protease in order to expose antigenic determinants that may be masked. This is particularly important when staining with monoclonal antibodies. Depending on the antigen to be studied, sections may be treated with different enzymes. In general sections are treated with 0.0025% pronase in Tris buffer (pH 7.6) for 4 minutes, or with pepsin in HCl buffer (pH 2.5) for 30 minutes. The tissue sections are washed several times in PBS, and then incubated with the appropriate supressor serum for 20 minutes. The supressor serum is drained off and the sections incubated

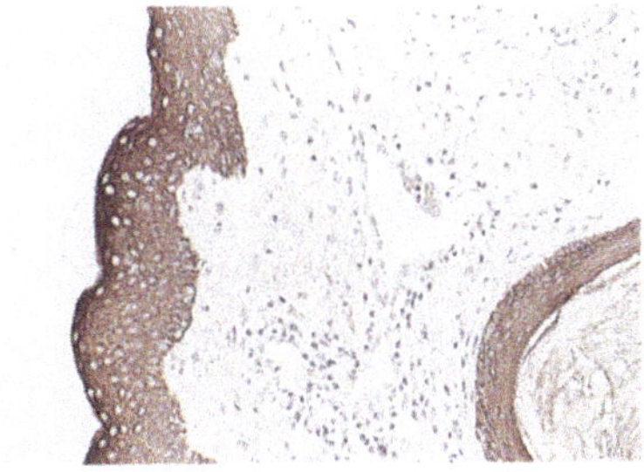

A

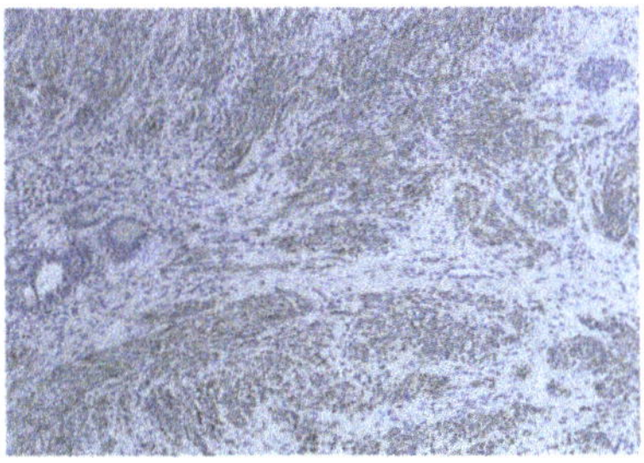

B

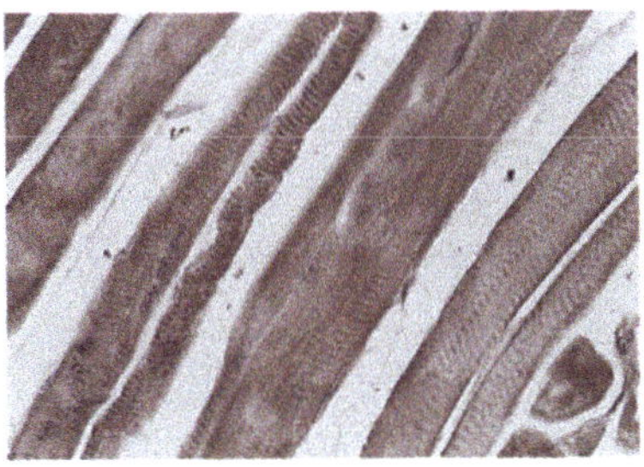

C

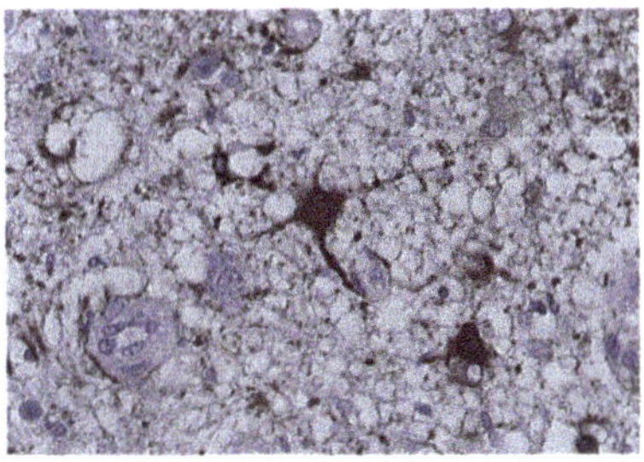

D

Figure 1. Intermediate filament expression in normal tissues. A) Normal adult skin stained with a rabbit antisera specific for cytokeratins. Epidermis and epithelium of adnexa are positively stained; the connective tissue of the dermis is negative. B) Connective tissue of adult ovary stained with antisera specific for vimentin. Ovarian follicular epithelium is negative. C) Skeletal muscle stained with monoclonal antibody reactive with desmin. Note increased staining in Z bands. D) Antisera to GFAP staining astrocytes and their projections in human brain.

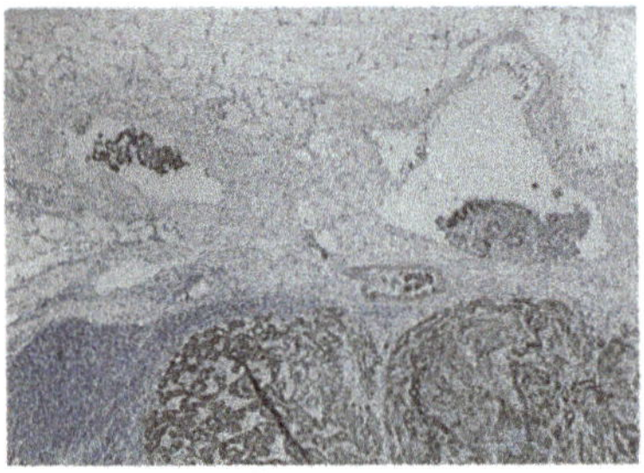

A

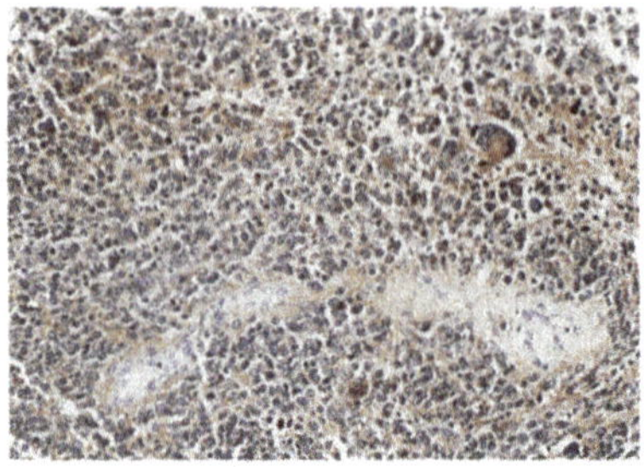

B

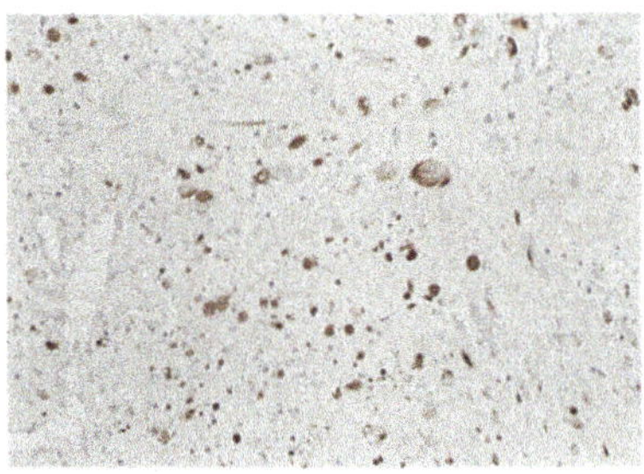

C

Figure 2. Intermediate filament expression in human tumors. A) Metastatic cancer invading lymph node and tumor emboli in blood vessels stained with a monoclonal antibody specific for low molecular weight cytokeratins. Final diagnosis was metastatic carcinoma of the breast. B) Undifferentiated retroperitoneal tumor from a 5-year-old male, stained with a monoclonal antibody specific for neuro-filaments. Final diagnosis was neuroblastoma. C) Small cell retroperitoneal tumor of unknown origin arising in a 18-year-old female, stained with an antisera specific for desmin. Final diagnosis was rhabdomyosarcoma.

with appropriately diluted primary anti-intermediate filament antibody overnight at 4°C in the case of deparaffinized sections, or for one hour at room temperature in the case of frozen sections. Peroxidase-antiperoxidase and avidin-biotin methods are used, following protocols similar to those described by Hsu et al. (18) and Sternberger (19). The secondary antibodies are horseradish peroxidase-conjugated (Ortho, Carpinteria, CA) or biotinylated (Vector Labvoratories). The sections are then washed several times in PBS and rinsed with 0.05 M Tris buffer, 0.1 M NaCl, at pH 8.0. For the final step diaminobenzidine (DAB) is usually used. Five mg of DAB tetrahydrochloride (Sigma Chemicals, St. Louis, MO) are dissolved in 100 ml of Tris buffer and 100 μl of 0.3% hydrogen peroxide is added. The DAB solution is filtered through a 0.2μ filter and development of the peroxidase reaction is performed by incubation with the tissue section for periods of 6 to 12 minutes. Other chromogens can be used, such as aminoethylcarbazol (AEC) and naphtol acetate (NA). The DAB treated sections are washed with distilled water, briefly counterstained with hematoxylin, and mounted with permount. The AEC and NA-treated sections are washed with distilled water, counterstained with hematoxylin and wet-mounted in 90% glycerol in PBS or Gelvatol.

4.3 Controls: Frozen and paraffin-embedded cells and tissues always serve as controls for each of the experiments. Sections of selected organs or tissues that express the appropriate intermediate filament(s) should be used for titration of the antibodies and positive controls. Negative controls include substitution of the primary antibody by a similar antibody of the same species and immunoglobulin subclass, but different reactivity, and also substitution of the primary antibody by PBS. Positive and negative controls should be included in all procedures and immunostainings.

5. CONCLUSIONS

The distribution, biochemical and physical characterization of intermediate filaments has been well studied. However, little is known about the regulation of expression or the mechanisms controlling the discrete histogenically related distribution of these proteins. Intermediate filaments can be used as markers of the embryological origin of tissues, and in some cases can be used to define the type of cell or state of differentiation of a cell within a given lineage. Their expression is generally conserved during malignant transformation. Therefore, these proteins can be used to identify the histogenic origin of tumors _in vitro_. This feature can be particularly useful in the identification of tumors of unknown origin as is demonstrated in

Figure 2. Intermediate filament expression can however change when cells metastasize (e.g., vimentin-cytokeratin co-expression in malignant epithelial cells present in pleural or ascitic fluid), and when tumors are grown in cultures (e.g., loss of GFAP expression in cultured gliomas). With the development of monoclonal antibodies (of both mouse and human origin) to the individual members of this family of proteins, a new degree of precision and ease is being introduced in the analysis of intermediate filament proteins in normal and malignant tissues.

ACKNOWLEDGEMENTS

The authors wish to thank Drs. L.J. Old, M.R. Melamed and H.F. Oettgen for their support.

REFERENCES

1. Lazarides E: Ann Rev Biochem 51:219-250, 1982.
2. Sun T, Eichner R, Schermer A, Cooper D, Nelson WC and Weiss RA: In: The Cancer Cell (eds., A. Levine, W. Topp, G. Vande-Woude and J.D. Watson), Cold Spring Harbor Laboratory, 1984.
3. Moll R, Franke WW, Schiller DL, Geiger B and Krepler R: Cell 31:11-24, 1982.
4. Osborn M and Weber K: Cell 31:303-306, 1982.
5. Steinert P, Zackroff R, Agnardi-Whitman M and Goldman RD: Meth Cell Biol 24:399-419, 1982.
6. Hynes RO and Destree AT: Cell 13:151-163, 1978.
7. Ishikawa H, Bischoff R and Holtzer H: J Cell Biol 38:538-555, 1968.
8. Willard M and Simon C: J Cell Biol 89:198-205, 1981.
9. Sun T, Eichner R, and Nelson WG, Tseng SG, Weiss RA, Jarvinen M and Woodcock-Mitchell J: J. Invest Derm 81:109-115, 1983 (suppl).
10. Ramaekers FCS, Haag D, Kant A, Moesker O, Jap PHK and Vooijs GP: Proc Natl Acad Sci, USA 80:2618-2622, 1983.
11. Lane EB, Hogan BLM, Kurkinen M and Garrels JI: Nature 303:701-704, 1983.
12. Franke WW, Schmid E, Osborn M and Weber K: Proc Natl Acad Sci, USA 75:5034-5038, 1978.
13. Thomson TM, Cote RJ, Houghton AN, Oettgen HF and Old LJ: Fed Proc 43:1513, 1985.
14. Gabbiani G, Schmid E, Winter S, Chaponnier C, de Chastonay C, Van de Kerckhove J, Weber K and Franke WW: Proc Natl Acad Sci, USA 78:298-302, 1981.
15. Bachman S, Kriz W, Kuhn C and Franke WW: Histochem 77:365-394, 1983.
16. DeLellis RA: In: Diagnostic Immunohistochemistry, Masson Publishing, USA, Inc., New York, 1981.
17. Erlandson, RA, Cordon-Cardo C, and Higgins PJ: Am J Surg Pathol 8:803-820, 1984.
18. Hsu, SM, Raine L, Fauger H: Am J Clin Pathol 75:734-738, 1981.
19. Sternberger LA: Immunochemistry, Second Edition, John Wiley & Sons, New York, 1979.

7

IMMUNODIAGNOSIS OF LYMPHOID AND MONONUCLEAR PHAGOCYTIC NEOPLASMS

E.S. JAFFE
J. COSSMAN

1. INTRODUCTION

The malignant lymphomas represent multiple diseases with diverse morphologic and clinical expressions. Morphologic classification schemes have been shown to be useful in delineating natural history, prognosis and response to therapy (1). However, in some instances distinctive morphologic entities may be very closely related clinically and/or biologically, whereas other diseases that share morphologic similarities may be clinically and biologically quite distinct. The application of modern immunologic techniques and concepts has permitted the development of a conceptual framework which may be used to decipher the morphologic diversity of these neoplasms, and has shown the relationship of lymphoid and mononuclear phagocytic neoplasms to the normal immune system (2).

The malignant lymphomas are fascinating and instructive models when viewed as neoplasms of the immune system. The spectrum of B-cell lymphomas reflects the functional and anatomic heterogeneity of the normal humoral immune system. The neoplastic cells often retain the morphologic, functional, and migratory characteristics of their normal counterparts. Likewise, the functional heterogeneity of the T-cell system is reflected in its malignant expressions and, indeed, malignant clonal expansions have been useful in the identification of normal cellular phenotypes not previously recognized (3).

2. TECHNIQUES USED TO CHARACTERIZE MALIGNANT LYMPHOMAS

The techniques used to characterize the malignant lymphomas are in principal identical to those used to characterize normal mononuclear cells. In this chapter we will emphasize those aspects unique to the study of malignant cells. The following techniques are recommended and their specificities are summarized in Tables 1 and 2.

1. Detection of surface immunoglobulin (sIg) individual light and heavy chain classes using $F(ab')_2$ affinity-purified goat-anti-human immunoglobulins (Tago Inc. Burlingame, CA.). Murine monoclonal (hybridoma) antibodies may be used as well, but should not be relied upon exclusively since selected B-cell clones may be negative with these specific reagents. SIg can be detected by indirect immunofluorescence with the fluorescence-activated cell sorter (FACS) or in frozen sections or cytocentrifuge smears using the ABC immunoperoxidase technique (see below).
2. EAC prepared with whole serum from AKR mice (EACmo) for detection of C3d (CR2) receptors and EAC prepared with human complement components (EAC4-b-hu) for detection of C3b (CR1) receptors. Quantify with rosette assay and evaluate morphologically with cytocentrifuge smears.
3. Detection of Fc receptors with OxIgGEA. Quantify with rosette assay and evaluate morphologically with cytocentrifuge smears.
4. E rosette technique for the detection of sheep erythrocyte receptors. Evaluate morphology with cytocentrifuge smears.
5. Detection of terminal deoxynucleotidyl transferase (TdT) by enzymatic assay or immunoassay using rabbit anti-calf TdT (BRL, Kensington, MD.) and ABC immunoperoxidase methodology. TdT is a feature of immature lymphoid cells (lymphoblasts) (Fig. 1). (4).
6. Monoclonal antibodies for the detection of lymphocyte differentiation antigens (Figs. 2 and 3; Table 2).
   a. Analysis with the fluorescence-activated cell sorter (FACS) for cells in suspension.
   b. Analysis using the ABC immunoperoxidase technique for imprint and cytocentrifuge smear preparations and frozen sections.
7. Phagocytic assays, e.g., latex.
8. Enzyme cytochemistry and histochemistry for: acid phosphatase (AP), tartrate-resistant acid phosphatase (TRAP), α-naphthyl butyrate esterase (B-EST),α-naphthyl acetate esterase (A-EST), β-glucuronidase (BG), alkaline phosphatase (ALP), peroxidase (PER), and ASD-chloroacetate esterase (ASDCL) (5).

Enzyme cytochemical and histochemical reactions are useful principally for the detection of mononuclear phagocytes (MP) and myeloid cells. MP are characterized by diffuse reactivity for most lysozomal enzymes: AP, B-EST, and A-EST. While punctate reactivity for these enzymes may be found in lymphocytes, most often T lymphocytes, in lymphoproliferative disorders these enzymes are not reliable indicators of a T- or B-cell origin. Myeloid cells, mainly of the neutrophilic series, are postive for ALP, PER, and ASDCL. Although negative for A-EST and B-EST, myeloid cells will show AP reactivity. Membrane ALP activity is characteristic of certain normal and neoplastic B lymphocytes (6). TRAP reactivity is characteristic of hairy cell leukemia but is found in some low-grade B-cell lymphomas associated with monoclonal gammopathy and some cases of adult T-cell leukemia/lymphoma.

Table 1. Markers of mature human mononuclear cells.

Cell Type	sIg	CR1	CR2	Fc	E	Phagocytosis
B cell	+	+	+	+	-	-
T cell	-	-	-	+/-	+	-
Monocyte/ histiocyte	-	+	+/-	+ +	-	+

Abbreviations: sIg, surface immunoglobulin; CR1, complement receptor for C3b; CR2, complement receptor for C3d; Fc, receptor for the Fc portion of IgG; E, receptor for sheep erythrocytes.

Table 2. Selected monoclonal antibodies for the characterization of T and B lymphocytes.

MoAb	Source	Antigen (MW, reduced)	Specificity
T200	Hybritech	200 kD	all hematopoietic cells (common leukocyte antigen)
Lyt 3	New England Nuclear	45-50 kD	sheep RBC receptor (T cells)
OKT4 T4 anti-Leu 3a	Ortho Coulter BD	60 kD	helper T cells
OKT8 T8 anti-Leu 2a	Ortho Coulter BD	33 kD	suppressor T cells
anti-Leu 1 Lyt 2	BD New England Nuclear	65 kD	Pan-T-cell
T101	Hybritech		some low-grade B-cell lymphomas

Table 2. (Continued).

MoAb	Source	Antigen (MW, reduced)	Specificity
OKT3 anti-Leu 4	Ortho BD	20/25 kD	Pan-T-cell (linked to T cell receptor)
3A1 or anti-Leu 9	BD	40 kD	Pan-T-cell
OKT6	Ortho	49 kD	cortical thymocytes
B1	Coulter	35 kD	Pan-B-cell
B2	Coulter	140 kD	C3d (CR2) receptor
B4	Coulter		Pan-B-cell
BA-1	Hybritech		Pan-B-cell
J5 BA-3	Coulter Hybritech	100 kD	common-ALL antigen (CALLA)
BA-2	Hybritech	24 kD	selected B-cell malignancies and neuroendocrine cells*
OKT9	Ortho	94 kD	transferrin receptor
anti-Tac	Dr. Thomas Waldmann NCI	53 kD	TCGF (IL-2) receptor
anti-HLA-DR	BD	28-34 kD	B cells, mononuclear
anti-Ia	Coulter	non-polymorphic antigen	phagocytes, activated T cells
PCA-1			plasma cells
OKT10	Ortho		immature T cells, activated lymphocytes

2.1. <u>General principles of lymphoma characterization</u>

Neoplastic lymphoreticular cells can be characterized in cell suspensions, frozen sections, or cytocentrifuge smears prepared from cell suspensions. Cell suspension techniques

* stains neuroblastomas, oat cell carcinomas

offer the opportunity for more precise quantitation, whereas frozen section techniques offer the ability to study lymphoid cells in the intact tissue environment. Since both methods have certain advantages, under ideal circumstances they should both be employed.

Malignant lymphomas are usually an admixture of neoplastic and normal and/or reactive elements. A cell suspension prepared from a malignant lymphoma will consist of a mixture of benign and malignant cells, and the malignant cells may not necessarily be in the majority. Therefore, in order to determine the phenotype of the malignant tumor, it is necessary to identify those markers associated with the neoplastic cells.

The malignant cells will usually be larger than normal cells. Therefore, when studying cells in suspension using the FACS, if the population is not homogenous, one should use the dual parameter mode or live gating and study both cell size (light scatter) as well as the fluorescence of the marker in question. Using these analyses one can identify the markers associated with either the "small" or "large" cell population.

Cytocentrifuge preparations can also be prepared from a cell suspension. The ABC immunoperoxidase technique can be used to identify sIg and cell surface antigens and, when counterstained, morphological correlations can be drawn. A cytocentrifuge preparation stained only with Wright-Giemsa can be used to better evaluate the cell population under study. Cytocentrifuge smears should also be prepared from the rosetted cell suspensions (EAC, IgGEA, or E), and when counterstained with Wright-Giemsa, the morphology of the rosetted cells can be determined.

The ABC technique can be applied to frozen sections for detection of sIg and lymphocyte differentiation antigens. Because of the abundance of interstitial immunoglobulins, it is often difficult to evaluate sIg in frozen sections, especially if the neoplastic cells are admixed with normal cells. On the other hand, most other cytoplasmic and membrane antigens are readily detected in frozen sections. Counterstaining with hematoxylin or methyl green permits some correlation with morphology. An "untreated" parallel frozen section can be stained with hematoxylin and eosin, as well.

Only a few antigenic determinants can be detected in paraffin-embedded sections, and the tissue must be optimally processed. Antigens preserved in paraffin sections include: cytoplasmic Ig (if abundant), Leu M1, and T200 under some circumstances. Obviously, paraffin-embedded sections should be studied only if other material is not available.

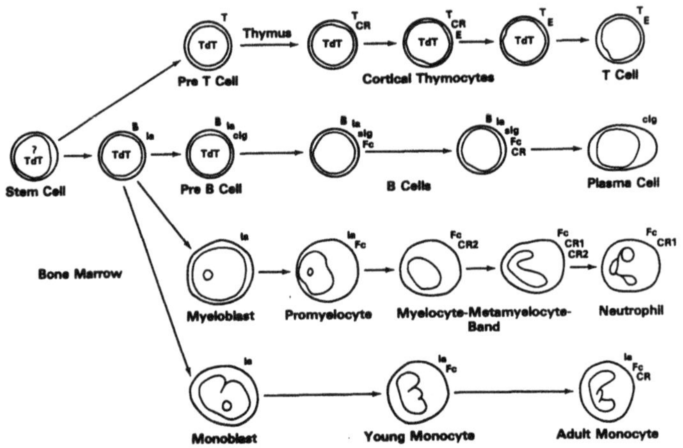

FIGURE 1. Scheme of normal lymphoid, myeloid, and monocyte differentiation. Presence of conventional cell surface markers is correlated with sequential stages of maturation. TdT is a feature of immature B and T lymphocytes (lymphoblasts) and is also characteristic of all lymphoblastic malignancies. Most non-Hodgkin's lymphomas have the phenotype of mature B or T lymphocytes. Reprinted with modifications from Ann Intern Med(94):218-235, 1981.

2.2. Preparation of lymphoma tissues for surface markers

2.2.1. Reagents and materials.

*1. Petri dishes, pipettes
*2. Stainless steel mesh
*3. 3 ml syringes
*4. Forceps, scalpel
5. Microscopic slides (12)

* = sterile.

*6. 50 ml conical tubes
*7. RPMI 1640 + antibiotics (1% Pen-Strep-gentamycin, 1% Fungizone)
*8. Fetal calf serum (FCS) (37°C)
*9. Dimethyl sulfoxide - freezing solution: RPMI + 20% FCS + 20% DMSO on ice
10. OCT Compound (Lab-Tek Products, Naperville, IL)
11. Freezing chuck
12. 2-methyl butane mixed with dry ice

2.2.2. Equipment.

1. Biological hood
2. 37°C water bath
3. Centrifuge
4. Programmed cell freezer
5. Liquid nitrogen storage

2.2.3. Methods - cell suspension and frozen tissue blocks.

*1. For solid tissue (lymph nodes, etc.), cut open in Petri dish containing RPMI and perform thorough gross inspection.
2. Place thin representative slice(s) on paper towel:
   a. blot dry
   b. imprint ten slides
   c. place at least one slice in B5 (7)
   d. snap-freeze remainder in OCT on chuck in 2-methyl butane dry ice mixture, label, wrap in foil, and store at < -70°C.
*3. Mince remaining tissue in RPMI.
*4. Pour minced fragments into stainless steel mesh over Petri dish.
*5. Gently press tissue through mesh with flat end of syringe handle.
*6. Pour cell suspension into 50 ml conical tube, count: if > 100 million go to step 7, if < 100 million go to step 10.
*7. Incubate 37°C for 30 min. This step allows shedding of cytophilic antibody on the surface of cells and should be performed if at all possible. Cytophilic antibody may be abundant on many B-cell lymphomas, due to the presence of Fc receptors on the neoplastic cells, and it will mask monoclonal sIg staining, producing an apparent polyclonal pattern.
*8. Carefully layer cells over warmed (37°C) FCS (25 ml cells to 8 ml FCS).
*9. Centrifuge at 400G for 10 min at room temp.
*10. Wash cells 2X in RPMI, count, and determine viability.
*11. Freeze cells in RPMI + 10% FCS + 10% DMSO (final concentration):
   a. 20 million to 200 million cells/ml (optimum = 100 million)

---
* = sterile.

b. add equal volume, freezing solution,* DROPWISE on ice to cells
c. freeze in programmed cell freezer
d. store in vapor phase over liquid nitrogen

2.3. Analysis of cell surface antigens using the fluorescence-activated cell sorter (FACS).

Although a conventional epifluorescent microscope can be used to detect cell surface antigens, the FACS or an equivalent cytofluorograph offers many advantages. The optical detection system of the automated equipment offers an unbiased eye, is more sensitive, allows for precise quantification of surface fluoresence with computer analysis and data storage, and permits the evaluation of tens of thousands of cells, and a large number of samples. The additional use of a microtiter plate (96-well, U-shaped bottom, Linbro Titertek), allows for efficient staining and washing of a large number of samples.

2.3.1. Immunofluorescence for cell sorter using microtiter plate.

1. Make cell suspension at 10 million cells/ml in RPMI 1640 medium.
2. Add 50 1 diluted antibody to each well.
3. Add 20-50 µl (200,000-500,000 cells) of cell suspension to each well.
4. Cover and incubate 30 min on ice.
5. Centrifuge plate at 1500 rpm for 2-4 min at 4°C. Remove supernatant by inverting plate and flicking. Wash cells two times: add 100-125 µl cold PBA,** resuspend pellet on a microtiter plate shaker, centrifuge as above and remove supernatant.
6. After removing PBA from pellets after last wash, add 50 µl goat-antimouse Ig (fluorescein labeled).*** Resuspend pellets.
7. Incubate on ice for 30 min. Be sure to keep plate covered from light.
8. Centrifuge plate at 1500 rpm for 2-4 min at 4°C. Remove supernatant. Wash cells three times as above (step 5).

---

* = sterile.

**PBA
  Phosphate-buffered saline
    9 g NaCl/liter
    pH 7.4
  2% BSA (bovine serum albumin)
  0.2% sodium azide

***goat anti-mouse IgG (heavy and light chains) (Kirkegaard and Perry, Gaithersburg, Md.).

9. After removing supernatant from third wash, resuspend cells in 100-150 µl cold PBA. Cells are ready to be read on FACS. Keep on ice and covered from light.

2.4. ABC immunoperoxidase technique for frozen sections or cytocentrifuge smears.

1. Prepare cytopreps or frozen sections. Slides should be kept in a compact closed box for 2 days at 4°C before staining.
2. Slides are fixed in acetone for 5 min (TdT slides should be fixed in 10% formalin for 30 min).
3. Quickly transfer slides to Tris buffered saline (TBS) to be washed (ten dips).
4. Second wash is in TBS for 3 min.
5. Third wash is in TBS and 5% horse serum for 5 min.
6. Primary antibody incubation: wipe carefully around the cells, apply primary antibody using the proper dilution, incubate in a humid chamber at room temperature for 2 hr.
7. Wash slides in TBS three times, 3 min each.
8. Secondary antibody incubation: wipe carefully around cells, apply biotin-labelled horse anti-mouse IgG 1:200 dilution for 1/2 hr. (for TdT and immunoglobulins use goat anti-rabbit IgG 1:100 dilution) for 1/2 hr.
9. Wash twice with TBS.
10. Block endogeneous peroxidase: methanol 200 ml + H_2O_2 50% 3 ml for 1/2 hr. This step is not usually needed with cytopreps. It is only done with frozen tissue sections with high endogeneous peroxidase, e.g., spleen.
11. Wash two times with TBS.
12. ABC incubation: 100 µl A + 62.5 µl B in 10 ml TBS. Or 50 µl A + 31 µl B in 5 ml TBS. Incubate for 1/2 hr.
13. Wash three times with TBS.
14. Incubate in diaminobenzidine hydrochloride *(DAB, Sigma, St. Louis, Mo.). and observe reaction under microscope. Usually takes 10-20 min. Solution: 100 mg DAB + 1 ml 8% nickel chloride + 2 drops H_2O_2 3% in 200 ml TBS.
15. Wash, counterstain, dehydrate, and mount. Use 1% methyl green or hematoxylin as a counterstain. When staining for TdT, use eosin as a counterstain so as not to mask the nuclear localization of the TdT enzyme.
16. Controls: use mouse, rabbit, or goat serum instead of 1° antibody.

3. NEOPLASMS OF THE IMMUNE SYSTEM

Sections 4, 5, and 6 summarize the malignancies which have been shown in a significant number of cases to be of B-cell, T-cell, or histiocytic or reticulum cell origin. Each of these three systems will be discussed addressing particular criteria for assigning the designated immunotype and unique phenotypic characteristics of individual entities. The terminology used for the non-Hodgkin's lymphomas is that of the Working Formulation; synonyms in other classification schemes are provided in that reference (1).

4. B-CELL LYMPHOMAS AND LEUKEMIAS

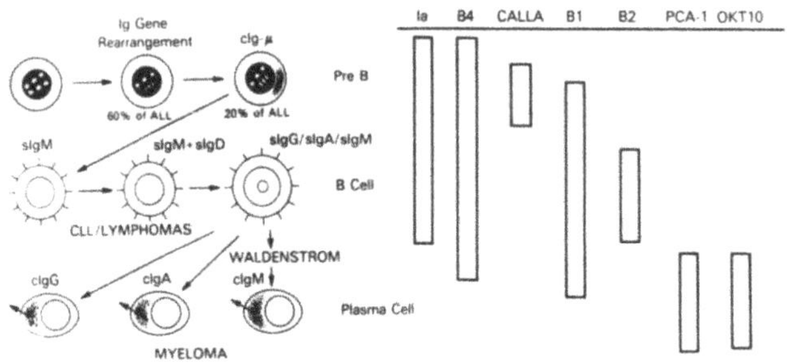

FIGURE 2. Schematic diagram shows stages of B-cell differentiation correlated with cell surface phenotype. Neoplasms of B-cell origin can be related to sequential stages of B-cell development: precursor B cells, mature B cells, and terminally differentiated or secretory B cells.

4.1. Neoplasms of precursor B-cell origin

Neoplasms of precursor B-cell origin include those leukemias and lymphomas with the phenotype of common-acute lymphoblastic leukemia (C-ALL) and pre-B-cell ALL. Although lacking conventional markers of T- or B-cell origin (Table 1), recent work investigating the rearrangement or deletion of immunoglobulin DNA in normal and neoplastic cells indicates the cells derived from common-ALL in nearly all instances show immunoglobulin gene rearrangement characteristic of B lymphocytes (8). Although spontaneous synthesis of Ig does not occur in C-ALL cells, they are irreversibly committed to differentiation in the B-cell pathway. Moreover, they can be induced to synthesize Ig in vitro (9). Pre-B-cell ALL is at a later stage of differentiation than C-ALL since neoplastic cells from this disorder have cytoplasmic heavy chains, but have not yet begun to synthesize light chains (10).

As with all lymphoblastic malignancies the cells are TdT-positive, although activity may be reduced in pre-B-cell ALL, correlating with its more differentiated status. Most (80%) cases of C-ALL and pre-B-cell ALL express the CALLA antigen detected by the monoclonal antibody J5, initially described as a potential "tumor-specific antigen" in this disorder (11, 12). Nearly all cases are Ia-positive. The B1 monoclonal antibody stains 50% of C-ALL and all pre-B-ALL (13). B4 has broader reactivity and is detected at an earlier stage of differentiation, reacting with cells from most cases.

These precursor B-cell phenotypes are seen in 70% of all cases of ALL. These phenotypes occur in only 10-15% of lymphoblastic malignancies with a lymphomatous presentation, i.e., lymphoblastic lymphomas (LBL) (14). Such precurser B-LBL do not present with mediastinal masses typical of T-LBL but have presented with either generalized lymphadenopathy or lytic bone disease (14).

4.2. Neoplasms of mature B-cell origin.

The essential feature of a mature B-cell malignancy is the presence of monoclonal sIg. The identification of a single light chain type is usually considered adequate evidence of the monoclonal nature of the proliferation. More than one heavy chain class may be demonstrable. Further evidence of monoclonality may be obtained by showing restricted staining of all cells by an anti-idiotypic antibody (15), or the presence of a single rearranged band on a genomic blot (Southern) hybridized with Ig gene probes (16).

4.2.1. Small lymphocytic lymphoma (SLL) and chronic lymphocytic leukemia (CLL). Nearly all of these low-grade lymphoproliferative disorders are monoclonal B-cell proliferations (17).

The predominant sIg is IgM with either κ or λ light chains. IgD frequently coexists with IgM. The sIg is of low density, often difficult to detect, and the density of sIg in a given case is usually very homogenous. In some patients spontaneous differentiation toward plasma cells with concomitant immunosecretion may occur, i.e., Waldenstrom's macroglobulinemia. Complement receptors are also present on the neoplastic cells with a predominance of receptors for C3d (18). Morphologically, clinically, and immunologically SLL and CLL are closely related (2).

Using monoclonal antibodies, typical CLL cells express a 65,000 dalton protein antigen (T65) normally found on T cells which can be identified with Leu 1, T101, and other similarly reactive antibodies (19). This antigen is on only very rare normal B cells and is not usually found on the cells of follicular lymphomas (17). It is also not found on the cells of Waldenstrom's macroglobulinemia.

Some cases of CLL and SLL express the so-called common acute lymphoblastic leukemia antigen, CALLA. CLL and SLL cells also react with monoclonal antibodies B1, BA1, and HLA-DR (Ia). We have recently determined that sIg, B1 and BA1, but not HLA-DR, are expressed in lower density in CLL-SLL than in lymphocytic lymphomas of intermediate differentiation (IDL) or follicular center cell lymphoma (FL) (17). In fact, there is a sequence of decreasing density of each of the first three markers proceeding as follows: FL > IDL > SLL. Those same three markers are progressively lost as normal B cells differentiate into plasma cells. This suggests a sequential differentiation pathway for these three types of low-grade B-cell lymphomas in man.

CLL/SLL appears to represent a block in B-cell differentiation. The non-neoplastic T lymphocytes in some patients with CLL have been shown to have a defect in helper-cell activity, a fact which may be related to the differentiation blockade (20). This helper-cell defect may also contribute to the hypogammaglobulinemia of CLL. In contrast to CLL, Waldenstrom's macroglobulinemia does not appear to be associated with a defect in helper cells. *In vitro* studies have shown that most cases of CLL and SLL tested are capable of proceeding to a stage of abundant immunoglobulin secretion when stimulated by phorbol ester (TPA) in culture (21). This indicates that these cells are frozen at a preterminal stage of B-cell differentiation but retain the capacity to differentiate when appropriate signals are provided. The reason why these cells don't differentiate *in vivo* is not known.

4.2.2. *Lymphocytic lymphoma, intermediate differentiation (IDL)*. Pathologically and immunologically lymphocytic lymphoma, intermediate differentiation (IDL) is intermediate between SLL and follicular lymphoma (FL) (22). This, too, is a B-cell malignancy with abundant monoclonal sIg and avid C3 receptors. The cells have membrane-associated alkaline phosphatase activity, a feature also seen in lymphocytes of the primary follicle and lymphoid cuff (6).

One can examine the ratio of the number of cells bearing only C3d receptors to the total number of cells bearing complement receptors. For normal B cells and the B cells of FL this ratio is approximately 0.3. However, for the cells of IDL and SLL/CLL this ratio is approximately 0.6. Thus, in this respect the cells of ML, INT resemble those of CLL/SLL (18).

Using monoclonal antibodies the cells of IDL express T65 found on CLL cells as well as CALLA found on the cells of FL. Thus, the cells of IDL have an intermediate antigenic phenotype. These cells also express B1, BA1, and BA2 (17).

Interestingly, a higher proportion of cases of IDL synthesize λ sIg than other B-cell lymphomas, which usually express monoclonal κ. This feature also has been described for centrocytic lymphomas in the Kiel classification, which share many morphologic and phenotypic characteristics with IDL (23). Thus, these lesions are probably closely related, if not identical.

4.2.3. *Follicular (nodular) lymphomas*. Follicular (nodular) lymphoma (FL) is the neoplastic equivalent of the lymphoid follicle (24). The cells have B-cell features, regardless of cytologic subtype. Moreover, different cytological subtypes show identical surface markers. The clinical and pathologic differences among subtypes appear to reflect kinetic differences of the various cell types. SIg is usually very abundant and the predominant immunoglobulin heavy chain class is IgM. The C3 receptor is easily detected both in cell suspensions and in frozen tissue sections, and receptors for both C3b and C3d are present. The cells are B1 and BA1 positive, and approximately 60% of cases express CALLA (with the J5 monoclonal antibody). The neoplastic cells do not react with Leu 1 or T101, in contrast to SLL, CLL, and IDL (17).

Variable numbers of cytologically normal T lymphocytes are present, and can be identified within, as well as between, the neoplastic follicles (22). The ratio of helper to suppressor T cells as identified by monoclonal antibodies does not differ from that in normal lymph nodes. Although the T cells are phenotypically normal, and do not appear to be a part of the neoplastic process, they may play a regulatory role vis-a-vis the neoplastic cells. Although the cells of FL usually do not spontaneously secrete Ig, after removal of autologous T cells and replacement with allogenic T cells, they can be induced to secrete <u>in vitro</u> (25).

4.2.4. <u>Diffuse aggressive lymphomas</u>. Diffuse aggressive lymphomas include, in the Working Formulation, tumors of the mixed, small and large cell, large cell, and small non-cleaved (non-Burkitt) subtypes and represent a morphologic end point for transformed cells of diverse origins (2). Clinically they are aggressive but, if a complete remission is obtained, it is likely to be sustained with a potential for longterm cure. In keeping with the transformed or dedifferentiated nature of the neoplastic cells, they fail to demonstrate the homing patterns characterstic of low-grade-B- or T-cell lymphomas and have a destructive growth pattern.

Approximately 65% of these tumors have B-cell markers. Cytologically, such tumors are often composed of the follicular center cell types described by Lukes and Collins: large cleaved, large non-cleaved, and small non-cleaved (26). These tumors may occur as a manifestation of progression of a FL or may apparently occur de novo. These B cell lymphomas do not have unique phenotypic characteristics. They usually stain with the pan-B-cell monoclonal antibodies B1, B4, and BA-1, but do not express complement receptors and are usually B2 negative. J5 is often positive and Ia is invariably present.

4.2.5. Burkitt's lymphoma (ML, small non-cleaved, Burkitt's type). Burkitt's lymphomas in endemic and non-endemic areas are identical pathologic processes (2). They are similar with respect to morphology, pattern of spread, and response to therapy. Whereas EBV is closely linked to Burkitt's tumor in Africa, and is present in 95% of endemic cases; it does not appear to play a role in Burkitt's lymphoma in non-endemic regions and is found in only 15% of cases. The tumor tends to involve germinal centers in both lymph nodes and Peyer's patches but rarely demonstrates a nodular growth pattern (27). Whether it homes to germinal centers or arises in germinal centers is not known.

Immunologic characteristics of endemic and non-endemic cases are similar and have B-cell features. Cells bear monoclonal sIg with IgM being the predominant heavy chain class. C3 receptors are present in EBV-positive cases, but not in EBV-negative cases. However, expression of C3 receptors can be induced in vitro (28).

Burkitt's lymphoma stains with the pan-B-cell monoclonal antibodies B1 and BA-1 and anti-Ia (HLA-DR). CALLA is virtually always present (29). TdT is negative, a feature which is helpful in distinguishing this common childhood tumor from lymphoblastic lymphoma (LBL), which is invariably TdT-positive (30).

Interestingly, specific chromosomal abnormalities in Burkitt's lymphomas occur at or near the sites of the genes for immunoglobulin (31). The most common translocation is 8q-14q+ and two other variants are also observed involving chromosome 8 and chromosomes 2 and 22. The Ig heavy chain gene locus is on 14q whereas the κ gene is on 2p and the λ gene on 22q. The translocation correlates with light chain type produced when chromosomes 2 and 22 are involved; e.g.,

8q/22q+ Burkitt's lymphomas produce λ light chain. Notably, the portion of the 8q chromosome involved in the translocation includes the so-called c-myc oncogene, which inserts in the area of the immunoglobulin gene near the "switch" region and may well be related to the activation of this gene and perhaps proliferation of the cell.

4.2.6. Hairy cell leukemia (leukemic reticuloendotheliosis). Tartrate-resistant acid phosphatase (TRAP) is a useful but not entirely specific marker for the neoplastic cells. The cells have some unusual features which initially were interpreted as suggestive of a monocytic origin. These include: 1) limited phagocytosis of inert particulate matter (latex beads), 2) avid Fc receptors, and 3) cell surface appearance as seen by scanning electron microscopy (32). However, indicative of a B-cell origin is the presence of monoclonal sIg, which reappears following capping or trypsinization indicating endogenous synthesis (33). IgG is the most common heavy-chain class. In some cases, the sIg appears cytophilic, bound via Fc receptors, and attempts at *in vitro* synthesis are unsuccessful. However, further proof of a B-cell origin is the presence of rearranged Ig genes (34). The cells express Ia and the usual pan-B-cell antigens B1 and BA-1, but are negative for CALLA. An unusual feature is the presence of the TAC antigen, which represents the receptor for T-cell growth factor (TCGF). However, the cells do not respond functionally to TCGF *in vitro* (34).

4.3. Neoplasms of differentiated B-cell origin.

Neoplasms at this terminal stage of B-cell differentiation synthesize and *secrete* monoclonal immunoglobulin. Thus, one can usually detect monoclonal immunoglobulin in the serum by protein or immunoelectrophoresis. Characteristiically, the cells have diminished sIg but abundant monoclonal cytoplasmic Ig (cIg). Due to the abundance of the cIg it can be detected even in paraffin sections by immunoperoxidase techniques.

At this terminal stage of B-cell differentiation, the cells lose many B-cell-associated antigens such as Ia, B1, B2, and

B4. However, the cells acquire reactivity with PCA-1 and OKT10 (35).

Most mature B cells and most B-cell lymphomas synthesize predominantly IgM. However, with terminal differentiation the the cells undergo heavy chain class switching to produce IgG or IgA. Waldenstrom's macroglobulinemia is a neoplasm of plasmacytoid lymphocytes, which clinically resembles a low-grade (SLL) lymphoma and involves primarily lymphoid organs (2). The cells retain many lymphoid characteristics and have a phenotype intermediate between SLL and multiple myeloma.

Multiple myeloma, in contrast, is a disorder of terminally differentiated plasma cells and is associated with production of IgG, IgA, IgM, IgD, and IgE in decreasing order of frequency. Interestingly, this corresponds to the normal amounts of these Ig classes synthesized on a daily basis. Thus, each individual plasma cell is probably at an equivalent risk for neoplastic transformation.

5. T-CELL LYMPHOMAS AND LEUKEMIAS

5.1. Neoplasms of precursor T-cell origin

T-ALL and T-LBL represent neoplasms at the earliest stages of T-cell differentiation (3, 14). Approximately 20% of ALL have T-cell markers. E+ or T-cell ALL and lymphoblastic lymphoma (LBL) are closely related disorders, clinically and immunologically; approximately 80% or more of cases of lymphoblastic lymphoma have a T-cell phenotype. The most consistently detected pan T-cell marker is 3A1 or Leu 9 (Becton-Dickinson, Sunnyvale, CA). The cells form E rosettes, have other T-cell antigens, and are frequently positive for acid phosphatase with a punctate distribution. Common ALL cells are usually negative for AP. The presence of C3 receptors may indicate a relationship to fetal thymocytes (3). LBL and T-ALL share many clinical features, including a high male: female ratio, poor prognosis, age distribution older than that of common-ALL, and the presence of a mediastinal mass.

Using monoclonal antibodies T-LBL usually has a more mature antigenic phenotype than T-ALL, although in both instances the cells will be positive for TdT (which is weaker in T-LBL) (30). The cells of T-LBL do not coexpress OKT4/OKT8 or Leu 3a/Leu 2a, whereas in T-ALL these antigenic markers are frequently coexpressed (14, 36). The cells of T-LBL are usually negative as well for OKT6. Conceptually, one can consider T-ALL to represent the earliest stage of T-cell differentiation equivalent to a bone marrow-derived pre-thymic T cell, whereas T-LBL relates to sequential stages of cortical intrathymic differentiation.

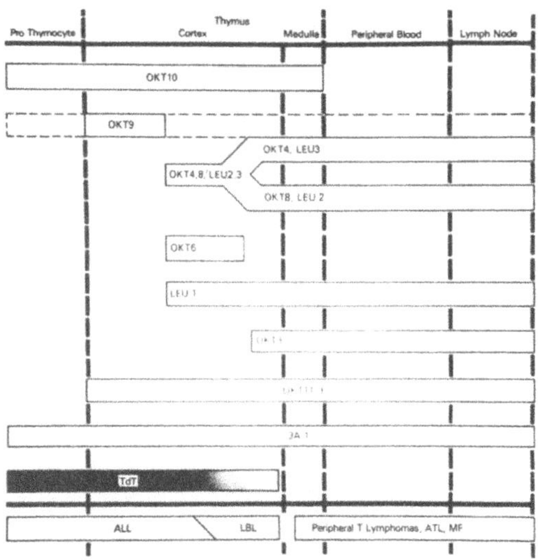

FIGURE 3. Schematic diagram indicates antigenic phenotype of T cells at sequential stages of differentiation. T-cell malignancies are related to specific stages of T-cell development. Reprinted with modification from Cancer Res(43):4486-4490, 1983.

5.2. Neoplasms of mature T-cell origin.

5.2.1. T-Cell chronic lymphocytic leukemia (T-CLL). Only 2% or less of all cases of chronic lymphocytic leukemia have been shown to be of T-cell origin. The demonstration of T-lymphocyte markers in a lymphoma of the small lymphocytic type is an even rarer event. Approximately 60% of cases of T-cell chronic lymphocytic leukemia (T-CLL) have distinctive morphologic features (37). Cytoplasmic azurophilic granulation on Wright-Giemsa stained smears is the most easily recognized feature and such granulation has not been observed in B-CLL. Almost all cases have a high content of β-glucuronidase and acid phosphatase activity, regardless of the presence of recognizable granules by light microscopy. It should be noted, however, that certain rare cases of B-CLL also may have increased β-glucuronidase and acid phosphatase activity. Such enzymatic activity in B-CLL has correlated with plasmacytoid differentiation and immunosecretory activity.

The degree of lymphocytosis reported in T-CLL has been highly variable with absolute lymphocyte counts ranging from 3,000 to 500,000 cells/μl. Some cases characterized by increased cell size, cytoplasmic basophilia, hepatosplenomegaly, markedly elevated white blood cell counts, and an acute clinical course would fit the description of acute prolymphocytic leukemia.

The potential for retained function in the proliferating cells of T-CLL accounts for a number of interesting clinical syndromes in this disorder. Normal helper and suppressor T cells regulate not only immunoglobulin production, but also erythropoiesis and myelopoiesis. Instances of T-CLL derived from the suppressor T-cell subset have been associated with neutropenia, pure red cell aplasia, and hypogammaglobulinemia, with increased susceptibility to infection. The neoplastic cells have been shown to function as suppressor cells in *in vitro* assays and can perform antibody-dependent cytoxicity (ADCC). Production of γ immune interferon has also been documented (38-39).

A number of these patients with proliferations of suppressor T cells (or T-γ cells as they were described in some reports) have had only modest elevations in their lymphocyte counts, which have remained stable, sometimes for many years. Thus, some authors have questioned whether or not such cases represent a truly neoplastic disorder and have termed the disorder chronic T-cell lymphocytosis (40).

Table 3. Immunologic phenotype of T-cell CLL.

All cases share the following features:

Sheep red blood cell rosettes (E)	+
Acid phosphatase	+
β-glucuronidase	+
Pan-T antigens	
Leu 4, OKT3	+
Leu 1*	+
TdT	-
OKT6	-
SIg	-

Subtypes of T-CLL	Helper (Tμ)	Suppressor (Tγ)
OKT8 (Leu 2a)	-	+
OKT5	-	+
OKT4 (Leu 3a)	+	-
ADCC	-	+
NK	-	-

5.2.2. Mycosis fungoides/Sezary syndrome. Mycosis fungoides/Sezary syndrome (MF/SS) are primarily cutaneous lymphoid malignancies, usually with a chronic clinical course and slow evolution with time (41). Most consider MF/SS to represent different stages of manifestations of the same neoplastic process. In SS the predominant cell is small, has the capacity to circulate or peripheralize, and patients clinically exhibit generalized exfoliative erythroderma and peripheral blood involvement. In MF a mixture of small and large abnormal lymphoid cells are present, and the large transformed cells, as in other nonHodgkin's lymphomas, have less of a tendency to circulate. Thus, the disease is associated with more discreet or localized lesions, plaques in early stages, and tumors in later stages. In late stages, systemic involvement of lymph nodes and other organs may also occur, and is considered to represent the same pathologic process.

Both phenotypically and functionally most cases have helper T-cell characteristics (42). The cells are OKT4/Leu 3a+ and OKT8/Leu 2a-. Although the cells react with the pan-T-cell monoclonal antibodies Leu 1 and OKT3, the cells are usually negative with 3A1 or Leu 9. Hypergammaglobulinemia noted clinically may be related to helper function *in vivo*. The neoplastic T cells

*Leu 1: also found in B-CLL

follow the same circulatory pathways as normal T cells, migrating through post-capillary venules to enter lymph nodes. Cytochemical stains usually demonstrate strong positivity for AP and BG, enzymes with low levels of activity in B-cell lymphomas and leukemias.

5.2.3. Peripheral T-cell lymphomas. Up to 25% of diffuse aggressive lymphomas have mature T-cell markers and would be included in the broad category of peripheral T-cell lymphomas (PTL) (43,44). In the Working Formulation, most PTL are included within the categories of diffuse mixed small and large cell and large cell, immunoblastic lymphomas. Although morphologically heterogeneous, common histologic features include a polymorphous inflammatory background, a prominent vascular component, and the presence of marked variation in cell size and shape.

When characterized by monoclonal antibodies, the cells of PTL are mature T lymphocytes. They lack TdT and usually express either a helper or suppressor phenotype (44). However, these antigens are not clonal markers and should not be interpreted as such. For reasons not understood, the majority of PTL express the antigens identified by OKT4 and/or anti-Leu 3a, indicative of the helper sub-type.

A characteristic and useful diagnostic feature is that the cells of PTL often express aberrant T-cell phenotypes. For example, they may react with only one of several pan-T monoclonal antibodies. For example, 3A1, (or Leu 9), an antibody that reacts with the vast majority of normal T cells, is negative in most cases of PTL. Thus, when searching for evidence of a T-cell origin, a panel of anti-T-cell monoclonal antibodies (e.g., anti-Leu 4, anti-Leu 1, anti-Leu 9, and Lyt 3) should be employed. Moreover, the demonstration of an aberrant T-cell phenotype provides supportive evidence that the T cells are neoplastic and not reactive, a feature helpful in distinguishing PTL from atypical reactive hyperplasias and B-cell lymphomas containing numerically predominant but normal T cells.

5.2.4. Adult T-cell leukemia/lymphoma. This acute lymphoid malignancy has distinctive clincial, pathologic, and epidemiologic features and it should not be included in the broad category of diffuse aggressive lymphomas (45). It is associated with the unique human retrovirus HTLV, Type I, and indeed the presence of antibodies to HTLV-I coincides with a distinct clinico-pathologic syndrome characterized by generalized lymphadenopathy, hepatosplenomegaly, skin and peripheral blood involvement, and hypercalcemia. The disease is aggressive with a median survival of only 9 months (46).

The most characteristic diagnostic feature is the presence of highly pleomorphic and polylobated lymphoid cells in the peripheral blood. The pathologic spectrum of the associated lymphomas is broad and encompasses several diffuse histologic subtypes in the Working Formulation. However, differences in survival cannot be correlated with differences in histologic subtype. In two-thirds of patients with cutaneous involvement, epidermal infiltration resembling Pautrier microabscesses was observed. However, most cases can be readily distinguished from mycosis fungoides/Sezary syndrome on clinical and epidemiologic grounds. The cells of ATL have a mature T-cell phenotype. Although they react with OKT4/anti-Leu 3a, they function in vitro as suppressor cells. A characteristic feature is reactivity with anti-Tac, a monoclonal antibody directed against the T-cell growth factor receptor. The hypercalcemia and osteolytic bone lesions frequently observed are probably secondary to a lymphokine produced by the malignant cells, either osteoclast-activating factor (OAF) or an OAF-like substance.

5.2.5. Angiocentric immunoproliferative lesions (AIL) and angiocentric lymphomas. Angiocentric immunoproliferative lesions (AIL) are a related group of lymphoproliferative disorders for which several diagnostic terms have been employed: lymphomatoid granulomatosis, polymorphic reticulosis, and atypical lymphocytic vasculitis. These lesions are all angiocentric and angiodestructive lymphoid proliferations comprised of an admixture of lymphocytes and other inflammatory cells.

Despite the polymorphic character of the infiltrate, the lymphocytes may show some cytologic atypia, and approximately 30% of patients go on to develop frank malignant lymphoma. Therefore, it has been argued that, in at least some patients, the disease may be neoplastic at the outset (43). Although only a small number of cases has been studied phenotypically, in both AIL and angiocentric lymphomas, the cells have had mature T-cell characteristics. The AIL are also often associated with a hemophagocytic syndrome which may be a consequence of lymphokine production by the neoplastic cells (47, 48).

6. TUMORS OF HISTIOCYTIC AND RETICULUM CELL ORIGIN

A histiocyte is a fixed-tissue monocyte and is essentially the same as a macrophage. The role of these cells is phagocytosis, antigen processing and presentation of antigen to lymphocytes. Their function is regulated to some degree by secreted substances from T lymphocytes. These cells possess large numbers of Fc receptors (for IgG) and also have complement receptors (primarily for C3b-C4b). Activated monocytes appear also to bear receptors for C3d. Ia antigens are present on monocytes and histiocytes. These cells contain lysosomal enzymes such as α-naphthyl acetate esterase (A-EST) and α-naphthyl-butyrate esterase (B-EST), so-called non-specific esterases (22).

Related cells which subserve an antigen-presenting function are the so-called reticulum cells. These cells are not phagocytic. Dendritic reticulum cells (DRC) are the antigen-presenting cells of the B-cell system and are found in follicles. Interdigitating reticulum cells (IRC) are the antigen-presenting cells of the T-cell system and are found in the paracortex of lymph nodes and other T-cell dependent zones. Closely related to IRC are the Langerhans cells (containing Langerhans or Basset granules) found in skin as well as lymphoid organs. DRC and IRC have Ia antigens and Fc receptors, as well as punctate weak activity for non-specific esterase and acid phosphatase.

Table 4. Markers of mononuclear phagocytes and related cells.

	FcR	CR	Ia	AP	NSE	Phagocytosis	Lyso	α-1-AT
MP	+	+	+	+D	+D	+	+	+
DRC	+	+	+	+P	+P	-	-	-
IRC	+	±	+	+P	+P	-	-	-

Abbreviations: MP, mononuclear phagocytes; DRC, dendritic reticulum cells, IRC, interdigitating reticulum cells and Langerhans cells; FcR, Fc receptors for IgG; CR, complement receptors; Ia, Ia or HLA-DR antigens; AP, acid phosphatase; P, punctate; D, diffuse; NSE, non-specific esterase; Lyso, lysozyme; α-1-AT, α-1-anti-trypsin.

6.1. Acute monocytic leukemia

Acute monocytic leukemia (AMOL) is a bone-marrow-derived neoplasm with monoblastic and monocytic features. Although the neoplastic cells have immunological markers characteristic of mononuclear phagocytes, the diagnosis in the clinical setting is made by characteristic enzyme cytochemical activity for A-EST and B-EST and an absence of the myeloid enzymes PER and ASDCL.

6.2. Malignant histiocytosis

Malignant histiocytosis (MH) is a systemic malignancy of mononuclear phagocytes that involves the entire reticuloendothelial system (49). The cells retain the functional properties (phagocytosis) as well as the surface markers characteristic of histiocytes. Since a number of hemophagocytic syndromes may simulate MH, to make the diagnosis one should observe cytologic features of malignancy, as well as evidence of a histiocytic derivation (47, 50). In contrast with AMOL, peripheral blood involvement is inconspicuous.

6.3. True histiocytic lymphoma (histiocytic sarcoma)

True histiocytic lymphomas (THL) are localized tumefactions which may or may not progress to disseminated disease. Some have preferred the term histiocytic sarcoma because of the potential confusion of THL with "histiocytic" lymphoma in the Rappaport scheme for tumors of transformed lymphocytes, and the apparent contradiction in the use of "lymphoma" for a tumor of histiocytic, and not lymphoid origin (51). These are stylistic choices and the term true histiocytic lymphoma appears to have gained wide acceptance in the literature.

In the vast majority of cases of THL it will be necessary to document the histiocytic derivation of the cells with immunologic and cytochemical markers (Table 4). Enzyme cytochemical stains can be performed on air-dried smears or imprints and/or frozen sections. The former are preferable for discerning the pattern of reactivity within the cytoplasm of the cells. Mononuclear phagocytes have diffuse reactivity for A-EST and B-EST. The activity is usually partially or totally inhibited by fluoride. Diffuse activity for AP and BG is also present. THL are negative for alkaline phosphatase and chloroacetate esterase. Peroxidase activity is minimal in extent as compared with myeloid cells.

NSE, AP, and BG activity are certainly not specific for THL. In particular, tumors of T-cell origin usually manifest punctate or perinuclear reactivity for the above enzymes, in contrast to the diffuse activity seen in mononuclear phagocytes. Tumors of transformed B cells also can have reactivity similar to that seen in T cells (44). A number of epithelial malignancies can demonstrate diffuse reactivity for these enzymes as well.

Using immunologic markers the cells of MH/THL have the phenotype of mononuclear phagocytes or monocytes. They have receptors for complement and the Fc fragment of IgG and will form rosettes with EAC and IgGEA. In addition, they will frequently phagocytose the bound red blood cells after rosetting. Due to strong Fc receptors the cells may manifest abundant cytophilic antibody and will demonstrate cytoplasmic and surface staining for IgG with both light chains present in proportion to their serum distribution. Phagocytic assays may also be helpful.

Monoclonal antibodies have been less useful in identifying MH/THL than in identifying tumors of the T- or B-cell lineages. The cells of MH/THL express Ia or HLA-DR antigens. However, these antigens are not specific for mononuclear phagocytes and are found on B cells, activated T cells, Langerhans cells, and even some non-lymphoid cells such as melanoma and seminoma cells. Most monoclonal antibodies reactive with monocytes and macrophages also react with the cells of the granulocytic series. Included in this category are the monoclonal antibodies MO1 and anti-Leu M1 (52). Antibodies with greater specificity for the monocyte-macrophage fraction include MO2 and anti-Leu M2. However, we have found these reagents to be of limited utility in the diagnosis of THL. It should be noted that anti-Leu M1 reacts with the malignant cells of Hodgkin's disease (53). Its reactivity with THL is unknown.

Heteroantisera against lysozyme (muramidase) and α-1-antitrypsin have been employed in paraffin sections for the identification of benign and malignant MP (54). Lysozyme is present in high concentration in epithelioid histiocytes and non-phagocytic histiocytes but cells undergoing active phagocytosis usually demonstrate minimal activity. It has been inconsistently present in the cells of MH/THL. It also has a broad distribution outside the lymphoreticular system and is found in myeloid cells, Paneth cells, serous cells of salivary and bronchial glands, proximal renal tubular epithelium, and alveolar lining cells, as well as the malignant derivations of the same. α-1-antitrypsin binds to lysosomes and will be found in cells containing these structures. Histiocytes usually have diffuse granular reactivity. Most but not all cases of THL are positive for α-1-antitrypsin (54).

Ultrastructural studies may also be of help in identifying features of mononuclear phagocytic origin, such as phagolysosomes, residual bodies, and primary lysosomal granules. Variable features include ribosomes and polyribosomes and polyribosomes and rough endoplasmic reticulum.

6.4. Histiocytosis X

Histiocytosis X is a proliferative lesion related to Langerhans cells. The neoplastic cells have the characteristic cell organelle, the Langerhans granule, when examined by electron microscopy. Other features characteristic of antigen-presenting cells can also be identified. An unusual feature of normal and neoplastic Langerhans cells is reactivity with OKT6, a monoclonal antibody which also stains cortical thymocytes. The cells are also reported to be positive for the S-100 protein, an antigen primarily associated with neural tissues.

6.5. Hodgkin's disease

Hodgkin's disease is unusual for a neoplastic disorder, because in tissues involved by this process the neoplastic cells may constitute the minority of the cells present. The neoplastic cells, the Reed-Sternberg cells and their mononuclear variants, are admixed with normal lymphocytes, histiocytes, eosinophils, neutrophils, plasma cells, and fibroblasts. The disease is characterized by functional deficits in T-cell-mediated immune responses, often early in the course and prior to therapy (55-56). Decreased levels of E-rosette-forming cells may be found in peripheral blood and may be due, in part, to the presence of serum factors acting on T cells (57). The lymphocytes within Hodgkin's lesions are usually identifiable as T cells, predominately T-helper cells. The nature of the malignant cell in HD is not established, but most favor a histiocytic or reticulum origin. In the past, a B-cell origin has been proposed based on the presence of either surface and/or cytoplasmic immunoglobulins (58). In addition, the nodules of nodular sclerosing Hodgkin's disease contain a large component of complement receptor B cells in frozen section studies (59). However, evidence of monoclonality and/or synthesis of Ig associated with Reed-Sternberg cells is lacking. The Ig is most likely passively absorbed via IgG Fc receptors present on the neoplastic cells, and later internalized into the cytoplasm. Internalization of cytophilic antibody has been shown in vitro, and similar binding in vivo might result in the presence of Ig on the surface of and within the neoplastic cells (60).

Recent observations have suggested that if the RS cell is related to the "histiocytic" system, it may be more closely related to an antigen-presenting cell, rather than a phagocytic cell (61). Although RS cells have Ia antigens and Fc receptors, they have never been observed to be phagocytic. They also lack the lysosomal enzymes characteristic of phagocytic cells. Rather, the cytochemical profile of RS cells resembles that of interdigitating reticulum cells, cells involved in antigen presentation to T cells usually identified in the lymph node paracortex. An interesting feature is the tendency of RS cells to be rosetted by normal lymphocytes, particularly T cells. This simulates a phenomenon normally demonstrated by T cells and histiocytes.

Uninvolved tissues in HD may show follicular hyperplasia with plasmacytosis. Increased IgG synthesis has been demonstrated in vitro by spleens from patients with HD (62). This Ig may have anti-lymphocyte activity. HD has been characterized as a lymphocyte "civil war" with self attacking self, analogous to graft vs. host disease (63). It is speculated that neoantigens are induced on lymphocytes, perhaps by a virus, which render them foreign as seen by the host's normal lymphocytes.

Attempts at long-term continuous cell culture of Hodgkin's disease have been variable in their success. For example, some lines having histiocytic characteristics proved to be short-term lines derived from contaminating monocytes and not of tumor cell origin. Recent insight into the origin of the Hodgkin cell has been provided by studies from Diehl and his colleagues in Germany (64). They have been able to culture putative Hodgkin's cells in long-term culture in vitro. These cells have some of the characteristics of "reticulum" cells and do not appear to be either T or B cells or phagocytes. Further, a monoclonal antibody (Ki-1) has been prouced against the cell line and this antibody stains Hodgkin's mononuclear cells and Reed Sternberg cells in tissue sections of Hodgkin's disease (65). The only normal cell so far identified by this antibody is a rare mononuclear cell with abundant cytoplasm that occurs near normal germinal centers. The origin and function of this cell is not known at present.

A useful diagnostic feature, which does not necessarily shed light on the cell of origin of Hodgkin's disease, is the reactivity of RS cells and their mononuclear counterparts with LeuM1, a monoclonal antibody which reacts with normal granulocytes (53). This reagent works in paraffin-embedded sections and thus has considerable clinical utility. It is positive in the vast majority of cases, with the exception of the lymphocyte predominant variant which is usually negative. LeuM1 detects a sugar sequence containing lacto-N-fucopentaose.

REFERENCES

1. Rosenberg SA, Berard CW, Brown BW, Burke J, Dorfman RF, Glatstein E, Hoppe RT, Simon RT: National Cancer Institute sponsored study of classification of non-Hodgkin's lymphomas: summary and description of a Working Formulation for clinical usage. Cancer(49):2112-2135, 1982.
2. Mann RB, Jaffe ES, Berard CW: Malignant lymphomas: a conceptual understanding of morphological diversity. Am J Pathol(94):105-192, 1979.
3. Jaffe ES, Braylan RC, Frank MM, Green I, Berard CW: Heterogeneity of immunologic markers and surface morphology in "childhood lymphoblastic lymphoma." Blood(44):930, 1974.
4. Bollum FJ: Terminal deoxynucleotidyl transferase as a hematopoietic cell marker. A review. Blood(54):1203-1215, 1979.
5. Shibata A, Bennett JM, Castoldi GL, Catovsky D, Flandrin G, Jaffe ES, Katayama I, Nanba K, Schmalzl, F Yam LT: International Committee for Standardization in Hematology (ICSH). Recommended methods for cytochemical procedures in hematology. Clin Lab Haematol, in press.
6. Nanba J, Jaffe ES, Braylan RC, Soban EJ, Berard CW: Alkaline phosphatase positive malignant lymphomas. A subtype of B-cell lymphomas. Am J Clin Pathol(68):535-542, 1977.
7. Bowling MC: Histopathology Laboratory Procedures of the Pathologic Anatomy Branch of the National Cancer Institute. U.S. Govt. Printing Office, Washington, D.C., 1967.
8. Korsmeyer SJ, Hieter PA, Ravetch JV, Poplack DG, Waldmann TA, Leder P: Developmental hierarchy of immunoglobulin gene rearrangements in human leukemic pre-B cells. Proc Natl Acad Sci USA(78): 7096-7100, 1981.
9. Cossman J, Neckers L, Arnold A, Korsmeyer S: Induction of differentiation in a case of common acute lymphoblastic leukemia. N Engl J Med(307):1251-1254, 1982.
10. Vogler LB, Crist W, Bockman DE, Pearl ER, Lawton AR, Cooper MD: Pre-B-cell leukemia. A new phenotype of childhood lymphoblastic leukemia. N Engl J Med(298):872-878, 1978.

11. Greaves MF, Janossy G, Roberts M, Rapson NT, Ellis RB, Chessels J, Lister TA, Catovsky D: Membrane phenotyping: diagnosis, monitoring and classification of acute "lymphoid" leukemias. In: Thierfeler S, Rodt H, Thiel, E (eds) Immunological Diagnoses of Leukemias and Lymphomas. Springer Verlag, New York, 1977, pp. 61-75.
12. Ritz J, Pesondo JM, Notis-McConarty J, Lazarus H, Schlossman SF: A monoclonal antibody to human acute lymphoblastic leukemia antigen. Nature(283):583, 1980.
13. Korsmeyer SJ, Arnold A, Bakhshi A, Ravetch JV, Siebenlist U, Hieter PA, Sharrow SO, Le Bien TW, Kersey JH, Poplack DG, Leder P, Waldmann TA: Immunoglobulin gene rearrangements and cell surface antigen expression in acute lymphocytic leukemias of T-cell and B-cell precursor origins. J Clin Invest(71):301-313, 1983.
14. Cossman J, Chused T, Fisher R, Magrath I, Bollum FJ, Jaffe ES: Diversity of immunologic phenotypes of lymphoblastic lymphoma. Cancer Res(43):4486-4490, 1983.
15. Miller RA, Maloney DG, Levy R, Warnke R: Treatment of B-cell lymphoma with monoclonal anti-idiotype antibody. N Engl J Med(306): 517-522, 1982.
16. Arnold A, Cossman J, Bakhshi A, Jaffe ES, Waldmann TA, Korsmeyer SJ: Immunoglobulin gene rearrangements as unique clonal markers in human lymphoid neoplasms. N Engl J Med (309):1593-1599, 1983.
17. Cossman J, Neckers LM, Hsu SM, Longo D, Jaffe ES: Low grade lymphomas: Expression of developmentally regulated B-cell antigens. Am J Pathol(114):117-124, 1984.
18. Cossman J, Jaffe ES: Distribution of complement receptor subtypes in non-Hodgkin's lymphomas of B-cell origin. Blood(58):20-26, 1981.
19. Royston I, Majda JA, Baird SM, Meserve BL, Griffiths JC: Human T-cell antigens defined by monoclonal antigens: The 65,000 dalton antigen of T cells (T65) is also found on chronic lymphocytic leukemia cells bearing surface immunoglobulin. J Immunol(125):725-731, 1980.
20. Fu SM, Chiorazzi N, Kunkel HG, Halper JP, Harris SR: Induction of in vitro differentiation and immunoglobulin synthesis of human leukemic B lymphocytes. J Exp Med(148): 1570-1578, 1978.
21. Cossman J, Neckers LM, Braziel RM, Trepel JB, Korsmeyer SJ, Bakhshi A: In vitro enhancement of immunoglobulin gene expression in chronic lymphocytic leukemia. J Clin Invest(73):587-592, 1984.
22. Jaffe ES, Braylan RC, Nanba K, Frank MM, Berard CW: Functional markers: A new perspective on malignant lymphomas. Cancer Treat Rep(61):953-962, 1977.
23. Swerdlow SH, Habeshaw JA, Murray LJ, Dhaliwal HS, Lister TA, Stansfield AG: Centrocytic lymphoma: A distinct clinicopathologic and immunologic entity. Am J Pathol (113):181-197, 1983.
24. Jaffe ES, Shevach EM, Frank MM, Berard DW, Green I: Nodular lymphoma: Evidence for origin from follicular B lymphocytes. N Engl J Med(290):813, 1974.

25. Braziel RM, Neckers LM, Jaffe ES, Cossman J: Induction of immunoglobulin secretion in follicular non-Hodgkin's lymphomas: Role of immunoregulatory T cells. Blood, in press.
26. Jaffe ES, Strauchen JA, Berard CW: Predictability of immunologic phenotype by morphologic criteria in diffuse aggressive non-Hodgkin's lymphomas. Am J Clin Pathol(77): 46-49, 1982.
27. Mann RB, Jaffe ES, Braylan RC, Nanba K, Frank MM, Ziegler JL, Berard CW: Non-endemic Burkitt's lymphoma. A B-cell tumor related to germinal centers. N Engl J Med(295):685-691, 1976.
28. Jaffe ES, Smith SA, Magrath IT, Freeman CB, Alabaster O: Induction of complement receptors in human cell lines derived from undifferentiated lymphomas. Lab Invest (45):295-301, 1981.
29. Ritz J, Nadler LM, Bhan AK, Notis-McConarty J, Pesando JM, Schlossman SF: Expression of common acute lymphoblastic leukemia antigen (CALLA) by lymphomas of B- and T-cell lineage. Blood(58):648-652, 1981.
30. Braziel RM, Keneklis T, Donlon JA, Hsu SM, Cossman J, Bollum FJ, Jaffe ES: Terminal deoxynucleotidyl transferase in non-Hodgkin's lymphoma. Am J Clin Pathol(80):655-659, 1983.
31. Croce CM, Tsujimoto Y, Erikson J, Nowell PC: Chromosomal translocation and B-cell neoplasia. Lab Invest(51):258-267, 1984.
32. Braylan RC, Jaffe ES, Triche JJ, Nanba K, Fowkles BJ, Metzger H, Frank MM, Dolan MS, Yee CL, Green I, Berard CW: Structural and functional properties of the "hairy" cells of leukemic reticuloendotheliosis. Cancer(41):210-227, 1978.
33. Cohen HJ, George ER, Kremer WB: Hairy cell leukemia: Cellular characteristics including surface immunoglobulin dynamics and biosynthesis. Blood(53):764, 1979.
34. Korsmeyer S, Greene W, Cossman J, Hsu SM, Neckers L, Marshall S, Jensen J, Bakhshi A, Leonard W, Jaffe ES, Waldmann T: Rearrangement and expression of immunoglobulin genes and expression of TAC antigen in hairy cell leukemia. Proc Natl Acad Sci USA(80):4522-4526, 1983.
35. Anderson KC, Bates MP, Slaughenhoupt BL, Pinkus GS, Schlossman SF, Nadler LM: Expression of human B-cell-associated antigens on leukemias and lymphomas: A model of human B-cell differentiation. Blood(63):1425-1433, 1984.
36. Bernard A, Boumsell L, Reinherz EL, Nadler LM, Ritz J, Coppin H, Richard Y, Valensi F, Dausset J, Flandrin G, Lemerle J, Schlossman SF: Cell surface characterization of malignant T cells from lymphoblastic lymphoma using monoclonal antibodies: Evidence for phenotypic differences between malignant T cells from patients with acute lymphoblastic leukemia and lymphoblastic lymphoma. Blood(57): 1105-1110, 1981.
37. Brouet JC, Flandrin G, Sasportes M, Preud'homme JL, Seligmann M: Chronic lymphocytic leukemia of T-cell origin. Lancet(ii)890-893, 1975.

38. Pandolfi F, Strong DM, Slease RB, Smith ML, Ortaldo JR, Herberman RB: Characterization of a suppressor T-cell chronic lymphocytic leukemia with ADCC but not NK activity. Blood(56):653-660, 1980.
39. Hooks JJ, Haynes BF, Detrick-Hooks D, Diehl LF, Gerrard TL, Fauci AS: Gamma (immune) interferon production by leukocytes from a patient with T γ -cell proliferative disease. Blood(59):198-201, 1982.
40. Aisenberg AC, Wilkes BM, Harris NL, Ault KA, Carey RW: Chronic T-cell lymphocytosis with neutropenia: Report of a case studied with monoclonal antibodies. Blood(58):818-822, 1981.
41. Broder S, Bunn PA Jr: Cutaneous T-cell lymphomas. Semin Oncol(7):310-331, 1980.
42. Broder S, Waldmann TA: Helper activity by lymphocytes derived from patients with the Sezary syndrome. J Clin Invest(58):1297-1306, 1976.
43. Jaffe ES: Pathologic and clinical spectrum of post-thymic T-cell malignancies. Special article. Cancer Investigation 2(5), 1984.
44. Cossman J, Jaffe ES, Fisher RI: Immunologic phenotypes of diffuse aggressive non-Hodgkin's lymphomas: Correlation with clinical features. Cancer(54):1310-1317, 1984.
45. Jaffe ES, Blattner WA, Blayney DW, Bunn PA Jr, Cossman J, Robert-Guroff M, Gallo RC: The pathologic spectrum of HTLV-associated leukemia lymphoma in the United States. Am J Surg Pathol(8):263-275, 1984.
46. Blayney D, Jaffe E, Blattner W, Cossman J, Robert-Guroff M, Longo D, Bunn P, Gallo R: The human T-cell leukemia/lymphoma virus (HTLV) associated with American adult T-cell leukemia/lymphoma (ATL). Blood(62):401-405, 1983.
47. Jaffe ES, Costa J, Fauci AS, Cossman J, Tsokos M: Malignant lymphoma and erythrophagocytosis simulating malignant histiocytosis. Am J Med(75):741-749, 1983.
48. Simrell CR, Crabtree GR, Cossman J, Fauci AS, Jaffe ES: Stimulation of phagocytosis by a T-cell-lymphoma-derived lymphokine. In: Vitetta E (ed) B- and T-Cell Tumors. UCLA Symposia in Molecular and Cellular Biology. Vol 24. Academic Press, New York, 1982, pp. 247-252.
49. Jaffe ES, Shevach EM, Sussman EH, Frank MM, Green I, Berard CW: Membrane receptor sites for the identification of lymphoreticular cells in benign and malignant conditions. Br J Cancer(31(Suppl II)):107-120, 1975.
50. Risdall RJ, McKenna RW, Nesbit ME, Krivit W, Balfour HH, Simmons RL, Brunning RD: Virus-associated hemophagocytic syndrome, a benign histiocytic proliferation distinct from malignant histiocytosis. Cancer(44):993-1002, 1979.
51. Van der Valk P, Meijer CJLM, Willemze R, Oosterom AT, Spaander PJ, Te Velde J: Histiocytic sarcoma (true histiocytic lymphoma) a clinico-pathological study of 20 cases. Histopathology(8):105-123, 1984.
52. Breard J, Reinherz EL, Kung PC, Goldstein G, Schlossman SF: A monoclonal antibody reactive with human blood monocytes. J Immunol(124):1943-1948, 1980.

53. Hsu SM, Jaffe ES: Leu M1 and peanut agglutinin stain the neoplastic cells of Hodgkin's disease. Am J Clin Pathol (82):29-32, 1984.
54. Isaacson P, Wright DH, Jones DB: Malignant lymphoma of true histiocytic (monocyte/macrophage) origin. Cancer (51):80-91, 1983.
55. Young RC, Corder MA, Haynes HA, DeVita VT: Delayed hypersensitivity in Hodgkin's disease. A study of 103 cases. Am J Med(52):63-72, 1973.
56. Levy R, Kaplan HS: Impaired lymphocyte function in untreated Hodgkin's disease. N Engl J Med(290):181-186, 1974.
57. Fuks Z, Strober S, Kaplan HS: Interaction between serum factors and T lymphocytes in Hodgkin's disease. N Engl J Med(295):1273-1278, 1976.
58. Garvin AJ, Spicer SS, Parmley RT, Munster AM: Immunohistochemical demonstration of IgG in Reed-Sternberg and other cells in Hodgkin's disease. J Exp Med(139):1077-1083, 1974.
59. Cossman J, Deegan MJ, Schnitzer B: Complement receptor B lymphocytes in nodular sclerosing Hodgkin's disease. Cancer(39):2166-2174, 1977.
60. Kadin ME, Stites DP, Levy R, Warnke R: Exogenous immunoglobulin and the macrophage origin of Reed-Sternberg cells in Hodgkin's disease. N Engl J Med(299):1208, 1978.
61. Kadin ME: Possible origin of the Reed-Sternberg cell from an interdigitating reticulum cell. Cancer Treat Rep(66): 601-608, 1982.
62. Longmire RL, McMillan R, Yelenosky R, Armstrong S, Lang JE, Craddock CG: In vitro splenic IgG synthesis in Hodgkin's disease. N Engl J Med(289):763-767, 1973.
63. DeVita VT: Lymphocyte reactivity in Hodgkin's disease: A lymphocyte civil war. N Engl J Med(289):801-802, 1973.
64. Diehl V, Kirschner HH, Burrighter H, Stein H, Fonatsch C, Gerdes J, Schaadt M, Heit W, Uchanska-Ziegler B, Ziegler A, Heintz F, Sueno K: Characteristics of Hodgkin's-disease-derived cell lines. Cancer Treat Rep(66):615-632, 1982.
65. Stein H, Gerdes J, Schwab U, Lemke H, Mason DY, Ziegler A, Schienle W, Diehl U: Identification of Hodgkin and Sternberg-Reed sternberg cells as a unique cell type derived from a newly detected small cell population. Int J Cancer(30):445-459, 1982.

8

IMMUNOHISTOCHEMISTRY OF LYMPHOMAS IN FROZEN TISSUE SECTIONS

Raymond R. Tubbs, D.O.

This paper will briefly review the history and perspective of an immunohistologic approach to lymphomas, specimen handling and processing, methods that are utilized, the rationale for immunophenotyping, review normal lymphocyte development and maturation, and then outline typical phenotypes of lymphoproliferative disease.

Cell suspension studies have been used for two decades and continue to be one of the cornerstones for immunologic characterization of lymphomas (1). Tissue section immunostaining of lymphomas was initiated by Taylor who used the peroxidase-antiperoxidase technique on paraffin sections to define the distribution of immunoglobulin phenotypes in Hodgkin's disease and in some non-Hodgkin's lymphomas (2). Warnke et al documented in 1978 the false negative immunoglobulin staining in paraffin sections and the utility of frozen tissue section immunohistology using immunofluorescence (3), and further demonstrated the denaturation of immunoglobulin or loss of antigenicity induced by a variety of fixatives (4). In 1980, immunoglobulin phenotypes defined by immunoperoxidase techniques were described using frozen tissue sections (5), and staining of T and B cell antigens was accomplished using monoclonal antibodies and frozen tissue sections with biotin-avidin and unlabeled immunoperoxidase techniques (6,7). In 1981, the concordance was verified between frozen section immunoperoxidase techniques and cell suspension studies (8). Epstein et al recently developed a series of monoclonal antibodies that detect differentiation antigens in paraffin sections of fixed material, and that are specific in part for individual subgroups of B-cell tumors (9).

It should be emphasized that immunophenotyping is not at this time a primary mode of diagnosis, but is rather one of several tools providing information that should be integrated together to form a final pathologic diagnosis.

SPECIMEN PROCESSING

Key to processing lymphoid tissue is the development of a comprehensive accession protocol (10,11). Fresh tissue received should be divided into several different aliquots. Well-fixed, thinly sectioned material for light microscopy remains the cornerstone of pathologic classification. The few monoclonal antibodies active in paraffin sections seem to work best in Bouin's or B5 solutions (9,11). Formalin fixed paraffin sections are helpful in recognition and subclassification of Hodgkin's disease, since lacunar cells are best visualized this way. For optimal cellular detail, particularly nuclear detail, B5 is the preferred fixative. If the quantity of tissue is limited, B5 is preferred, if enough material for only one fixative is available. B5-fixed tissue is also used for morphometry in plastic sections. A small piece of tissue should be embedded and held for electron microscopy, but not routinely processed.

Touch preparations from the freshly cut surface of the node are helpful in terms of evaluating the Wright's stain. In the pre-monoclonal antibody era, identification of T cells other than with sheep erythrocyte rosettes depended on cytochemical profiles and were very valuable at that time. Currently, the Wright's stain can be used to make some decisions about the extent of immunophenotyping at the time of specimen accession and to recognize macrophages.

A fresh cell suspension should also be prepared from the tissue. A comparatively large volume of tissue (>1 cm^3) is usually required to extract enough cells to do all the markers. Generally, 1 x 10^6 cells per antigen desired are required for ease of flow cytometry analysis. The derived cell suspension is stained by direct and/or indirect immunofluorescence and analyzed by manual immunofluorescence or flow cytometry. In selected cases, DNA analysis may also be performed; and cytogenetics may be done using the cell suspension to look for marker chromosomes (e.g. Burkitt's lymphoma) or in borderline cases of atypical hyperplasias. It may also be necessary to look for abnormal gene rearrangements in extracted DNA (suspension or frozen tissue) in such cases. Cytocentrifuge preparations should also be prepared from the ficoled cell suspension using 2-3 x 10^6 cells/ml and air dried overnight prior to immunoperoxidase staining (12).

Frozen tissue should always be obtained from a lymph node submitted from a patient without an established tissue diagnosis, or when lymphoma is being considered. The frozen tissue can be kept indefinitely, and if needed, can be retrieved. If only a small amount of material is available, and only one immunophenotyping method can be used, frozen section/cytocentrifuge immunohistochemistry is preferred over flow cytometry.

IMMUNOPHENOTYPING REAGENTS & METHODS

For at least two decades cell suspension studies have been and still continue to be important in establishing immunophenotypes. More recently, frozen and paraffin section methods have also assumed an important role in immunophenotyping lymphoproliferative disease.

There are a variety of tissue techniques now which can be used for immunophenotyping. The term "immunohistology" is used here for immunologic procedures applied to tissue sections (paraffin or frozen sections) (11). "Immunocytology" is used here to refer to individually immunostained cells in derived cell suspensions, usually in cytocentrifuge preparations (11). For heavy and light chain immunoglobulin (Ig) phenotypes, the direct immunoperoxidase technique is preferred (10). In this procedure, an antibody (e.g. $F(ab)'_2$ goat anti-human κ) is conjugated directly with the enzyme peroxidase and binds to its corresponding antigen in the tissue. Following incubation the tissue section is exposed to the chromogen and substrate and a color reaction product is produced at sites of antigen/enzyme localization.

Direct methods are generally not sufficiently sensitive to permit detection of non-Ig differentiation antigens in tissue. There are certainly some directly-conjugated fluorescent markers that work well in the cell suspension. But amplification is usually necessary for detection of differentiation antigens in tissue sections. Indirect immunoperoxidase or immunofluorescent techniques, unlabeled (e.g. peroxidase-antiperoxidase), or biotin-avidin systems have been used. Most of the indirect systems that have been devised do not have sufficient sensitivity to obtain reliable, reproducible results. There are few exceptions (some antibodies have very favorable conjugation ratios with enzyme), but generally, a more sensitive technique is needed. The avidin-biotinylated peroxidase complex (ABC) technique is preferred (10). The secondary reagent, biotinylated anti-mouse IgG, forms a molecular bridge between the mouse monoclonal primary antibody and a soluble preformed complex of avidin and biotinylated peroxidase. The net effect is localization of many enzyme molecules for a given antigen focus in the tissue section, and consequently amplification of the color reaction product.

Many monoclonal antibodies are currently available for phenotyping lymphoproliferative disorders (Table I) (11). The antibodies identify cell-associated surface and cytoplasmic antigens and do not directly measure or necessarily imply specific immunoregulatory function. Some are Pan-T markers, that is, they are broadly reactive in T cell populations. Generally, T11 has been the most useful in our experience. This antibody labels cells forming spontaneous rosettes with sheep erythrocytes. T3 or Leu4 also mark all peripheral T cells and detect antigens independent of the sheep erythrocyte receptor molecule. T1 and Leu1 are also broadly reactive Pan-T markers, labeling intrathymic as well as peripheral T cells; curiously, they

TABLE I - IMMUNOPHENOTYPES OF LYMPHOCYTE POPULATIONS

Cell Population Maturation Stage	Expressed T Cell Antigens* T10	T9	T1/L1	T11/L5	T3/L4	T6	T4/L3	T8/L2	Corresponding Neoplasms
T cell stages:									
Early Thymocyte	+	+	+	+	-	-	-	-	Lymphoblastic lymphoma, T cell ALL
Immature Cortical Thymocyte	+	-	+	+	+	+	+	+	Thymoma, T cell ALL
Mature Thymocyte	+	-	+	+	+	-	+	+	Lymphoblastic lymphoma, T cell ALL
Peripheral T Cells*									
Inducer/Helper	-	-	+	+	+	-	+	-	Cutaneous T cell lymphoma, some large cell & mixed non-Hodgkin's lymphomas, T CLL
Cytotoxic/Suppressor	-	-	+	+	+	-	-	+	T CLL, peripheral T cell lymphoma

	Expressed B Cell Antigens* Ia	J5	B4	L2	C	SIg	CIg(δ,γ)	B1	B2	L14	L1	PCA	
B cell stages:													
Pre-pre-B	+	+	+	+	-	-	-	+/-	-	-	-	-	"Common" ALL
Pre-B	+	+	+	+	+	-	-	+/-	-/+	-	-	-	Pre-B ALL, some lymphoblastic lymphomas
Immature	+	-	+	+	+	+	+	+	+	+	+	-	Small lymphocytic lymphoma, CLL
Virginal	+	+w	+	+	+	+	+	+	+	+	+	-	Follicular small cleaved lymphoma
B Blast	+	-	+	+	+	+	+	+	-	+	+	-	Large cell & small non-cleaved lymphoma
Plasma cell	-	-	-	-	-	-/w+	+	-	-	-	-	+	Plasma cell myeloma

Abbreviations: + = present; - = absent; -/+ & +/- = variable; c = cytoplasmic heavy chain; ALL = acute lymphocytic leukemia; CLL - chronic lymphocytic leukemia; +w = weakly positive

* Designations refer to antigens detected by monoclonal antibodies, which identify cellular populations and do not directly profile function.

also label the neoplastic B lymphocytes of most cases of B cell chronic lymphocytic leukemia (11,13-16).

T cells are antigenically and functionally heterogeneous (1). Mature T cells can be broadly grouped as the T4/Leu3 inducer and helper population, and the T8/Leu2 population of cytotoxic and suppressor T cells. Subpopulations within these groups can be further defined with other monoclonal antibodies. The suppressor fraction within the T8/Leu2 population can be identified with Leu15 (17). Immature cortical thymocytes are labeled by T6, and earlier intrathymic subsets labeled by T9 and T10.

The development of non-Ig B cell markers defined by monoclonal antibodies has lagged behind the development of T cell markers somewhat. Broadly reactive B cell markers include Leu14, Leu10, B1 and B4, LN2, and HLA-Dr reagents (11). B cell subsets can also be identified with monoclonal antibodies, e.g. J5/CALLA for pre-pre B cells, B2 for immature and virginal B cells. Recently, monoclonal antibodies LN1, LN2, and LN3 were developed and detect antigens that survive fixation and paraffin embedding (9). LN3 is an Ia equivalent that requires B5 sections for optimum staining (9). LN1 is essentially a follicle center cell and macrophage marker and LN2 is a B cell and dendritic reticulum cell broadly reactive monoclonal antibody (9).

Macrophage markers include LeuM3, HLA-Dr, LN3, and others. However, sinus macrophages are most completely labeled with antibodies to α-1-chymotrypsin (11). The natural killer cell population are probably best detected with Leu11 (18). Leu7 detects large granular lymphocytes, but not all of the NK population is detected by Leu7 (19). Leu15 is broadly expressed on natural killer cells as well as the suppressor fraction of T cells (17).

There are obviously relative merits accorded cell suspension and tissue section methods (Table II) (11). Quantitation, especially via flow cytometry, is easily generated from derived cell suspensions. Immunohistologic preparations are generally more difficult to quantitate; one

TABLE II
RELATIVE MERITS OF
CELL SUSPENSION AND IMMUNOHISTOLOGIC METHODS

	Suspensions	Immunohistology
Quantitation	Easily accomplished	Difficult
Sample size	$\geq 1 \times 10^6$ cells/Ag preferred	Very small representative sample adequate
Sample storage & retrieval	Possible	Easily accomplished
Morphologic correlation	Difficult for immunofluorescence (sorts, panning)	Usually good, esp. cytocentrifuge preps

can currently only easily do semiquantitation or subjective evaluations. Quantitation using an image analyzer may soon be possible. Generally, about 1 x 10^6 cells per antigen are preferred for flow cytometry analysis of cell suspensions. On the other hand, a very small amount of representative frozen tissue will suffice for immunohistology. In terms of sample storage and retrieval, it is obviously easy to keep frozen sections and to bring them out as needed and evaluate them. Storing a cell suspension is a bit more difficult, but can be accomplished by freezing cells under nitrogen and DMSO with 10-30% cell loss after thawing. Morphologic correlation for most cell suspension methods is very difficult; cytocentrifuge preparations of rosettes or flow cytometry minisorts can be used. In immunohistology, the morphologic correlation is usually good. In frozen sections, there may be some problems with resolution. Immunoperoxidase-stained cytocentrifuge preparations give excellent resolution. One other artifact is sometimes a problem in immunohistologic preparations: collagen, and sometimes vascular endothelium, are associated with adherence of antibodies. Ordinarily, this is just a problem with anti-immunoglobulin reagents in frozen tissue sections and is not a problem with antibodies to differentiation antigens or any antigen in cytocentrifuge preps.

Each approach has different relative merits. The best approach at this time is to use both cell suspension methods and immunohistologic methods together to formulate the immunophenotype by integrating the information from both procedures. If the biopsy size is small, frozen section immunohistology and immunoperoxidase-stained cytospins are preferred.

At this time, phenotyping requires the use of fresh cell suspensions, acetone-fixed cytocentrifuge prep, and/or frozen tissue sections. Paraffin sections of fixed material, at least at the present time, are inadequate. The only exceptions are plasma cell myeloma and plasmacytoid lymphocytic lymphoma. Monoclonal antibodies with specificity for differentiation antigens surviving fixation and paraffin embedding are being developed (e.g. the LN series) (9).

THEORETICAL APPROACH TO IMMUNOPHENOTYPING

Four basic concepts underlie the approach to phenotyping. Generally, these are assertions for which there is considerable evidence (1,11): 1) lymphocyte development is not a random haphazard event, but proceeds through distinct, predictable maturation stages; 2) at each of these maturation stages there are combinations of expressed cellular antigens that are peculiar to an individual differentiation stage; 3) lymphomas are neoplastic clonal expansions of the immune system, arrested at certain points in lymphocyte maturation that generally correspond to these distinct maturation stages for normal development, and 4) lymphomas display combinations of antigens that correspond to the phenotype of the maturation stage at which they are arrested.

Immunophenotyping should not be the primary sole method of diagnosis. Its proper role in most instances is the corroboration of the histopathologic diagnosis. The parameters that can be evaluated include clonality as an index of malignant vs reactive hyperplasias for B cell populations (10), and to establish phenotypes for lymphomas known to be characterized by antigenic restriction (11). For example, if a lymphoma has been classified as cutaneous T cell lymphoma, then the immunophenotype should in most instances reflect the immunophenotype most commonly associated with cutaneous T cell lymphoma (T11+ B1- T4+ T8- Leu9-). One group has shown that differential expression of κ/λ isotypes and C3 receptors are associated with different biologic potentials independent of histopathology (20). Otherwise, there is no convincing evidence that there is independent clinical relevance for any immunologic marker at this time for non-Hodgkin's lymphomas (21). Finally, anti-idiotypic reagents can be assayed for avidity for tumor cells using immunohistology (22).

LYMPHOCYTE ONTOGENY

Normal lymphocyte development maturation stages, expressed cellular antigens, and corresponding neoplasms are summarized in Table I (1,11,13-19,23-30). Lymphoid stem cells that migrate to the thymus mature through early thymocyte and immature cortical common thymocyte stages. Mature thymocytes differentiate along two separate pathways, as mature inducer/ helper or cytotoxic/suppressor cellular pathways. At each of these stages there are combinations of antigens peculiar to that stage. None are absolutely specific, with perhaps the exception of T6, which seems to be restricted to the immature cortical thymocytes. But for most stages, there are selective combinations of antigens: e.g., in the early thymocyte stage mature markers like Leu3/T4, and Leu2/T8 are absent, but T9 and T10, broadly reactive monoclonals like Leu1, T11/Leu5, and TdT are present. At the later immature cortical stage, T6, T4 and T8 are expressed. Mature peripheral T cells selectively express only T8/Leu2 or Leu3/T4.

Normal B lymphocyte development is still being elucidated and defined (1,11,13-19,23-30). B cells also progress through distinct maturation stages. Pre-pre-B cells arise from committed lymphoid stem cells and then give rise to pre-B cells that are characterized by cytoplasmic μ heavy chains independent of κ and λ light chains or surface Ig synthesis. Isotope diversity characterizes the development of virginal B lymphocytes from immature B cells; a switch in the expression of heavy chains (μ to δ & γ) occurs. At the virginal B cell stage, there is also weak expression of the early B cell markers J5/Calla. The switch to IgG production is accompanied by readily detectable cytoplasmic immunoglobulin and deletion of B2. Maturation to the plasma cell is characterized by loss of many B cell antigens (Ia, B4, LN1, LN2, B1, Leu14); cytoplasmic immunoglobulin is prominent, but most of the B cell non-immunoglobulin markers are lost at the plasma cell stage.

For each T or B cell stage, there are combinations of antigens peculiar to that particular stage, and neoplasms which correspond to these differentiation stages (1,11,13-19, 23-30). For example, follicular small cleaved cell lymphoma displays an array of antigens that corresponds best to the virginal B cell stage (24). Common acute lymphocytic leukemia corresponds best to the pre-pre B cell stage and the observed antigenic phenotype is usually that of pre-pre B cells (Ia+ J5/Calla+ B4+ SIg- CIg- LN1- LN2+). Similarly, the lymphocyte component of thymomas usually bears Leu1, T11 and Leu5 (pan-T markers), with variable expression of subset antibodies T4, T8, Leu2, Leu3 and uniform expression of T6. This array of antigens is most peculiar to the immature cortical or common thymocyte stage of T cell development. Mycosis fungoides (cutaneous T cell lymphoma) is usually charcterized by broadly reactive Pan-T cell antigens with the single exception of Leu9 or 3A1 (Leu1+ T11+ T3+ Leu9-) (31). Mycosis fungoides is also characterized by restricted subset antigen distribution (T4/Leu3+, T8/Leu2-). This combination of antigens corresponds most closely to the mature inducer/helper peripheral T lymphocyte.

SPECIFIC IMMUNOTYPES OF LYMPHOPROLIFERATIVE DISORDERS

Immunophenotypes of reactive hyperplasias

In excess of 500 cases phenotyped with frozen tissue section immunohistochemistry were recently reported (7). 207 reactive hyperplasias had polyclonal (both κ and λ Ig) staining, and a physiologic distribution of lymphocyte differentiation antigens (LDA). Four cases were classified as atypical hyperplasias; three displayed monoclonal staining, one showed polyclonal κ and λ staining. Of three cases without definite histopathologic evidence of malignancy by light microscopy that had a monoclonal B cell proliferation, one progressed clinically and a histologic dianosis of lymphoma was subsequently established. A second patient's lymph nodes showed follicular hyperplasia by light microscopy and monoclonal immunostaining; but other nodes showed typical follicular lymphoma. The third case, an intramammary mass excised with a clinical diagnosis of carcinoma, was an intramammary lymph node with diffuse plasmacytosis (monoclonal κ) in the medullary cords. The patient remains disease-free at three years post-biopsy. The fourth case of atypical hyperplasia had polyclonal immunostaining and has not developed lymphoma.

Follicular hyperplasia is characterized by infrequent κ and λ light chain bearing cells in the interfollicular zone. The follicles are outlined by a variable amount of immunoglobulin staining. Follicle centers show highly variable expression of immunoglobulins, ranging from negative to strongly positive. However, the mantle zones are invariably positive for immunoglobulin light chains. In frozen tissue sections, anti-immunoglobulin antibodies adhere to endothelium or collagen network supporting the endothelium. In some follicles a peculiar segregation of staining to one pole within the follicle center is sometimes observed.

Immunoglobulin heavy chains are distributed in different anatomic domains. Mantle zone lymphocytes and primary follicles uniformly express IgD. There is essentially no IgD present in follicle center cells or on interfollicular lymphocytes. IgM is the major heavy chain associated with the cortical follicle and is expressed on both mantle zone lymphocytes and follicle center cells.

The distribution of T cells in follicular hyperplasia as defined by differentiation antigens T11 and Leu1 is principally in the paracortex and interfollicular zone (10,11). There are some T11+ T4+ cells in follicle centers often segregated to one pole and often in apposition to the interface between the mantle zone and the follicle center. This distinctive distribution may be the morphologic manifestation of the immunoregulatory function of T4 (inducer/helper) lymphocytes, facilitating the intrafollicular maturation of B cells. These T cell distributions are reproducible for peripheral lymphoid tissue regardless of site.

Most of the T cell dependent areas, the paracortex and interfollicular zone, are characterized by T4/Leu3 subset excess (10,11,32-34). The T cells within follicles are also principally of the T4/Leu3 subset (32-35). The T8/Leu2 antigen, expressed on cytotoxic/suppressor T cells, is identified on fewer cells, primarily in the T cell dependent zones (32-35). There are very few T8/Leu2+ cells within follicle centers (32-35). The overall lymph node ratio of T4/Leu3:T8/Leu2 roughly parallels that of the peripheral blood. "Reactive" lymph nodes that look very similar histologically are probably functionally quite different. Follicular hyperplasias may have a T4:T8 ratio of 3:1-6:1, whereas sinus histiocytosis may be 2 or less.

The T8/Leu2 distribution is somewhat different for cases of follicular hyperplasia that occur in patients with acquired immune deficiency syndrome and related illnesses (34). Despite an histopathologic appearance very similar to follicular hyperplasias of other causes, the immunohistology in this setting is unique in our experience. A peculiar striking increase of T8/Leu2+ lymphocytes is observed in T cell dependent zones, and especially within follicle centers (34).

The T8 monoclonal antibody also immunostains the splenic endothelium diffusely (36). Also, the T6 monoclonal antibody immunostains Langerhan's cells of skin and squamous mucous membrane (10).

The early intrathymic T cell markers, T9 and T10, are not restricted to the T cell series (10). T9 immunostains the follicle center cell population prominently in peripheral lymph node. T9 simply labels the transferrin receptor, which is a marker distributed widely in tissue. T10 is paradoxically also expressed by plasma cells (10).

Ia-like antigens in the peripheral lymph node show diffuse staining of B cell dependent areas including the mantle zones, larger cells in the interfollicular zone that has a dendritic morphology, and most sinus macrophages. LN2,

B1 & Leu10 immunostains about equally the follicle center cells, the mantle zone population, and some cells in the interfollicular zones. Leu14 labels cortical follicles. B2, B7, C3b, LN1 react preferentially with follicle center populations.

Tissue macrophages are probably at least as heterogeneous as T and B lymphocytes. There is no one single best reagent to selectively identify macrophages in lymph node. M1, MO2, LeuM3 and similar monoclonal antibodies, despite their utility in recognizing peripheral blood monocytes, are inconsistently expressed on nodal macrophages. α-1-chymotrypsin is certainly not specific for macrophages, but is broadly reactive with sinus macrophages and granuloma histiocytes. Many other antibodies developed for B cells (e.g. LN3, Leu10, LN1, LN2 and others) are also expressed on macrophages.

Natural killer/large granular lymphocyte (NK/LGL) populations can be identified by at least three reagents. The most specific for peripheral blood NK cells is probably Leu11 (18), which, in our experience, stains very few cells in the peripheral nodal tissue. Leu7, which stains LGL that are responsible for only part of NK activity (19), are restricted essentially to a follicle center cell population (10). Leu15 detects not only suppressor T cells but also a subpopulation of NK's (17).

IMMUNOPHENOTYPES OF NON-HODGKIN'S LYMPHOMAS (NHL)

Of 257 NHL recently reported, about 20% were T cell lymphomas (10). 67% had monoclonal staining (117 κ and 54 λ). A group of cases which in the past would have been called "null" cell lymphomas were shown to be Ig- B cell lymphomas by restricted expression of the non-Ig differentiation antigen B1. Using multiple monoclonal antibodies, the B cell lymphomas can be further phenotyped as to stage of B cell maturation (1,11, 13-19,23-29). Most lymph node based NHL are follicle center cell lymphomas with antigens peculiar to virginal or secretory B blast stage.

Two general immunohistologic patterns are observed in immunostained frozen tissue sections from non-Hodgkin's lymphoma, reflecting general architectural growth patterns of these tumors (Figure 1,2). Lymphomas in which there is a follicular component demonstrate monoclonal immunostaining within neoplastic follicles, i.e., the lymphomatous follicle demonstrates absent or very rare cells outlined by cell-associated immunoglobulin for one light chain (e.g., λ) and positive staining of the majority of cells in the lymphomatous follicle with the alternate light chain (e.g., κ). These findings are illustrated in Figure 1. Variable numbers of T cells defined by T11 or Leu1 are present within the neoplastic follicles, but generally are far more numerous in the intrafollicular zone. Diffuse lymphomas (Figure 2) are characterized by a diffuse architectural pattern of staining with individual tumor cells showing cell-associated monoclonal staining (κ or λ as opposed to essentially negative staining with the alternate light chain). The pattern may be difficult to interpret if extensive desmosplasia is present or if the cytologic pattern is mixed. We have found immunoperoxidase-stained cytocentrifuged preparations to be especially helpful in these settings, especially with respect to establishing an immunoglobulin phenotype.

The International Working Formulation for NHL is divided into four categories based upon biologic potential (35). Low grade, intermediate grade, and high grade designations imply less aggressive, intermediately aggressive, or highly aggressive clinical behavior, respectively. General immunophenotypes for NHL classified by the International Formulation have recently been described (10).

The low grade lymphomas consist of small lymphocytic lymphoma (SLL) (many of which represent the tissue phase of chronic lymphocytic leukemia), plasmacytoid lymphocytic lymphomas as a variant of SLL, and most of the follicular lymphomas (follicular small cleaved, follicular mixed). SLL is usually composed of B cells bearing both B2 and B1 monoclonal IgM SIg (and CIg in our experience using acetone-fixed cytocentrifuge preparations) and antigenically corresponds best to the immature B cell stage. Cases of SLL associated with chronic lymphocytic leukemia are usually also Leu1+ (38). Plasmacytoid lymphocytic lymphoma and extranodal small lymphocytic lymphoma not associated with CLL are usually Leu1- (38). Plasmacytoid lymphocytic lymphoma is also usually associated with monoclonal SIg (and CIg), most commonly IgM .

Follicular lymphoma, predominantly small cleaved cell type, displays B cell immunophenotypes. The most common phenotype expressed is that of the virginal B cell, i.e., monoclonal SIg/CIg, Leu10+ B1+ B2+ T11- Leu1- and weak staining with J5/Calla (26). Variable numbers of T cells and NK cells infiltrate the neoplastic follicles, and T cells predominante in interfollicular zones (32,33). The significant increase of T8+ immunoregulatory lymphocytes in neoplastic follicles suggests a potential role for biologic response modifiers as therapeutic agents in follicular lymphomas. Follicular lymphoma, mixed small cleaved and large cell, is always of B cell origin in our experience. Some are Ig-, but retain expression of B cell markers such as B1 and Leu14.

There are four intermediate grade lymphomas in the International Formulation. Follicular lymphoma, predominantly large cell type, is usually monoclonal Ig+ Leu14+ B1+ B2-. Malignant lymphoma, diffuse small cleaved cell type, and diffuse, mixed small cleaved and large cell type include both T cell and B cell phenotypes (10). Diffuse large cleaved and non-cleaved cell lymphomas differ somewhat from other lymphomas above with respect to phenotype in two ways: 1) only occasional T cell cases occur among these cases of predominantely B cell (follicular center cell) origin, and 2) Ig- T11- ("null") phenotypes are more common. The latter are Ig- B cell lymphomas for the most part, characterized by expression of Leu14 and B1 (10).

High grade lymphomas, namely large cell immunoblastic

(IBL), lymphoblastic, and small non-cleaved cell (SNC) types, show different phenotypes (10). Furthermore, morphologic subtypes of immunoblastic lymphoma (plasmacytoid, clear cell, and polymorphous), are often also of distinct immunophenotype (10). A relatively higher percentage of immunoblastic lymphomas (as compared to other large cell NHL) display T cell phenotypes (44% T, 56% B for the entire group of large cell, immunoblastic tumors) (10). Ig+ B cell phenotypes are much more common than Ig- B1+ Leu14+ cases. Plasmacytoid subtypes of IBL are, in our experience, always immunoglobulin positive and usually bear κ light chains. Clear cell types are usually of T cell origin, but B cell variants have also been observed. T cell phenotypes are more frequently observed with polymorphous immunoblastic lymphoma.

Lymphoblastic lymphoma is most often a T cell process (10). However, there are some cases described that have shown pre-B or other phenotypes (39-41). All intrathymic stages of T cell development can be observed, and some described phenotypes do not easily fit into T cell maturation niches (10).

The third high grade lymphoma in the International Formulation is small non-cleaved cell lymphoma. T cell variants are not identified. Readily detectable monoclonal surface and cytoplasmic immunoglobulin, usually of IgM class, is present. Non-Ig lymphocyte differentiation antigens, such as Leu14, Leu10, B1, and B2 are variably expressed. It is possible that variants of small non-cleaved cell lymphoma that would be previously classified as undifferentiated non-Burkitt's type may not reflect the same precise B cell developmental niche as typical Burkitt's cases. This issue has yet to be clarified.

Miscellaneous types of lymphoma in the International Formulation include composite lymphoma, mycosis fungoides (cutaneous T cell lymphoma, cerebriform cell lymphoma), true histiocytic lymphoma (malignant histiocytosis) and extramedullary plasmacytosis, as well as unclassifiable cases. Immunohistology may be helpful in identifying those cases which are currently acceptable as composite lymphomas, such as coexistent T and B cell tumors, or Hodgkin's disease associated with non-Hodgkin's lymphoma. Mycosis fungoides, in its cutaneous presentation (1), is most commonly of the helper/inducer subset phenotype (T11+ Leu1+ T4+ T8-), and curiously fail to express Leu9/3A1, which is a monoclonal antibody broadly expressed on lymphoblastic lymphoma/ leukemia, and reactive lymphocytosis (31). Whether the presence of a T4+ Leu9/3A1- cutaneous infiltrate is diagnostic of mycosis fungoides, as opposed to reactive hyperplasia, is a hypothesis that has yet to be tested.

IMMUNOHISTOLOGY OF HODGKIN'S DISEASE

The immunohistologic findings in Hodgkin's disase can sometimes be helpful in the differential diagnosis of high-grade polymorphous immunoblastic sarcoma vs Hodgkin's disease, and in confirming morphologic subtypes of Hodgkin's disease (11). The Reed-Sternberg cell and mononuclear variants do not express T cell markers, and selective immunostaining of the neoplastic population may be helpful in confirming polymorphous T cell IBS immunoblastic lymphoma (11,42,43). The small lymphocyte population in Hodgkin's disease is most commonly T11+ T4+, with only a few T8+ cells noted in a typical case (42,43). Reed-Sternberg cells and mononuclear variants are typically Leu-M1 and LN2+ with variable surface expression of Ia antigens (Figure 3) (11,44).

FUTURE PROSPECTS

Much work still needs to be done in the immunohistologic evaluation of lymphoproliferative disorders. Immunologic markers providing independent prognostic clinically relevant information are at best infrequent. Secondly, for the majority of follicle center cell lymphomas, there are very few parameters to selectively identify corresponding individual lymphomas of follicle center cell origin. Thirdly, there is a paucity of antibodies reactive with antigens preserved in fixed, paraffin-embedded tissue sections. The development of such reagents would greatly enhance the optical resolution of tissue sections when interpreting immunophenotyping preprations. Also, some promising results have been reported for anti-idiotypic monoclonal antibodies as therapeutic reagents (22), and clearly immunohistology can play a role in preliminary evaluation of such management decisions.

SUMMARY

Immunohistologic methods have been developed to detect cell-associated antigens in tissue sections. Currently, optimum use of the reagents requires frozen tissue sections, preferably interpreted in conjunction with immunoperoxidase-stained cytocentrifuge preparations and flow cytometry analysis of a derived cell suspension. At this time, immunologic markers which provide independent prognostic clinically relevant information are infrequent. The current role of immunophenotyping is the identification of T or B cell maturation stages for a given lymphoproliferative disorder, which in many but not all instances helps to corroborate a histopathologic interpretation. Future efforts should be directed at the development of more monoclonal antibodies detecting antigens preserved in paraffin sections to facilitate optical resolution, development of monoclonal antibodies which are stage-specific for individual follicle center cell lymphomas, and the development and expansion of anti-idiotypic antibodies and other potential therapeutic applications as part of management strategies for non-Hodgkin's lymphomas.

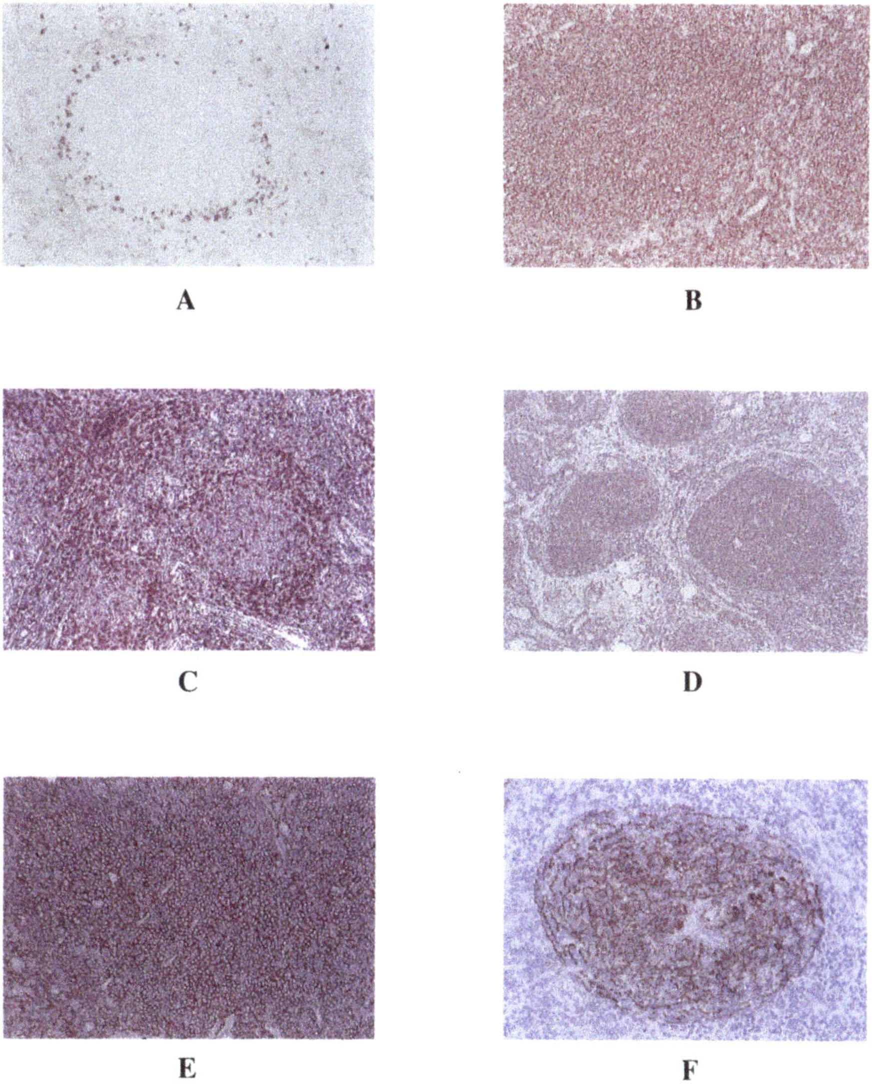

Figure 1. Photomicrographs, follicular lymphoma, predominantly small cleaved cell. A) Neoplastic follicles do not express cell-associated κ light chains. B) Lymphomatous follicles show individual cell-associated immunostaining for λ light chains. C-F) Most of the T11+ cells lie in the interfollicular zone, but the lymphomatous follicles also express LN2 (D), Leu-10 (E), and show B7+ follicular dendritic immunostaining (F). Immunoglobulin light chains were detected with the direct immunoperoxidase technique. Leu1, Leu-10, B7 and LN2 were detected with the avidin-biotinylated peroxidase complex technique followed by hematoxylin counterstain of acetone-fixed frozen sections (A-C, E-F) and paraffin sections of Bouin's-fixed tissue (D).

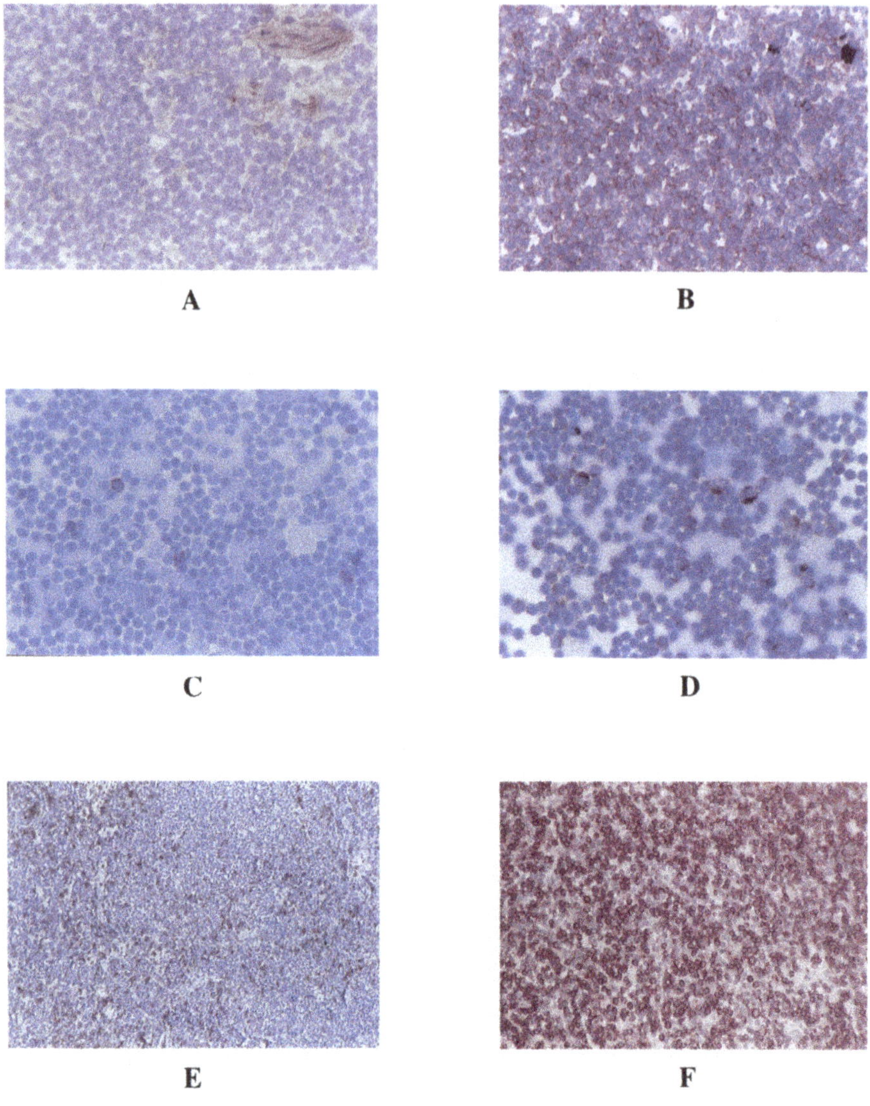

Figure 2. Photomicrographs, small lymphocytic lymphoma with Russell bodies. A) (Direct Technique) The collagen associated vessel walls is positive, but the individual cells are negative for κ light chains. B) (Direct Technique) Diffuse individual with cellular immunostaining for λ light chains, and CIg in Russell bodies, is identified. C) (Direct Technique) Cells in the cytocentrifuge preparations do not contain cytoplasmic κ light chains. D) (Direct Technique) Monoclonal λ cytoplasmic light chains are present in the majority of the cells in the derived cell suspension (acetone fixed cytocentrifuged cells). E) (Avidin-biotinylated Complex Method) Leu1 + cells are infrequent. F) (Avidin-biotinylated Complex Method) The neoplasm also demonstrates expression of LN2 in paraffin sections of Bouin-fixed material.

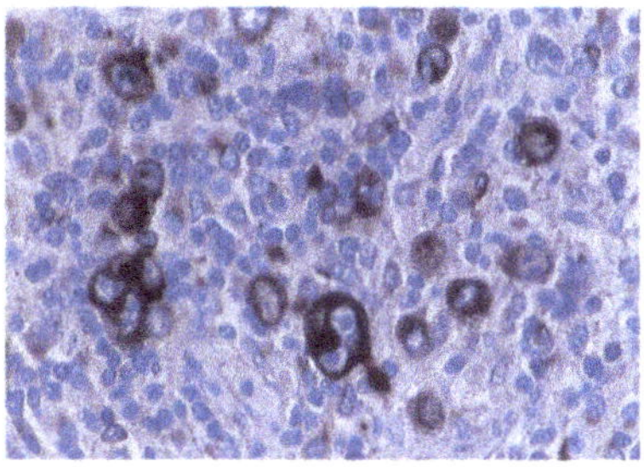

A

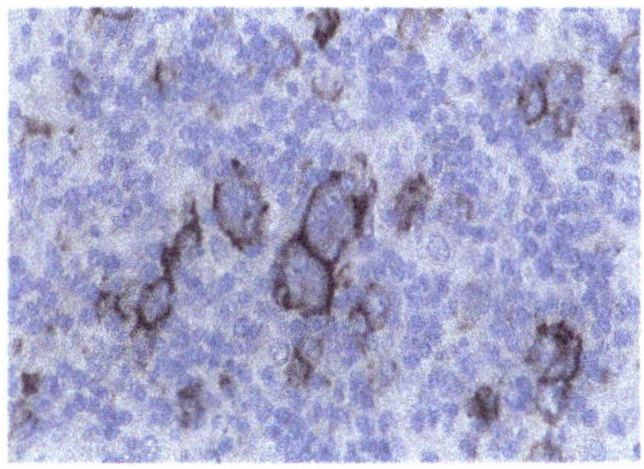

B

Figure 3. Photomicrographs, nodular sclerosing Hodgkin's disease. A) An LN2+ Reed-Sternberg cell is present. B) LN3 labels the surface of Reed-Sternberg cells and mononuclear variants. Avidin-biotinylated peroxidase complex technique and hematoxylin counterstain were applied to paraffin sections of Bouin's (A) and B5-fixed (B) tissue.

REFERENCES

1. Aisenberg AC: Current concepts in immunology: Cell-surface markers in lymphoproliferative disease. N Eng J Med (301):512-518, 1979.
2. Taylor CR: An immunohistological study of follicular lymphoma, reticulum cell sarcoma and Hodgkin's disease. Eur J Cancer (12):61-75, 1976.
3. Warnke R, Pederson M, Williams C, Levy R: A study of lymphoproliferative diseases comparing immunofluorescence with immunohistochemistry. Am J Clin Pathol (70): 867-875, 1978.
4. Warnke R: Alteration of immunoglobulin-bearing lymphoma cells by fixation. J Histochem Cytochem (17):1195-1196, 1979.
5. Tubbs RR, Sheibani K, Sebek BA, Weiss RA: Immunohistochemistry versus immunofluorescence for non-Hodgkin's lymphomas. Am J Clin Pathol (73):144-145, 1980.
6. Stein H, Bonk A, Tolksdorf G, Lennert K, Rodt H, Gerdes J: Immunohistologic analysis of the organization of normal lymphoid tissue and non-Hodgkin's lymphomas. J Histochem Cytochem (28):746-760, 1980.
7. Warnke R, Levy R: Detection of T and B cell antigens with hybridoma monoclonal antibodies: A biotin-avidin-horseradish peroxidase method. J Histochem Cytochem (28):771-776, 1980.
8. Tubbs RR, Sheibani K, Weiss RA, Sebek BA, Deodhar SD: Tissue immunomicroscopic evaluation of monoclonality of B-cell lymphomas: Comparison with cell suspension studies. Am J Clin Pathol (76):24-28, 1981.
9. Epstein AL, Marder RJ, Winter JN, Fox RI. Two new monoclonal antibodies (LN-1, LN-2) reactive in B5 fixed, paraffin embedded tissues with follicular center and mantle zone human B lymphocytes and derived tumors. J Immunol, in press.
10. Tubbs RR, Fishleder A, Weiss RA, Savage RA, Sebek BA, Weick JK: Immunohistologic cellular phenotypes of lymphoproliferative disorders. Comprehensive evaluation of 564 cases including 257 non-Hodgkin's lymphomas classified by the International Working Formulation. Am J Pathol (113):207-221, 1983.
11. Tubbs RR, Sheibani K: Immunohistology of lymphoproliferative disorders. In Santa Cruz D, Battifora H (eds) Seminars in Diagnostic Pathology. In Press, Nov 1984.
12. Fishleder A, Tubbs RR, Valenzuela J, Norris D: Immunophenotypic characterization of acute leuekemia by immunocytology. Amer J Clin Pathol (81):611-617, 1984.
13. Cossman J, Neckers LM, Hsu SM, Longo D, Jaffe ES: Low-grade lymphomas. Expression of developmentally regulated B-cell antigens. Am J Pathol (115):117-124, 1984.
14. Aisenberg AC, Wilkes BM, Harris NL: Monoclonal antibody studies in non-Hodgkin's lymphomas. Blood (61):469-495, 1983.
15. Burns BF, Warnke RA, Doggett RS, Rouse RB: Expression of T-cell antigen (Leu-1) by B cell lymphomas. Am J Pathol (113):165-171, 1983.

16. Knowles DM, Halper J, Azzo W, Wang CY: Reactivity of monoclonal antibody Leul and OKT1 with malignant human lymphoid cells. Cancer (52):1369-1377, 1983.
17. Landay A, Gartland L, Clement AT: Characterization of a phenotypically distinct subpopulation of Leu-2+ cells which suppresses T cell proliferative responses. J Immunol. In press.
18. Phillips JJ, Babcock GF: NKP-15: A monoclonal antibody reactive against purified human natural killer cells and granulocytes. Immunol Lett (6):143, 1983.
19. Lanier LL, Lee AM, Phillips JH, Warner NL, Babcock GF: Subpopulations of human natural killer cells defined by expression of the Leu-7 (HNK-1) and Leu11 (NK-15) antigens. J Immunol (131):1789-1796, 1983.
20. Gold EJ, Mertelsman RH, Filippa DA, Szatrowski TH, Koziner B, Clarkson B: Prognostic significance of receptors for the third component of complement and heavy chain phenotype in diffuse B cell lymphoma. Blood (62):107-111, 1983.
21. Horning SJ, Doggett RS, Warnke RA, Dorfman RF, Cox RS, Levy R: Clinical relevance of immunologic phenotype in diffuse large cell lymphoma. Blood (63):1209-1215, 1984.
22. Miller RA, Maloney BG, Warnke R, Levy R: Treatment of B-cell lymphoma with monoclonal anti-idiotypic antibody. New Engl J Med (306):517-522, 1982.
23. Foon KA, Schroff RW, Gale RP: Surface markers on leukemia and lymphoma cells: Recent advances. Blood (60):1-19, 1982.
24. Nadler LM, Anderson KC, Bates M, Park E, Slaughenhoupt B, Schlossman SF: Human B cell-associated antigens: expression on normal and malignant B lymphocytes. In Bernard A, Boumsell L, Dausset J, Milstein C, Schlossman SF (eds) Leukocyte typing. Springer-Verlag, New York, pp 354-363, 1984.
25. Zola H, Bradley JG, Brooks DA, Macardle PJ, McNamara PJ, Moore HA, Nikoloutsopoulos A: The human B cell lineage studied with monoclonal antibodies. In Bernard A, Boumsell L, Dausset J, Milstein C, Schlossman SF (eds) Leukocyte typing. Springer-Verlag, New York, pp 363-371, 1984.
26. Anderson KC, Bates MP, Slaugherhoupt BL, Pinkus GS, Schlossman SF, Nadler LM: Expression of human B cell-associated antigens on leukemias and lymphomas: A model of human B cell differentiation. Blood (63):1424-1433, 1984.
27. Aisenberg AC, Wilkes BM, Long JC, Harris NL: Cell surface phenotype in lymphoproliferative disease. Am J Med (68):206-213, 1980.
28. Hsu S-M, Jaffe ES: Phenotypic expression of B-lymphocytes. 1. Identification with monoclonal antibodies in normal lymphoid tissues. Am J Pathol (114):387-395, 1984.
29. Hsu S-M, Jaffe ES: Phenotypic expression of B-lymphocytes. 2. Immunoglobulin expression of germinal center cells. Am J Pathol (114):396-402, 1984.

30. Reinherz EL, Kung PC, Goldstein G, Levey RH, and Schlossman SF: Discrete stages of human intrathymic differentiation: Analysis of normal thymocytes and leukemic lymphoblasts of T cell lineage. Proc Natl Acad Sci (77):1588-1592, 1980.
31. Haynes BF, Metzgar RS, Minna JD, Bunn PA: Phenotypic characterization of cutaneous T-cell lymphoma. Use of monoclonal antibodies to compare with other malignant T cells. New Engl J Med (304):1319-1323, 1981.
32. Dvoretsky P, Wood GS, Levy R, Warnke RA: T-lymphocyte subsets in follicular lymphomas compared with those in non-neoplastic lymph nodes and tonsils. Hum Pathol (13):618-625, 1982.
33. Miller ML, Tubbs RR, Fishleder A, Savage RA, Sebek BA, Weick JK: Immunoregulatory Leu-7+ and T8+ lymphocytes in B cell follicular lymphomas. Human Pathol (15):810-817, 1984.
34. Mangkornkannok-Mark M, Mark AS, Dong J: Immunoperoxidase evaluation of lymph nodes from acquired immune deficiency patients. Clin Exp Immunol (55):581-586, 1984.
35. Poppema S, Bhan AK, Reinherz EL, McCluskey RT, Schlossman SF: Distribution of T cell subsets in human lymph nodes. J Exp Med (153):30-40, 1981.
36. Tubbs RR, Savage RA, Sebek BA, Fishleder A, Weick JK: Antigenic phenotype of splenic hairy cells. Am J Med (76):199-205, 1984.
37. Rosenberg SA, Berard CW, Brown BW, Burke J, et al: Non-Hodgkin's Lymphoma Pathologic Classification Project, National Cancer Institute sponsored study of classification of non-Hodgkin's lymphomas: Summary and description of a working formulation for clinical usage. Cancer (49):2112-2135, 1982.
38. Harris NL, Bhan AK: Relationship between chronic lymphocytic leukemia, lymphocytic lymphoma, plasmacytoid lymphoma, and plasmacytoma: Immunohistologic characterization with monoclonal antibodies. Lab Invest 25A, 1984.
39. Cossman J, Chused TM, Fisher RI, Magrath I, Bollum F, Jaffe ES: Diversity of immunological phenotypes of lymphoblastic lymphoma. Cancer Research (43):4486-4490, 1983.
40. Link MP, Roper M, Dorfman RF, Crist WM, Cooper MD, Levy R: Cutaneous lymphoblastic lymphoma with pre-B markers. Blood (61):838-841, 1983.
41. Borowitz MJ, Croker BP, Metzgar RS: Lymphoblastic lymphoma with the phenotype of common acute lymphoblastic leukemia. Am J Clin Pathol (79):387-391, 1983.
42. Poppema S, Bhan AK, Reinherz EL, Posner MR, Schlossman SF: In situ immunologic characterization of cellular constituents in lymph nodes and spleens involved by Hodgkin's disease. Blood (59):226-232, 1982.
43. Martin JME, Warnke RA: A quantitative comparison of T-cell subsets in Hodgkin's disease and reactive hyperplasia. Frozen section immunohistochemistry. Cancer (53):2450-2455, 1984.
44. Hsu SM, Jaffe ES: Leu M1 and peanut agglutinin stain the neoplastic cells of Hodgkin's disease. Am J Clin Pathol (82):29-32, 1984.

9

THE USE OF IMMUNOCYTOCHEMICAL TECHNIQUES IN THE DIAGNOSIS OF LYMPHORETICULAR PROLIFERATIONS

ALVARO A. GIRALDO, M.D. and JEANNE M. MEIS, M.D.

1. INTRODUCTION

The numerous advances in immunology during the last decade have given origin to a variety of new immunological techniques that have become available in clinical laboratory practice. The "lymphoreticular" proliferations are perhaps the most extensive area in human immunology that have been studied recently by all these new techniques.[1,2,3] At the authors' hospital, considerable experience has been gained during the last six years, in which 405 cases have been thoroughly studied by a diversity of immunological techniques. These cases included studies done on cell suspensions of solid tissues (lymph nodes, gastric lymphomas, etc.), as well as studies on markers on lymphoid cells of various body fluids (pleural effusion, CSF, etc.) and peripheral blood. These studies have facilitated diagnosis in many cases. They have also helped to confirm or rule out certain histologic impressions. This review will relate the authors' experiences regarding immunocytochemical techniques in the diagnosis of lymphoreticular proliferations. However, we will not review the details of every technique used. A reference to a well established technique will always be given. If a modification of any technique is used in the authors' lab, mention will be made with the proper notations. Points of critical importance and interpretation of studies will be emphasized throughout this review. We hope this will be a comprehensive review, useful to those ready to embark upon the development of these studies in their own laboratories. We also hope it will be useful to those with less specimen volume who are looking for answers to frustrating failed techniques and to those interested in interpretation of more unusual problems.

2. SPECIMEN COLLECTION AND PREPARATION

Perhaps the most important starting point for an adequate immunological evaluation of a specimen is the proper collection of the material. The reliability of a diagnosis based on immunological evaluation of tissue or a cell suspension depends on percent cellular viability and on antigen preservation of the tissue. It is frustrating to have a surgical specimen mishandled, resulting in a cellular viability of only 30% to 40% and rendering the specimen useless for immunological evaluation. Carefully made instructions for the clinician, surgeon, paramedical and laboratory personnel should be made in order to maximize the use of the tissue obtained. These instructions should be very explicit with practically no room left for last minute improvisations. Modifications may occasionally be made by an expert, preferably the immunopathologist, in unusual cases. Different types of specimens requiring immunological work-up should be handled differently, depending on the techniques to be used in the evaluation of each case. One should also be prepared to perform additional immunological studies in the event that unexpected results arise during the work-up of a case. Hence, it is important to allocate the specimen in such a manner, so that frozen tissue, cell suspensions, cytospins, etc. are available for further studies if necessary. Sometimes the tissue sample is very small, allowing only a limited number of studies. In these cases, one has to select the most important immunological tests based on other clinical and laboratory information, and proceed to prepare the specimen accordingly. Let's analyze the different types of specimens and their proper handling.

2.1 Peripheral Blood and Bone Marrow

After the introduction of cellular immunological techniques, such as E rosettes, the peripheral blood lymphocytes were the most commonly studied and the most frequent type of specimen handled in the immunology laboratory. However, the contribution of B and T lymphocyte enumeration in the patient care was minimal. We are still looking for clinical applications of these studies. They are occasionally used in cases of suspected congenital or acquired immunodeficiency syndromes. The lymphocytic leukemias, however, are an exception. Acute lymphoblastic leukemia (ALL) and T cell chronic lymphocytic leukemia (CLL) require immunological evaluation for optimal treatment.

The peripheral blood and bone marrow are collected under sterile conditions in a preservative free of heparin, since stimulation studies may be desirable in certain immunodeficiency syndromes. The amount of peripheral blood to be collected should be calculated, based on the patient's lymphocyte count and on the projected studies for the case, i.e., B & T surface markers, cytoplasmic markers, stimulation studies. According to conventional techniques,[4] gradient centrifugation with Ficoll-Hypaque is performed, isolating the mononuclear cells. Once the interphase is collected, a cytospin is prepared and stained with Wright Giemsa. This specimen is compared to the mononuclear cells in the peripheral blood smear to assure that the interphase cells are representative. It is important to note that in cases of leukemia, the abnormal cells do not necessarily accumulate at the interphase with the normal lymphocytes. Occasionally, we have had to recover the abnormal cell population in the bottom or in the supernatant of the gradient.

The percent viability of a cell suspension collected properly is usually in the high 90's. A viability of less than 80% is an indication for a new specimen collection. This is usually due to trauma to the tube of blood, defective solutions for cell washings (acid pH or contaminated RPMI, etc.), delay in specimen processing, excessive heat, contamination of the specimen, and other miscellaneous events.

2.2. Effusions

Pleural fluids are also collected in a manner similar to peripheral blood to prevent clotting of the specimen. Occasionally, gradient centrifugation is not needed, and only regular spinning of the fluid is required to isolate a cell bottom. This is usually more representative of the cellular composition of malignant effusions, especially in certain types of lymphoma. However, if the fluid is bloody, gradient centrifugation with Ficoll-Hypaque is required as with peripheral blood. The same precautions are observed in discarding the supernatant and button only after the evaluation of the cytospin isolate by the pathologist. One can also concentrate the initial sample by regular centrifugation and then proceed to perform a gradient centrifugation on the concentrated specimen diluted in RPMI or HBSS.

2.3. CSF.

One rarely has to collect this fluid in heparin. Leukemic and lymphomatous infiltration of CNS produces a cellular fluid which is usually not hemorrhagic. The cellular composition of this fluid is usually homogeneous. It is best evaluated by centrifugation and isolation of the cell button. We have found that the studies of the cellular composition of this fluid without any gradient centrifugation are more rewarding.

2.4. Solid Tissues

A great deal of solid tissue has been studied in our laboratory. Cooperation between the surgeon and the immunopathology laboratory is crucial in this area. This ensures tissue viability, promptness of processing for cell suspension studies and freezing. Since most of our tissues are from lymph nodes, we will concentrate mostly on comments about this technique. However, these principles also apply to most solid tissues, with minor variations. These will be noted when essential.

The lymph nodes are always collected promptly from the operating room in a fresh state and with an intact capsule. They are brought to the laboratory wrapped in saline gauze. The lymph node is stripped of fat, and with the capsule intact, it is flooded with RPMI fluid. The lymph node is loafed at 2 mm. intervals. The pathologist examines the lymph node carefully for gross areas of involvement. The grossly involved areas of the lymph node should be sampled and submitted for cell suspension studies. A fragment of the lymph node, usually an entire slice of it, is taken for immunological studies. One-half of this slice is placed in aluminum foil, covered with OCT compound, wrapped, labeled and snap frozen by dipping it in liquid nitrogen for 20-30 seconds. We do not use isopentane since we have found it does not offer any advantage over our procedure and is also more cumbersome and time consuming. The tissue is properly stored in a Revco freezer at -70°C. Frozen tissue is used for immunoperoxidase stains for T cell antigens and other antigens, because they are well preserved after deep freezing. Just before the tissue is ready to be sectioned, it is taken from the freezer to the cryostat, which is maintained at -22°C, and allowed to equilibrate a period of ½ hour to 2 hours. Sections 4-7 microns thick are made on glue-covered slides (Sobo glue to water 1:10) and immediately fixed in acetone (reagent grade) by one quick dip and allowed to dry overnight. The sections can be wrapped individually in aluminum foil and stored in the refrigerator for up to 2 weeks (perhaps longer) for future studies. The majority of the tissue sections, however, are stained the day following sectioning. Just before the immunoperoxidase staining is begun, the sections are fixed in acetone for 10 minutes.

The other half of the slice of the lymph node is again covered in RPMI solution and sliced into 2 cubic mm. fragments. The entire fluid with the fragments of lymph nodes is collected. The cell suspension is made by teasing the tissue into fine fragments and gently squeezing these fragments through a stainless steel mesh. The cells are washed in the conventional way. A viability of at least 80% is required in order to complete the entire immunological work-up of this material. We do not use Ficoll-Hypaque gradient separation in this case, since the cell suspension is usually entirely representative of the lesional tissue. If a considerable amount of blood is present, ammonium chloride treatment is used to lyse the red blood cells. Cytocentrifuge preparation of the suspensions are also made and stained with Giemsa in order to evaluate cell morphology and to determine the type of markers to be performed. Representative portions of the lymph node are also placed in buffered formalin and B5 fixative. Sections from the latter are usually prepared for immunoperoxidase stains since antigen preservation is usually better than in formalin fixed tissue. Touch imprints are also prepared from a fragment of lesional tissue, air dried and fixed in acetone for 10 minutes. These imprints may be very valuable in the performance of additional markers if needed.

We usually realize the need for immunological studies of non-nodal tissues at the time of frozen section. Therefore, the immunological laboratory should constantly be prepared to perform these studies on short notice. We have found that the workload of a day can be shifted to accommodate these "emergency" studies. However, there is always a rare case that comes in the very late afternoon or night. In these cases, one can prepare the cell suspension and store it in the refrigerator overnight and sometimes even over the weekend if it is placed in McCoy medium. We try to schedule cases within our daily workload when we are advised by the surgeon, the clinician or other pathologist of an upcoming "lymphoreticular" case.

We have studied a great variety of lymphoid lesions from several organs such as salivary gland, lung, gastrointestinal tract, soft tissue, etc. The protocol that we follow for collection of the specimen is the same one that we have for lymph nodes. In a few cases, the lymphoid elements are within a fibrous stroma and very difficult to isolate. Only in this case do we use enzyme digestion with collagenase. No interference with the evaluation of conventional markers has been found. We always keep in mind the possibility of stripping off or modification of antigens by this enzyme, although we have not found a case in which we suspect this has happened.

3. IMMUNOLOGICAL TECHNIQUES

Once the sample has been collected, the choice of which immunological techniques to use has to be made. This choice depends upon the amount of tissue available, the type of lesion that is most likely to be present or ruled out, and the urgency of the diagnosis. Under the best circumstances, a "full" work-up of the specimen would include all of the modalities to be discussed.

3.1. Immunofluorescence

This technique[4] can be applied to tissues, cytospins, and cell suspensions. In general, if one is searching for surface markers, the cell suspension technique must be used. To evaluate cytoplasmic markers (i.e., cytoplasmic immunoglobulin in multiple myeloma or TdT in ALL), cell suspensions and frozen tissue sections are used. The simultaneous search for surface and cytoplasmic markers, most commonly immunoglobulin, requires the initial use of cell suspensions for surface analysis, followed by cytoplasmic stain of the same specimen. This is performed on the cytospin of the surface-labeled specimen. It is important to properly label the tubes and slides so that each pair of them is stained for the same antigen or immunoglobulin chain. The purpose of initially staining surface immunoglobulins for a specific chain is to entirely block this surface antigen. Then the cytoplasm is stained for the same specific chain. Different fluorochromes must be used for surface and cytoplasmic immunoglobulin detection. Double staining is the only desirable method to evaluate combined surface and cytoplasmic immunoglobulin.

Two different fluorochromes are mainly used. They are fluorescein and rhodamine. The fluorescent microscope should have the capability of reading these two fluorochromes as well as allowing transillumination. Among the different systems commercially available, we use the Zeiss epifluorescence microscope with a double set of filters. One is for fluorescein and the other is for rhodamine. We also have a special attachment slide projector within the fluorescent field that allows us to compare intensity of fluorescence to a projected control kodachrome slide of known fluorescent intensity. This special attachment is necessary to eliminate subjective assessment of the intensity of fluorescence, especially in cases where intensity of fluorescence is an important parameter. The reagents should be calibrated with the control kodachromes, since the intensity of fluorescence may decrease significantly with storage or handling. We have not encountered this problem in our laboratory due to the high volume of tests performed. Quality control and titrations of these reagents should always be performed. These are the same as for any conventional immunofluorescent assay.

It is important to point out that rhodamine is much less impressionable to the human eye than fluorescein. Therefore, if the possibility exists that the intensity of your assay will be very low, fluorescein should be used and the reading should be done after the observer's eyes have become accustomed to darkness. These points are best illustrated in cases of well differentiated (also called small lymphocytic) lymphocytic lymphoma with plasmacytoid differentiation. In these cases, the amount of surface immunoglobulin is very scant[5], resulting in very pale fluorescence which can be easily missed by the observer or even be discarded as "faint background" or "just the shadow of the cells". Fluorescence may not be detected with rhodamine in these cases. Even though fluorescence with fluorescein may be pale, a monoclonal proliferation of cells can be recognized by the exclusive presence of either kappa or lambda chains on the cell surface. If one stains simultaneously for cytoplasmic immunoglobulin, rhodamine is the fluorochrome to be used. The intensity of cytoplasmic fluorescence with rhodamine is greater because immunoglobulin in the cytoplasm is more abundant than on the surface and therefore easier to read. However, if one is dealing with a case of acute lymphoblastic leukemia and wants to rule out a pre-B cell type, the detection of mu chains in the cytoplasm is best achieved by the use of fluorescein labeled anti-IgM on cytospin preparations, since the amount of immunoglobulin present in this type of leukemia is rather scant and finely granular.

Fluorescent surface marker analysis for B cells includes a panel of individual light and heavy chains except E. When the number of cells available is rather low, we restrict our studies to search for kappa and lambda in order to demonstrate or rule out the presence of a monoclonal proliferation of B cells. It has also become routine to search for surface B-1 antigen in our laboratory, since we have found large cell lymphomas with no detectable surface or cytoplasmic immunoglobulin, but only B-1 antigen. The reagents used for the detection of surface immunoglobulins are polyclonal antibodies, preferably fluorescent labeled Fab_2 fragments. This avoids any nonspecific attachment of labeled antibody via the Fc receptor. To detect B-1 antigen, specific monoclonal antibody of mouse origin and indirect fluorescent staining are used to visualize the reaction. Once the cell preparations are stained, wet mounts are made and read immediately. If there is any short delay in the reading, the slides should be kept in the refrigerator and protected from light until reading is performed. If delayed reading is anticipated, the cell suspensions are treated with formalin prior to making the slide. This type of preparation can be preserved for up to 2-3 weeks if kept in a humid chamber and protected from light in the refrigerator. This type of preparation is advantageous, since it allows us to go back and review or rectify the cell counts or seek additional information that may have been missed or overlooked initially.

We recommend that a cytospin of the cell suspension be made, stained with Giemsa and studied prior to counting to identify the possible neoplastic cell population. The reading of each fluorescent stained slide is done manually, counting 200 cells or more, if needed. These slides are also reviewed by the immunopathologist who assesses qualitative characteristics of the abnormal cell population, such as cell size, intensity and pattern of fluorescence (such as capping). All of this information is recorded on a special form and interpreted by the immunopathologist.

At this point, we should also mention the use of the fluorescent activated cell sorter (FACS). We have no experience in the use of automatic instrumentation for human diagnostic purposes, although we have some experience with its use in experimental lymphomas with the mouse SJL model.[6] We have not purchased a FACS due to the high cost of the machine and the need for highly trained personnel dedicated almost exclusively to the operation of it. In a busy immunology laboratory, diversity of the technical personnel is essential for smooth operation. Even though the accuracy on a count of 10,000 cells is higher than one of 200 cells, this is not crucial in a diagnostic immunopathology laboratory as it is in a research laboratory. The diagnostically significant features of a lymphoid population can be completely appreciated by a good pair of trained eyes looking through a fluorescent microscope and observing multiple features simultaneously in a count of 200 cells per slide. These findings can be integrated and interpreted by an experienced observer rather than computer analysis based on only two or three parameters. I also doubt the practical value of discovering a very small monoclonal proliferation of B cells in the peripheral blood when morphological or numerical findings cannot support the diagnosis in any way.[7] A clinician should always hesitate in starting treatment for a condition that cannot be supported by a morphological diagnosis. The contribution of the FACS, however, cannot be denied in experimental animal and human cellular immunology. It can also be a great asset to the immunopathology laboratory but should not be considered an indispensable instrument in the evaluation of cell suspensions used for diagnostic purposes.

With advanced technology, sophisticated instrumentation will appear and be capable of analyzing combined surface and cytoplasmic fluorescence as well as the presence of capping and simultaneous morphological evaluation. For the time being, the lack of a FACS in the immunopathology laboratory should not discourage the evaluation of cell surface markers by manual methodologies.

So far, we have referred to B cell markers. However, since the introduction and commercialization of monoclonal antibodies, a considerable number of reagents have also become available for the study of T cell surface markers by fluorescent methodologies. These assays have also come to replace the old and more conventional methodologies such as rosetting.

Some of these reagents have also been approved by federal regulatory agencies to be used for diagnostic purposes in the clinical laboratory.

In the evaluation of the T cell populations, we have become mostly accustomed to the OKT series.[8] Other series, mainly the Leu series, have also been evaluated by us and found to be quite satisfactory. I believe that it is best to become familiar with a group of monoclonal antibodies and always try to use the same ones. The interpretation of results in this way becomes much easier and more consistent. We are routinely staining for OKT-11 (pan-T), OKT-3 (peripheral-T), OKT-4 (helper-inducer-T), OKT-8 (suppressor-cytotoxic-T) and OKT-6 (thymocytes). With the use of these markers, one can establish the phenotype of a reactive or neoplastic T cell population. The principles of immunofluorescence, quality control and details of reading are essentially the same as the ones already discussed for B cells.

Other cytoplasmic markers frequently used include common acute lymphoblastic leukemia antigen (CALLA), on the surface of ALL cells as well as in lymphoblastic lymphoma (convoluted and non-convoluted) and cytoplasmic TdT. The MO series is also beginning to be most commonly used in the evaluation of lymphoproliferative disorders in which the monocyte-macrophage is the primary cell involved.

3.2. Immunoperoxidase

This technique is perhaps today the most widely used method for evaluation of lymphoid proliferations in the general pathology laboratory.[9] Ready to use kits have minimized difficulties that many of us encountered several years ago when only "purified" polyclonal antibodies were used and other reagents were made from "scratch". This experience allowed us to understand the pitfalls of this technique and to adequately interpret the results. With the development of monoclonal antibodies, immunoperoxidase staining grew even bigger, creating a bonanza for many laboratories engaged in the massive production of "histologic diagnostic kits". With numerous kits available on the market, it is very difficult to sort out which ones are diagnostically useful in the immunopathology laboratory. We recommend that each particular lab get acquainted very well with a limited number of suppliers, preferably no more than two, and learn to use their reagents in a meaningful, consistent and reproducible manner. In general, the manufacturer's recommendations should be followed and if changes are made, the reason for these changes should be well understood.

As previously mentioned, antigen preservation is essential for successful immunoperoxidase staining. Many of the technical difficulties are due to poor handling and collection of the specimen. Two main types of prepared tissue can be used for immunoperoxidase staining: Frozen section material and paraffin embedded material. To detect T cell antigens, frozen sections are required since these antigens are preserved only in properly frozen tissue. We routinely stain for OKT-3, OKT-4, and OKT-8, using monoclonal antibodies as the primary antibody and peroxidase-labeled goat anti-mouse as the secondary antibody. AEC is used for color development in our laboratory. The histoset kits are also used. If one is dealing with the Leu-series, there is a commercially available avidin-biotin system with peroxidase that uses DAB as a color developer. We have also had success with this method. The frozen tissue sections can also be used to detect cytoplasmic immunoglobulin and in surface immunoglobulin. Either monoclonal antibodies for kappa and lambda chains or purified polyclonal antibodies for the different light and heavy chains can be used. Two other antigens that we have recently become familiar with are the common leukocyte antigen (CLA) and common epithelial membrane antigen (CEMA). These two antigens have helped us to identify undifferentiated carcinomas within lymph nodes and other organs, as well as to confirm the leukocytic origin of a neoplasm. It is preferable to search for these antigens in frozen tissue sections.

Paraffin sections can also be used for immunoperoxidase staining. The tissue should be preferably fixed in B5, Zenker's or Bouin's fixative, and "de-Zenkerized" as usual. Tissues fixed in buffered formalin usually have significant antigen deterioration, rendering them inadequate for proper evaluation, even after enzymatic treatment with trypsin and papain. Deparaffinization of the tissue sections should be complete, otherwise the intensity of the background precludes any interpretation. Incomplete deparaffinization may also interfere with the penetration of antibody. Careful control of the oven temperature is also required, since antigen destruction occurs with overheating of tissue. To block endogenous peroxidase activity, especially in lymphoreticular lesions, we use 2% hydrogen peroxide in alcohol for 10 minutes. This step avoids the heavy background and prominent staining of granulocytes, histiocytes and blood elements. We have not found a loss of antigenic potency in the markers being studied. After immunoperoxidase staining, the slide is counterstained unless the case is going to be photographed for publication. In this case, black and white pictures can adequately demonstrate findings without counterstaining. When counterstain is used, we use Mayer's hematoxylin and mount with glycerol if AEC was used. Harris hematoxylin is acceptable when DAB is used. In this case, regular permount mounting can be used.

The use of immunoperoxidase techniques in tissue sections is preferred in many circumstances, since it allows the detection of the cellular antigens with simultaneous preservation of the architecture of the lymphoreticular lesion. Cellular morphology can also be appreciated facilitating the interpretation of the lesion.

Immunoperoxidase techniques can also be used on cell suspensions to detect cell surface antigens. The primary and secondary antibody reactions, as well as the peroxidase steps, are done in vitro on the cell suspension. Cytospin preparations are then made and the color is usually developed with AEC, followed by counterstaining with Mayer's hematoxylin and mounting with glycerol. This preparation offers the best cytological detail while simultaneously visualizing the cell surface marker. However, the lack of architectural arrangement limits its use and demands observer interpretation.

Many modifications of the immunoperoxidase technique have been used and excellent reviews on the subject are available. The use of different color reagents and double labelling has been advocated. However, the more complicated and complex the staining, the more difficult the interpretation becomes. More controls are required and the results become less reliable. We prefer to use the PAP, avidin-biotin peroxidase and the indirect staining for monoclonal antibody use. A new related technique utilizes glucose oxidase instead of peroxidase. The glucose oxidase has the advantage of not requiring blockage of endogenous activity in tissue sections since this activity is not normally present. Commercially available reagents for this technique are beginning to appear on the market at this time.

3.3. Rosette Techniques.

The use of these techniques have been abandoned in many laboratories since monoclonal antibodies to surface markers have become available. However, two types of rosettes offer a significant deal of information when properly used. E-rosettes allow us to study the morphology of the rosetting T cells on stained cytospins and to keep a permanent record that can be referred to if needed. The stained cytospin of EAC rosettes allows us to study the morphology of B cells. One must keep in mind, however, that other cells with C3 receptors, such as monocytes-macrophages, will also rosette. Evaluation and interpretation is then needed from the immunopathologist.

4. RESULTS

A total of 405 cases have been studied immunologically in the last six years. We will review the indications, findings and interpretation of these studies. The cases will be analyzed according to the source of the specimen studied.

4.1. Normal Values

Prior to the implementation of these techniques in the clinical immunopathology laboratory, the normal values were established. The peripheral blood of approximately 100 patients considered "normal" population was studied. The majority of these patients came from the outpatient laboratory. Mainly patients undergoing annual physical examination were selected. A large portion of this group was also represented by laboratory personnel who volunteered for these studies. The normal lymph node distribution of B and T cells was established mainly from patients undergoing radical surgery for carcinoma of head, neck, breast and colon. Lymph nodes of patients with no gross evidence of metastases and confirmed later by microscopic examination were selected. Although it can be argued that the presence of cancer in these patients may affect the distribution of the different subsets of lymphocytes, no differences were evident when we compared these values to values from lymph nodes of patients biopsied with no history of malignancy. Normal values from other sites, such as pleural effusions were never established since pleural effusions are always pathologic. However, a considerably large number of pleural effusions were studied initially during the development of the immunology lab, not as a diagnostic study, but to become accustomed to techniques used in handling these specimens.

4.2. Studies of Peripheral Blood

The normal established values for the peripheral blood are seen in Table 1. One hundred twenty-three cases from peripheral blood have been studied in the immunology laboratory for B and T cell enumeration and/or stimulation following the protocol in Table 1. The indications for these studies were varied. Table 2. Patients with a diversity of conditions thought to be related to immunological mechanisms such as collagen diseases, were among 19 cases included in a category which we call "immune diseases". The findings were nonspecific and too variable to have any diagnostic or prognostic significance. The most common finding was a mild leucopenia, with a polyclonal increase in the number of B cells and a decrease in the number of T cells. Most of these values could be considered within normal limits. We believe, and have also demonstrated experimentally,[10] that the distribution of lymphocyte subsets in infiltrated organs in autoimmune diseases does not parallel the changes in the peripheral blood.

Table 1. Lymphocyte Surface Markers in Peripheral Blood.

Absolute lymph count : Adult 1.0-4.9X10^3/mm^3

	Monoclonal Antibodies	
E-Rosettes 65-78%	OKT 3 (Pan-T)	- 64-80%
	OKT 11 (E-Rossette Receptor)	- 72-84%
	OKT 4 (Helpers)	- 32-50%
	OKT 8 (Suppressors)	- 22-36%
Surface Immunoglobulin:	Ratio Helpers/Suppressors	- 0.9-2.0
polyvalent 6-10%	OKT 6 Thymocytes	- 0-2%
anti-mu	Other ________	-
anti-delta	OKIal (B-Lymphs, activ. T	-
anti-epsilon	Lymphs, some monos)	- 9-27%
anti-gamma	BA-1 (B-Lymph lineage)	- 4-19%
anti-kappa	CALLA (Common ALL Ag)	2%
anti-lambda	Other ________	-

The next group of patients on whom B and T cell enumeration of peripheral blood lymphocytes was performed was a group of 10 patients with so-called "repeated infections". This group included cases of mucocutaneous candidiasis, recurrent herpes genitalis and tuberculosis. The great majority of these patients had stimulation studies with PWM, Con-A and PHA in time-dose related studies. In this group, the studies were considered within normal limits with normal stimulation indices. An exception was a patient with herpes which demonstrated a low stimulation response that returned to normal values six weeks after resolution of the acute epidose.

Table 2. Indications for Peripheral Blood B and T Cell Studies.

Benign	No. cases	Malignant	No. cases
Autoimmune diseases	19	C.L.L. - B type	26
Repeated infections	10	C.L.L. - T Type	2
Lymphopenia	6	C.L.L. non-B-non-T	2
Congenital immunodeficiency	10	P.D.L. - B type	4
Acquired immunodeficiency	8	Intermediate B type	2
Benign lymphocytosis	12	A.L.L.	10
		Hodgkin's disease	12

Another group of patients was evaluated for the presence of lymphopenia (less than 1000 lymphocytes/cubic ml). Six cases belonged to this group. Five patients were older than 65 years and showed a normal B and T cell distribution.

Four patients with immunodeficiency syndrome were also evaluated. Three of them had common variable immunodeficiency and one had congenital IgA deficiency. All showed normal T and B cell distribution.

A group of five newborns were also studied during the first few days of life to rule out congenital thymic aplasia. All of these patients presented with hypocalcemia and the thymic shadow on chest x-ray was not clearly evident; the peripheral blood of all of these patients had over 50% T cells excluding the diagnosis of Di George syndrome. We have had only one case of incomplete Di George syndrome in which the patient had 30% T cells at the time of birth associated with cardiac abnormalities. By the age of 2 years the T cell count was normal and the cardiovascular abnormalities had been partially corrected surgically. T cell enumeration in newborns suspected of having Di George syndrome is the only stat indication for T cell enumeration in our laboratory. The results are usually available in an hour utilizing the OKT-11 fluorescent assay.

The next group of patients studied were those with suspected acquired immunodeficiency syndrome (AIDS). In these cases, there was an absolute lymphopenia with an inverted H/S ratio. We have had only one classical case of AIDS in which the patient died within 6 months of diagnosis with Pneumocystis carinii pneumonia. Two other patients, both drug users, are being followed currently with a syndrome of pre-AIDS. One of them has progressive generalized lymphadenopathy and exhibits a mildly inverted H/S ratio with a normal lymphocyte count. The other patient is a homosexual male with a H/S ratio of 0.2 (normal 1-2) and a total lymphocyte count of 4200/cubic ml. This patient also has a positive HBSA in serum, a high titer of antibody to CMV (32,000) and a monoclonal gammopathy (IgG) in serum. The latter patient remains clinically asymptomatic. In five other high risk patients, the diagnosis of AIDS has been excluded due to a normal lymphocyte count and a normal H/S ratio.

The next group of patients studied were those in which enumeration and characterization of B and T cells was done because of lymphoproliferative disorder with suspected peripheral blood involvement or overt leukemia. Among this group of patients was an interesting subgroup with a diagnosis of Hodgkin's disease. Inhibitory T cell factor was proposed[11] as a new diagnostic test to aid in making or confirming a diagnosis of Hodgkin's disease. This inhibitory T cell factor masked the E-receptor on T lymphocytes, thereby lowering the number of T cells determined by E-rosettes in the peripheral blood of patients with active Hodgkin's disease. This factor was shed off during overnight incubation with fetal calf serum. If these lymphocytes were then exposed to the serum of another patient with active Hodgkin's disease, the inhibitory T cell factor would again mask the E-receptors of these lymphocytes. The masking of E-receptors by inhibiting T cell factor was believed to be specific for Hodgkin's disease. We decided to test this hypothesis. In the first three patients with active Hodgkin's disease, we demonstrated the presence of an inhibitory T cell factor in the peripheral blood that was responsible for a low T cell count with a large number of "null" cells and that shed off with overnight incubation in FCS. However, we were unable to demonstrate that this factor was specific for patients with active Hodgkin's disease. In one case of a patient with mediastinal lymphadenopathy and questionable pulmonary infiltrates, we found an inhibitory T cell factor, suggesting the possibility of Hodgkin's disease. A biopsy obtained through mediastinoscopy demonstrated Histoplasma capsulatum infection. Today, it is well known that inhibitory T cell factors are also present in the serum of patients with systemic fungal disease. We abandoned the use of this test as an aid in the diagnosis of Hodgkin's disease.

Eight additional patients with no clinical evidence of active Hodgkin's disease after therapy have been evaluated; four of these had mild lymphopenia and a low absolute number of T cells, the other 4 patients had normal values of B and T lymphocytes in the peripheral blood.

Twelve patients with benign lymphocytosis have been evaluated; seven of these had atypical forms that were finally classified as probably "viral" in etiology. Three additional patients had a previous history of lymphoma. One patient with no previous history of lymphoma had circulating cleaved lymphocytes which proved to be of polyclonal origin rather than a manifestation of small cleaved lymphocytic lymphoma (also called poorly differentiated lymphocytic lymphoma or PDL). Another patient was clinically thought to have a T cell chronic lymphocytic leukemia (CLL) but immunological studies did not support the diagnosis. We believe this group of 12 patients benefited from these studies since most of them were old and therefore more likely to have lymphocytic leukemia.

The peripheral blood of patients with possible CLL was characterized for B and T cell markers for three reasons. The first one was to establish a diagnosis without performing a marrow biopsy. The second reason was to detect the presence of a T cell CLL in clinically suspicious cases, i.e. where the course was aggressive, the patient was young and there was a family history of CLL. The third reason was to exclude the possibility of a leukemic phase of a poorly differentiated lymphocytic lymphoma (PDL) also termed lymphosarcoma cell leukemia. The differentiation of this leukemia from CLL is made easily with immunofluorescence[5], B cell CLL characteristically has a very low amount of monoclonal surface immunoglobulin with a very dim pattern of fluorescence, in contrast to PDL which has a very abundant and therefore bright pattern of fluorescent monoclonal surface immunoglobulin as well as a prominent degree of capping.

A total of 26 patients with B cell CLL have been studied. Nine of these patients expressed double heavy chains, characterized as IgMD

Kappa. This group of patients are being followed carefully to determine if there is any difference in prognosis from the CLL patients in which only one heavy chain has been detected. It is presently thought that the patients with double heavy chains of monoclonal surface immunoglobulin have a more favorable prognosis. Four additional patients were classified as lymphosarcoma cell leukemia. Another two patients had a T cell CLL. One was 28 years old and the other patient 50 years old at the time of diagnosis. Both of them died within five years. In two patients no markers could be demonstrated on the surface of the leukemic lymphocytes. One of them is alive three years after diagnosis. The other one was lost to follow up. Two additional patients had been classified as intermediate CLL of B cell type. Both of these patients had a rather abundant amount of monoclonal surface immunoglobulin with no evidence of capping and absence of complement receptors.

Finally, a group of 10 patients with acute leukemia, mostly children, have been studied by immunological surface markers of peripheral blood cells. The results of these studies have been conclusive, making bone marrow biopsy unnecessary in these patients. Four patients were classified as having acute lymphoblastic leukemia (ALL) non-T-non-B, CALLA positive and TdT negative. Two patients were classified as ALL, had negative immunological markers. Cytochemistry in these cases indicated acute myelogenous leukemia. The immunological characterization of patients with ALL is important for prognosis and treatment.

4.3. Studies of Bone Marrow.

A total of 19 aspirates have been characterized with immunological markers. Table 3. Most of these studies were diagnostic, and none of them repeated the studies performed on peripheral blood. We believe that once a diagnosis is reached by either peripheral blood or bone marrow immunological studies, there is no reason to repeat these studies in the bone marrow or blood, respectively.

In four cases, B and T cell studies were reported as "normal", meaning there was no evidence of a monoclonal proliferation of cells or abnormal markers within the cells populating the marrow. These studies were done on bone marrow aspirates from patients with anemia in which an occult lymphoma was suspected.

Table 3. Bone Marrow B and T Cell Studies.

	No. cases
Normal	4
A.L.L. non-B-non-T	7
A.L.L. T cell type	1
Convoluted T lymphoma	2
Lymphoma B cell	2
Malignancy non-lymphoid	3

The second group of patients had underlying malignancies. Seven patients were classified as acute lymphoblastic leukemia (ALL). In these patients, the peripheral blood did not contain a sufficient number of white blood cells for proper immunological evaluation. Seven patients had ALL which was classified as non-B, non-T, CALLA positive and TdT negative. One patient had T-ALL. There were two cases of convoluted T-cell lymphoma (lymphoblastic lymphoma), CALLA positive. A patient with B cell CLL and another patient with mixed lymphoma (large and small cleaved cell type) of B cell origin were also diagnosed by the presence of monoclonal surface immunoglobulin. Three patients did not exhibit any detectable markers for T or B cells. These were finally diagnosed as an undifferentiated carcinoma in one case and as acute myelogenous leukemia in the remaining two cases.

4.4. Studies in Pleural Effusion and CSF.

Among the eight cases of patients with pleural effusion, there were four with a concurrent mediastinal mass. Table 4. In three of these cases, the pleural fluid contained a neoplastic cell population with T cell markers, allowing us to make a definitive diagnosis and avoiding the need for a mediastinal biopsy. The E-rosette cytospins allowed us to simultaneously visualize the E-rosette around the neoplastic cells and their nuclear morphology. These three cases also exhibited CALLA antigen. The fourth patient with a mediastinal mass had a polyclonal proliferation of T and B cells within the pleural effusion. Biopsy of the mediastinal mass showed a teratocarcinoma.

Table 4. Pleural and C.S.F. B and T Cell Studies.

	No. cases	
	Pleural	C.S.F.
Benign	4	2
B cell malignancy	0	2
T cell malignancy	3	2
Non-lymphoid malignancy	1	0

Four additional cases with pleural effusion had a polyclonal proliferation of T and B cells. These cases were diagnosed as benign "inflammatory" or "reactive" pleural effusions. However, one of these patients underwent open pleural biopsy due to prominent thickening of the pleura visualized on CAT scan of the chest. This biopsy demonstrated a small cleaved cell lymphoma (PDL). The pleural effusion in this case was probably the result of lymphatic obstruction by the tumor, with no apparent shedding of the malignant cells into the pleural fluid. This case demonstrates that a polyclonal population of lymphocytes within a pleural effusion does not entirely exclude the diagnosis of a malignant lymphoreticular process involving the pleura.

Six cases from CSF have been studied with immunological markers. Two of these patients showed a convoluted T cell lymphoma in which the E-rosette/cytospins were again used to visualize the neoplastic characteristics of the rosetting cells. Two other patients with a previous diagnosis of B cell lymphoma were also studied, with both demonstrating CNS involvement by the presence of monoclonal surface immunoglobulin on CSF lymphocytes. One of these cases was a large cell lymphoma and the other was a well-differentiated lymphocytic lymphoma with CLL. The other two cases evaluated by immunological surface markers in CSF were finally diagnosed as reactive lymphocytosis rather than lymphoma. Clinical follow-up in both cases revealed no evidence of lymphoma. The patients probably had a form of aseptic meningitis.

4.5. Studies in Solid Tissues.

A large number of cases from solid tissues, mainly lymph nodes and tumor masses, have been studied and fully characterized by immunological methods in our laboratory. The majority of these studies were performed on cell suspensions, utilizing antibodies to surface immunoglobulin of all heavy and light chains, B1 antigen and a panel of T cell surface markers, including OKT 3, OKT 11, OKT 8, OKT 4, OKT 6. The presence of CALLA and TdT by immunofluorescence was also determined in the great majority of cases. Immunoperoxidase stains of frozen sections were also performed on most of the cases, searching for the presence of B1, Kappa, lambda, OKT 3, OKT 11, OKT 4, and OKT 8. Occasionally we used B5 or formalin-fixed tissue for immunoperoxidase staining for Kappa and lambda chains. However, we did not use formalin-fixed tissue for B or T cell markers. In the great majority of cases a diagnosis could be established with reasonable certainty with the above mentioned studies and when correlated with the light microscopic findings of the case. In difficult cases, additional studies were required, such as immunoperoxidase on frozen sections for common leukocyte antigen (CLA) and epithelial membrane antigen (EMA). Immunoperoxidase stains for CEA, keratin and other antigens were performed to exclude the diagnosis of a lymphoid lesion.

4.5.1. Lymph Nodes. The main purpose of immunologically characterizing the lymphocytes in lymph nodes is to distinguish between benign and malignant lymphoid proliferations.[12, 13] The distribution of different subsets may aid in the final characterization of lesion as well as have prognostic significance. Several groups can be recognized:

A. Benign or reactive proliferations: One hundred and two lymph nodes were finally characterized as benign, both immunologically and morphologically. The distribution of B and T cell subsets in a non-reactive lymph node was normal and paralleled the distribution of subsets in the peripheral blood (see Table 1).

Sixty-six lymph nodes belonged to the "normal" lymph node group. Table 5. All of these cases except one, had a normal T & B cell distribution with polyclonal surface immunoglobulin. The exception was a 71-year-old patient who had 25% B cells with a clonal excess of 22% Kappa and 3% lambda. The T cell markers were as follows: OKT 11, 59%; OKT 4, 61%; OKT 8, 15%; H/S ratio 4. The microscopic appearance of this lymph node was normal. This node was obtained during a cholecystectomy when the surgeon noticed several enlarged mesenteric lymph nodes. There was no evidence of peripheral lymphadenopathy. Subsequent studies including bone marrow biopsy have been unremarkable. This patient is being carefully followed.

Table 5. Lymph Node B and T Cell Studies in Benign Proliferations.

	No. cases
Normal B and T cell distribution	66
Polyclonal B cell increase	26
T cell decrease	11
Infectious process	6

The second group of benign lymph nodes were composed of 26 cases with a marked polyclonal increase of B cells (over 40%) and a normal number of T cells with a H/S ratio greater than 2. These lymph nodes usually had prominent follicular hyperplasia and/or expanded medullary regions in the lymph node. There was a lymph node from a 49 year old female with a suggestion of a clonal excess. She had 40% B cells with 31% Kappa and 8% lambda. No clinical or histological evidence of lymphoma was found in this case. Two year follow-up of this patient is presently unremarkable.

The third group of benign lymph nodes were mainly characterized by a normal number of polyclonal B cells with a significantly decreased number of total T cells (below 35%). The distribution of T cell subsets as well as the microscopic appearance of this group has been the most variable of all the benign lymph nodes. Only 11 cases have been recognized in this group. Due to the lower number of cases, no conclusions can be drawn. No association with viral infection or other diseases such as Hodgkin's has been noted in this particular group.

The fourth group was associated with infectious diseases: six cases had a final clinical diagnosis of toxoplasmosis and 3 cases were diagnosed as cat scratch disease. No distinctive immunologic pattern of reaction was noted. Most of these cases had a polyclonal increase of B cells (approximately 30%) with a slightly increased H/S ratio (approximately 3).

B. Non-Hodgkin's lymphoma of B cell type: A total of 63 cases of nodal lymphomas, B cell type, have been found in our series. Fifty-three of these have been classified as B cell lymphomas by the presence of a clonal excess of surface immunoglobulin. The definition of a clonal excess, according to Ligler[14], is as follows:

$$CE = \frac{\text{No. } K^{+} \text{ cells} - \text{No. } \lambda^{+} \text{cells}}{\text{No. } K^{-} \text{ cells} + \text{No. } \lambda^{-} \text{cells}}$$

The clonal excess value for lymph nodes, bone marrow, spleen and peripheral blood with lymphomatous involvement is greater than 0.4 for kappa positive tumors and less than 0.4 for lambda positive tumors.

The frequency of each type of lymphoma is summarized in Table 6.

Table 6. Nodal Lymphomas of B-Cell Type

Type of Lymphoma	Number of Cases
Well differentiated	7
Intermediate degree	7
Poorly differentiated lymphocytic (PDL)	16
Mixed (large cell and small cleaved cell)	7
Large cell	16

The well differentiated lymphocytic lymphoma, also called small lymphocytic (Figure 1), is characterized by the presence of a scant amount of surface immunoglobulin[5]. In the few cases seen with plasmacytic differentiation, the same type of immunoglobulin can be demonstrated in the cytoplasm of the cells. The demonstration of the surface immunoglobulin can also be accomplished by immunoperoxidase stains in cytospins or frozen sections. Six cases were of IgM Kappa. Of these, 3 expressed delta chains too. Another case expressed IgMD lambda surface immunoglobulin. Table 7. Follow-up in these cases is desirable to establish any possible correlation between the immunlogical findings (i.e., 2 heavy chains) and the course of this type of lymphoma which is usually rather long and mild.

The intermediate degree of differentiated lymphoma (Figure 2) is characterized immunologically by the presence of a rather bright monoclonal surface immunoglobulin, intermediate in brightness between well differentiated lymphocytic or small lymphocytic lymphoma and poorly differentiated or small cleaved lymphoma. They do not show any significant capping and usually do not exhibit complement receptor. Seven cases that belonged to this category were seen. Two cases were shown to have MD Kappa surface immunoglobulin. Three cases expressed IgG Kappa. The other two cases showed IgM Kappa and IgM lambda on their surfaces.

Table 7. Distribution of Surface Immunoglobulin and B-1 Antigen in B Cell Lymphomas.

Type of Lymphoma	Type of Surface Marker				
	MK or λ	MDK or λ	GK or λ	MGK or λ	B-1 only
W.D.L.L.	3	4			
Intermediate	2	2	3		
P.D.L.	13	2	1		
Mixed	3		3		1
Large Cell	9		3	1	3

The poorly differentiated or small cleaved cell lymphoma (Figure 3) was characterized by the presence of bright fluorescence of monoclonal surface immunoglobulin with a prominent degree of capping. Immunoperoxidase stains of frozen section tissues can also demonstrate the presence of the monoclonal immunoglobulin. This lymphoma is more frequently seen in the nodular or follicular form but can also be diffuse. No differences between the nodular and the diffuse forms were noted immunologically. Sixteen cases belonged to this group. Six cases were IgM Kappa type, seven cases IgM lambda type, one case MD Kappa type and another case IgG Kappa type.

The mixed lymphoma group (lymphocytic-histiocytic type) (Figure 4) was composed of small cleaved and large cells, both of which expressed the same type of surface immunoglobulin. The population of smaller cells expressed bright surface immunoglobulin with a prominent degree of capping, while the population of larger cells expressed bright surface immunoglobulin without evidence of capping. One mixed lymphoma did not express any surface immunoglobulin but was B1 positive. Histologically, the diagnosis of a nodular mixed lymphoma was evident. The surface immunoglobulin in the cell suspension was 0%; OKT 3, 30%; OKT 4, 20% and OKT 8, 6%. The most important point in this case is that in spite of the nodularity of the lymphoma, the cells did not express surface immunoglobulin as expected. Cytoplasmic immunoglobulin was also negative. Six other cases belong to the group of mixed lymphoma; three of these were IgM kappa and 3 IgG kappa.

The large cell lymphoma (Figure 5) is rather polymorphous and is called histiocytic lymphoma in the older classifications. They are usually diffuse but can be nodular. They can have monoclonal surface immunoglobulin but some do not express it. Histologically, they can be made up of different types of cells defined as large cleaved, large non-cleaved or immunoblastic. A total of 16 cases of large cell lymphoma of B cell type have been included in this category. Thirteen cases of these have shown monoclonal surface immunoglobulin in moderate amount. The cells can be recognized under fluorescence by their size and by the presence of bright monoclonal surface Ig. Eight cases showed M kappa surface immunoglobulin and one M lambda. Two cases expressed G kappa, one G lambda and one MG kappa. Three cases did not express any surface or cytoplasmic Ig. However, all of them showed B-1 antigen indicating their B cell nature.

The contribution to the diagnosis of this group of B cell lymphomas by immunological techniques is rather significant. The immunological studies in the great majority of the cases allowed us to determine with almost certainty that we were dealing with a monoclonal proliferation of B cells, and that the diagnosis of lymphoma was evident. We did not find any discrepancy between the immunological results and the histological diagnosis in any particular case. On the contrary, they complemented each other.

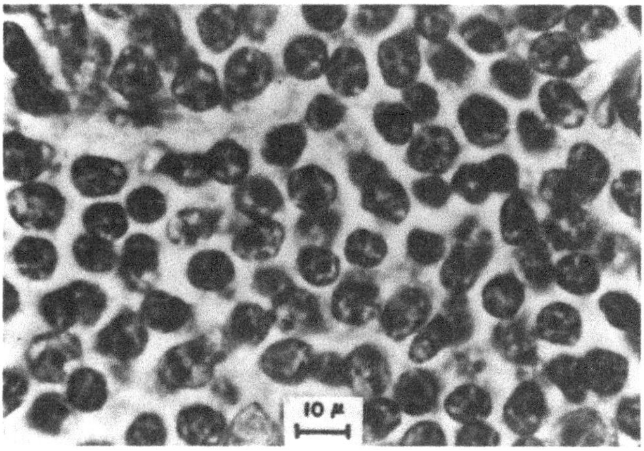

FIGURE 1. Well differentiated lymphocytic lymphoma (small lymphocytic lymphoma) H&E stain.

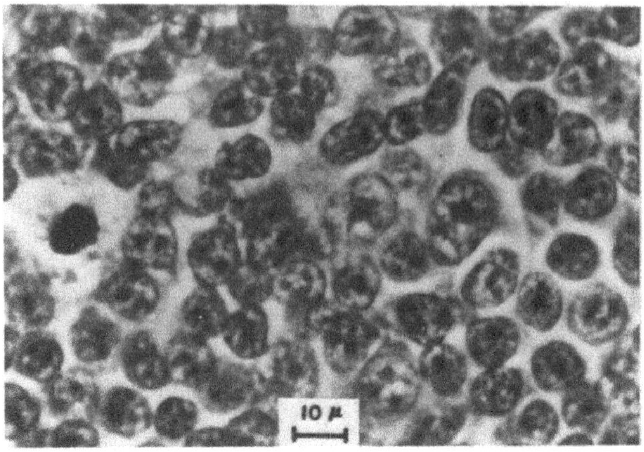

FIGURE 2. Lymphocytic lymphoma intermediate degree of differentiation. H&E stain.

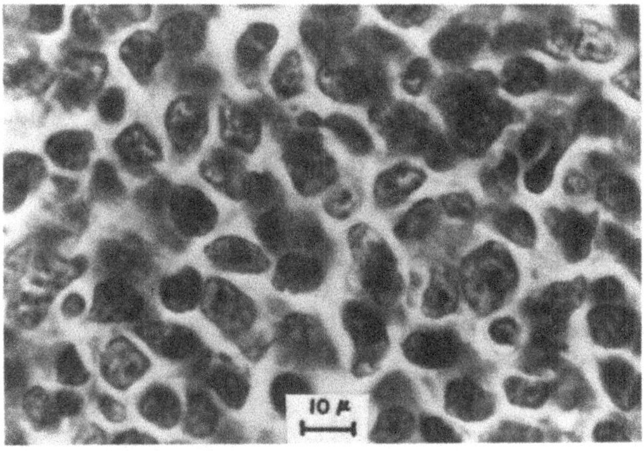

FIGURE 3. Poorly differentiated lymphocytic lymphoma (small cleaved cell lymphoma) H&E stain.

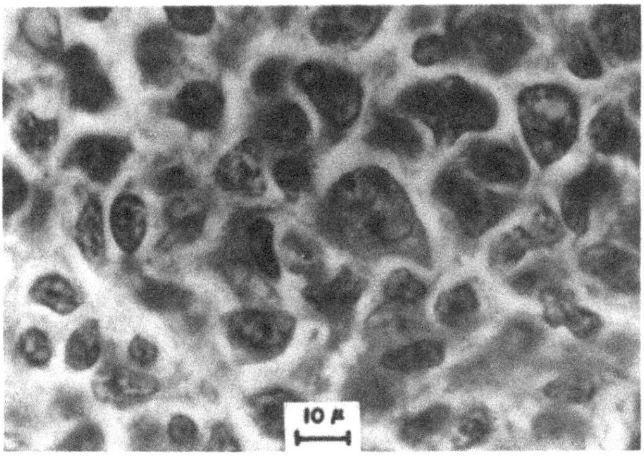

FIGURE 4. Mixed lymphoma, lymphocytic-histiocytic (small cleaved and large cell lymphoma) H&E stain.

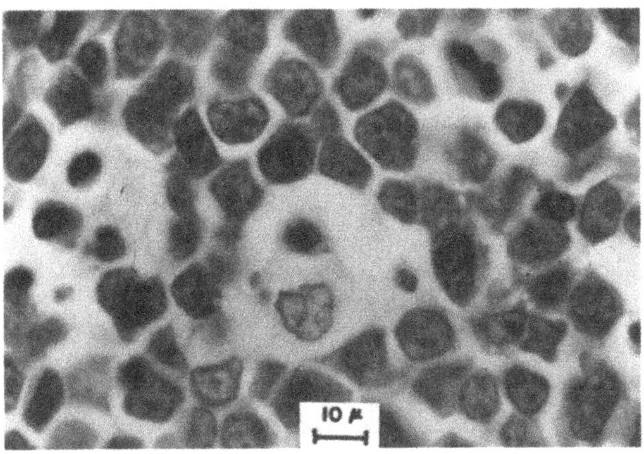

FIGURE 5. Histiocytic lymphoma (large cell lymphoma) H&E stain.

C. Non-Hodgkin's lymphoma of T cell type: The diagnosis of a T cell lymphoma is more difficult to make than B cell lymphoma. The monoclonal concept of this lymphoma cannot be established immunologically as for B cells with currently available techniques and reagents. A phenotype can be recognized as the predominant population in a T cell lymphoma, but predominance of one phenotype does not allow one to identify that particular group as monoclonal. The diagnosis of T cell lymphoma is made in our laboratory when two conditions are satisfied. First, the histological diagnosis of lymphoma has been firmly established by morphological criteria. Secondly, the previously determined malignant cell population must express T cell markers. The cell suspensions for surface T cell marker analysis are less helpful in the diagnosis of this lesion than with B cell lymphomas. However, usually one can see a predominance of a T cell subtype of a lack of expected T cell markers, such as the presence of OKT 3 with the absence of OKT 11, as well as high numbers of OKT 4, OKT 8, or OKT 6 with low numbers of OKT 3 and OKT 11. The cytospins of E-rosette preparations in the primary diagnosis of T cell lymphoma can be of help only if the neoplastic population of T cells has been previously determined by morphological criteria. Even under the best circumstances, these T cell marker findings are consistent with but not diagnostic of a T cell lymphoma. It should be noted that positive E-rosettes of large immunoblasts can also be seen in benign reactive immunoblastic proliferations. The morphology of E-rosetted cells, however, can be of great value in a recurrent lymphoma where one is looking for a specific type, such as in lymphoma involving the CSF. When the diagnosis of T cell lymphoma of well differentiated lymphocytes is suspected, a more difficult problem is encountered since the neoplastic cell cannot be distinguished morphologically from the normal T cell.

Immunoperoxidase stains for T cell antigens on frozen sections of tissues with a T cell lesion are important. They allow one to identify the markers of the neoplastic cell population in relationship of the morphology of the lesion.

We have encountered 7 cases of T cell lymphoma and 3 additional cases of convoluted lymphoma (also called lymphoblastic lymphoma). Table 8. In addition to positive E-rosettes, the convoluted lymphomas expressed CALLA on the cell surface. Among the 7 cases of T cell lymphoma were 2 of small lymphocytes and one composed of intermediate size lymphocytes. The other four cases have all been classified as nodal T cell lymphoma of immunoblastic type. The majority of the latter tumors expressed OKT 4 markers. In general, this group of lymphomas has been characterized clinically by a poor response to chemotherapy, frequent recurrences, B-symptoms, and a very short fatal clinical course in some. A more complete evaluation of these cases is being prepared for a future report by the authors.

Table 8. Nodal Malignancies of Non-B Cell Type.

Type of Malignancy	No. Cases
Non-Hodgkin's lymphoma of T cells	
Small lymphocytic	2
Intermediate lymphocytic	1
Immunoblastic	4
Convoluted	3
Hodgkin's lymphomas	20
Undifferentiated non-lymphoid tumor	10

D. Hodgkin's lymphoma: The diagnosis of Hodgkin's disease in our experience cannot be suspected, diagnosed or confirmed by immunological methods alone at the present time. The only contribution of the immunological characterization of lymphomas in the diagnosis of Hodgkin's disease is in the rare case in which a B cell lymphoma is the differential diagnosis in question. A positive or negative result for monoclonal B cells can assist in this differential diagnosis. The most common situation, in which this differential diagnosis is entertained is in the case of the lymphocytic predominant form of Hodgkin's disease versus well differentiated lymphocytic lymphoma. In this case, the lack of monoclonal surface immunoglobulin on the small lymphocytes would favor a diagnosis of Hodgkin's disease. The presence of monoclonal surface immunoglobulin would of course exclude Hodgkin's lymphoma. The second subtype of Hodgkin's disease that can be confused with a B cell lymphoma is the reticular variant of lymphocyte depleted versus immunoblastic lymphoma. The presence of monoclonal surface or cytoplasmic immunoglobulin in the larger cells would exclude the diagnosis of a Hodgkin's lymphoma.

We have characterized the nodal lymphocytes in 20 cases of Hodgkin's disease, aiming for patterns of reactions that would correlate with types of Hodgkin's, mainly lymphocytic predominance or not, and with response to therapy evolution and prognosis. The conclusion of these studies will take years to follow-up. At the present time, we do not see any specific pattern of reaction within these nodes, although a tendency for a high T cell count (over 85%), with a predominance of helper cells usually with a rate of H/S over 4, has been observed in over half of these cases. Similar findings have been observed in four additional cases of malignant lymphoma with high content of epithelioid histiocytes that has been classified as Lennert's lymphoma. It is also to be noted that some cases of malignant lymphoma with epithelioid histiocytes in which a monoclonal surface immunoglobulin has been demonstrated in a high percentage of the cell suspension, have been classified as B cell lymphomas by us.

E. Metastatic tumor of non-lymphoid origin: A total of 10 lymph nodes with metastatic lesions have also been studied. The great majority of these cases have been anyalyzed to rule out lymphoma. It is interesting that a suspension of single cells has been obtained in the great majority of cases without any enzyme digestion. Among the tumors encountered in this group were melanoma, seminoma, leukemia and undifferentiated malignant neoplasms. The lack of common leukocyte antigen was then noticed in cell suspensions examined by immunofluorescence or in frozen sections examined by immunoperoxidase. B and T cell markers were also absent. Some of these cases have expressed epithelial membrane antigen (EMA) by immunofluorescence on cell suspension or by immunoperoxidase on frozen sections. An interesting case of metastatic seminoma to a lymph node with small lymphocytic lymphoma was also found within this group.

4.5.2. Solid Tissues of Non-nodal Origin. Within this group, we are classifying large extranodal lymphoid tumors that could have initially originated in lymph nodes. We are also including lymphoid lesions from other organs, such as lung, stomach, etc. A total of 36 cases belonged to this category. Table 9. Seventeen presented as large mediastinal, abdominal or pelvic masses. Seven of these represented thoracic masses. One was classified as a large B cell lymphoma (histiocytic lymphoma) in a 30-year-old female with no evidence of pleural or peripheral lymphadenopathy. The large neoplastic cells composed 92% of the cell population and showed monoclonal IgG kappa surface immunoglobulin. The other six cases were all thymic in origin. One of them was a hyperplastic thymus and the other thymomas in which over 95% of the cells were of T cell origin and expressed OKT 6 surface antigen. We should point out that no convoluted lymphomas (lymphoblastic) were found in this group since mediastinal biopsies have been avoided in cases where marker studies were done on peripheral blood, bone marrow, peripheral lymph nodes, or pleural effusions.

Table 9. Solid Tissues of non-Nodal Origin B and T Cell Studies.

Organ	Benign Lymphoid	Benign Thymic	B-cell Malignancy	T-cell Malignancy	Hodgkin's Disease	Non-Lymphoid
Mediastinal		6	1			1
Pelvic	1		5	1		2
Other	4		9	1	3	2

Among the abdominal pelvic masses, ten patients were studied. Six patients were diagnosed as large cell lymphoma. One was a T cell lymphoma and the other five were B cell lymphomas. All of the B cell lymphomas expressed B-1 surface antigen, but only three of them expressed monoclonal surface immunoglobulin. All were kappa type. There were two cases in which no lymphoid neoplasm was finally diagnosed. One was benign reactive lymphoid tissue and the other was an inflammatory malignant fibrous histiocytoma.

The last 19 cases include lymphoid lesions from a great variety of organs in which the diagnosis of a lymphoproliferative disorder was suspected at the time of the frozen section. All of these cases represented primary organ lesions with no evidence of lymph node involvement. The B and T cell marker analysis in these cases was of great value in arriving at the final diagnosis. Primary extranodal lymphoma is usually more difficult to diagnose than nodal lymphoma when the diagnosis is based solely on morphology. There are extranodal lymphoid lesions that are morphologically identical to nodal lymphomas, further complicating the definition of extranodal lymphoma. Immunologic characterization of these lesions by surface markers can be decisive in determining the benign or malignant nature of these lymphoid infiltrates. A total of nine extranodal B cell lymphomas were diagnosed based on the presence of monoclonal surface immunoglobulin and according to the different morphological pattern that were previously discussed in lymph nodes. Single cases were diagnosed in the parotid gland, tonsil, lung, small bowel and soft tissues of the neck. Two cases each were diagnosed as B cell lymphoma in the stomach and in the spleen. A T cell lymphoma of the skin was also seen. There were three cases of Hodgkin's disease involving the parotid, spleen and soft tissues of the neck. The value of B and T cell markers in excluding the more common B cell neoplasms has already been discussed. Two non-lymphoid malignancies were diagnosed by exclusion. One of them was a glioma metastatic to a cervical lymph node and the leukemic infiltrate in the skin of a leukemic patient who was subsequently to have proven bone marrow involvement. Finally, there were three benign lymphoid lesions within the thyroid (all lymphocytic thyroiditis), one within the breast and one benign nodule in the subcutaneum. These were also diagnosed on the basis of morphology and B and T cell marker studies.

5. CONCLUSIONS

This review has shown the value of immunologic evaluation of B and T cell markers in the diagnostic immunopathology laboratory. A definite place has already been established by these techniques in the diagnosis of lymphoid lesions. The neoplasms that can be diagnosed are continually expanding with the development of new monoclonal antibodies and instrumentation. These studies have also contributed to understanding the pathogenesis of these lymphoproliferative lesions. The classification of lymphoproliferative lesions will ultimately depend upon both immunologic and morphologic parameters, which will further delineate prognostic and therapeutic categories.

Abreviations: RPMI - Rosswell Park Memorial Institute. HBSS - Hanks' Balanced Salt Solution. AEC - Amino-ethylcarbazole. PWM - Pokeweed Mitogen. CMV - Cytomegalo Virus.

REFERENCES

1. Lukes RJ et al: A morphologic and immunologic surface marker study of 299 cases of non-Hodgkin's lymphomas and related leukemias. Am J Pathol(90) 461-486, 1978.
2. Foon K, schroff RW, Gale, RP: Surface markers on leukemia and lymphoma cells: recent advances. Blood(60) 1-19, 1982.
3. Aisenberg, AC, Wilkes, BM, Harris, NL: Monoclonal antibody studies in non-Hodgkin's lymphomas. Blood(61):469-475, 1983.
4. Horwitz D: Enumeration of Human T, B and "L" Lymphocytes. In: Rose NR, Bigazzi PE(ed) Methods in Immunodiagnosis. John Wiley & Sons, New York, 1980, pp 1-13.
5. Aisenberg AC, Wilkes BM, Long JC, Harris, NL. Cell Surface Phenotype in Lymphoproliferative Disease. The Am J of Med(68) 206-213, 1980.
6. Rosloniec EF, Kuhn MH, Genyea CA, Reed AH, Jennings JJ, Giraldo AA, Beisel KW, Lerman, SP. Aggressiveness of SJL/J Lymphomas Correlates with Absence of $H-2D^{S}$-Antigens. The J of Immunology(132) 2:945-952, 1984.
7. Ault KA. Detection of small numbers of monoclonal B lymphocytes in the blood of patients with lymphomas. New Eng J of Med(300) 1401-1405, 1979.
8. Rowlans DT, Whiteside TL, Danielle RP. Cells of the immune system. In: Todd.Sanford.Davidsohn(ed) Clinical Diagnosis and Management by Laboratory Methods. WB Saunders Co, Philadelphia, 1984, pp 822-847.
9. Taylor CR. Immunoperoxidase Techniques. Archives of Pathology and Laboratory Medicine(102) 113-121, 1978.
10. Creemers P, Giraldo AA, Rose NR, Kong YM. T cell subsets in the thyroids of mice developing autoimmune thyroiditis. Cellular Immunology(87) 692-697, 1984.
11. Fuks Z, Strober S, Kaplan HS. Interaction Between Serum Factors and T Lymphocytes in Hodgkin's Disease. New Eng J of Med(295) 1273-1278, 1976.
12. Tubbs RR, Fishleder A, Weiss RA. Immunohistologic Cellular Phenotypes of Lymphoproliferative Disorders. Am J Path(113) 207-221, 1983.
13. Harris NL, Data RE: Distribution of neoplastic and normal B-lymphoid cells in nodular lymphomas: use of an immunoperoxidase technique on frozen sections. Hum Pathol(13) 610-617, 1982.
14. Ligler, FS. The Clonal Excess Method for Detecting B-cell Lymphoma. Clinic Immunology Newsletter(3)8 45-47, 1982.

10

IMMUNOHISTOCHEMISTRY OF NEUROENDOCRINE NEOPLASMS OF THE BRONCHOPULMONARY TRACT AND SKIN

I. LEE, W.W. FRANKE, V.E. GOULD

I. NEUROENDOCRINE NEOPLASMS OF THE BRONCHOPULMONARY TRACT:

Bronchopulmonary neuroendocrine (NE) neoplasms encompass a wide spectrum of pathologically and clinically distinct entities which include typical carcinoids, well-differentiated NE carcinomas, and NE carcinomas of intermediate and small cell type (1,2). Typical carcinoids are predominantly centrally located. Microscopically they exhibit the classical architecture of solid cellular clusters and/or ribbons with little, if any, cellular pleomorphism. Metastases are very rare and appear only late in the course of the disease. Well-differentiated NE carcinomas have received various vague designations such as "atypical carcinoids", and have sometimes been misinterpreted as "early oat cell carcinomas". These tumors are most often peripheral and display considerable cytological pleomorphism; however, they still retain an organoid pattern (Fig. 1a). Mitotic figures are readily found but the mitotic activity is not as brisk as in NE carcinomas of intermediate or small cell type. Metastases are frequent. We have observed 2 to 5 years survival in about 50% of cases. NE carcinomas of intermediate and small cell type have a similarly aggressive course: they differ only in the size and arrangement of their cells. The NE carcinomas of intermediate cell type show solid clusters of pleomorphic cells with frequent central necrosis and peripheral palisading. The nuclei are vesicular and are at least twice the size of their small cell counterparts. The NE carcinomas of small cell type display an ill-defined architecture and consist of small atypical cells with hyperchromatic nuclei. Necrosis is a prominent feature, as is the characteristic crushing artifact. The mitotic count is brisk. Mixed forms may occur. Focally, features of squamous and glandular diffentiation are not uncommon.

Ultrastructurally, bronchial carcinoids contain numerous neurosecretory granules. Although the granules are usually round and between 150 to 250 nm in size, the size, shape, and the density of their cores vary considerably. Aggregates of intermediate filaments often coexisting with clusters of neurosecretory granules are frequently observed. Well-differentiated NE carcinomas are not conspicuously granulated. NE carcinomas of intermediate and small cell type often show interlacing cytoplasmic processes where their rather scanty neurosecretory granules tend to aggregate. They generally lack delimiting basal lamina, although carcinoids regularly show a distinct basal lamina.

In the majority of the NE neoplasms of the bronchopulmonary tract, reactivity for neuron specific enolase (NSE), serotonin, and various neuropeptides, can be demonstrated immunohistochemically (Fig. 1b). Sections from paraffin blocks are usually adequate for this purpose. However, proper preservation and fixation of the tissue is critical. We have found that Bouin's is the fixative of choice for these materials. By the PAP technique, the overwhelming majority of bronchial carcinoids display reactivity for NSE, serotonin, bombesin, and leu-enkephalin. Some "ectopic" materials including gastrin, melanin- stimulating hormone, VIP, etc., are also found. The majority are immunoreactive for more than one hormone. Evaluation of single sections stained for two hormones and of step sections immunostained sequentially for multiple hormones has provided strong evidence that single cells may indeed secrete and store more than one hormone (3). This observation seemingly reflects the heterogeneity of the neurosecretory granules disclosed by electron microscopy. The intensity and distribution of the immunostaining are often notably heterogeneous (4). Well-differentiated NE carcinomas also produce similar materials as those of carcinoids. ACTH is often found in these tumors while it is not frequently found in bronchial carcinoids; this is at variance with the findings of others (5) and may reflect variable taxonomic criteria. In the NE carcinomas of intermediate cell type, the most frequently demonstrated material has been ACTH, followed by bombesin, leu-enkephalin, etc. Compared to the previous three tumors, the immunoreactivity for various hormone is less frequently demonstrated in the NE cell carcinomas of small cell type. The materials most frequently demonstrated are bombesin and ACTH. Occasionally immunoreactivity for serotonin, leu-enkephalin, calcitonin, somatostatin, and VIP may also be found. Immunoreactivity for more than one hormone is also observed as is the synchronous or asynchronous variability in the expression of hormones between the primary and its metastases.

Immunohistochemistry of intermediate filaments (IF) is having a tremendous impact on diagnostic surgical pathology in general (for review see, 6,7). In human tissue, the cytokeratin family encompasses at least 19 different polypeptides which display considerable cell-specificity (8). Recently, we studied the expression of IF in the bronchopulmonary NE neoplasm with immunofluorescence and two dimensional electrophoresis using monoclonal antibodies. Frozen tissue of carcinoids, well-differentiated NE carcinomas, and NE carcinomas of intermediate and small cell types were examined. By immunofluorescence, every NE carcinomas studied was positive for cytokeratins 8, 18, and 19(9) (Fig. 1c). These cytokeratin polypeptides have been described in diverse simple epithelia and in certain carcinomas such as adenocarcinomas of the lung. Immunoreactivity for desmoplakin (demosomal plaque proteins) was also demonstrated in every case (Fig. 1d). Two dimensional gel electrophoresis conformed the presence of the said cytokeratin polypeptides.

These bronchopulmonary NE neoplasms were negative for other types of IF's including neurofilaments (Fig.1e). These results were contradictory to some previous reports using paraffin sections (10). We concluded that bronchopulmonary neoplasms express cytokeratins instead of possibly in addition to neurofilaments. This also indicates that the strict equation of the cytokeratin or possibly other types of IF's with traditional concepts of tumor histogenesis should be avoided.

In surgical pathology, we frequently come across pulmonary neoplasm with multidirectional differentiation. Recently, Gazdar et al. have reported that 6% of untreated small cell pulmonary carcinomas showed "mixed" histologic feature; subsequent to therapy, 39% of the tumors displayed "mixed" histology some of which was radically at variance with that of the primary (11). This parallels our observations. Thus, it is very likely that bronchopulmonary neoplasms derive from "stem" cells which, during and subsequent to neoplastic transformation, may show squamous, mucosubstance producing or NE features or mixtures thereof. Indeed, this notion may be applicable to the general understanding and taxonomy of neoplasms.

2. NEUROENDOCRINE CARCINOMAS OF THE SKIN:

Recently there have been numerous reports of NE carcinomas of the skin, which would seemingly indicate that these previously under-recognized neoplasms may not be rare. However, the literature of NE skin carcinomas has been very

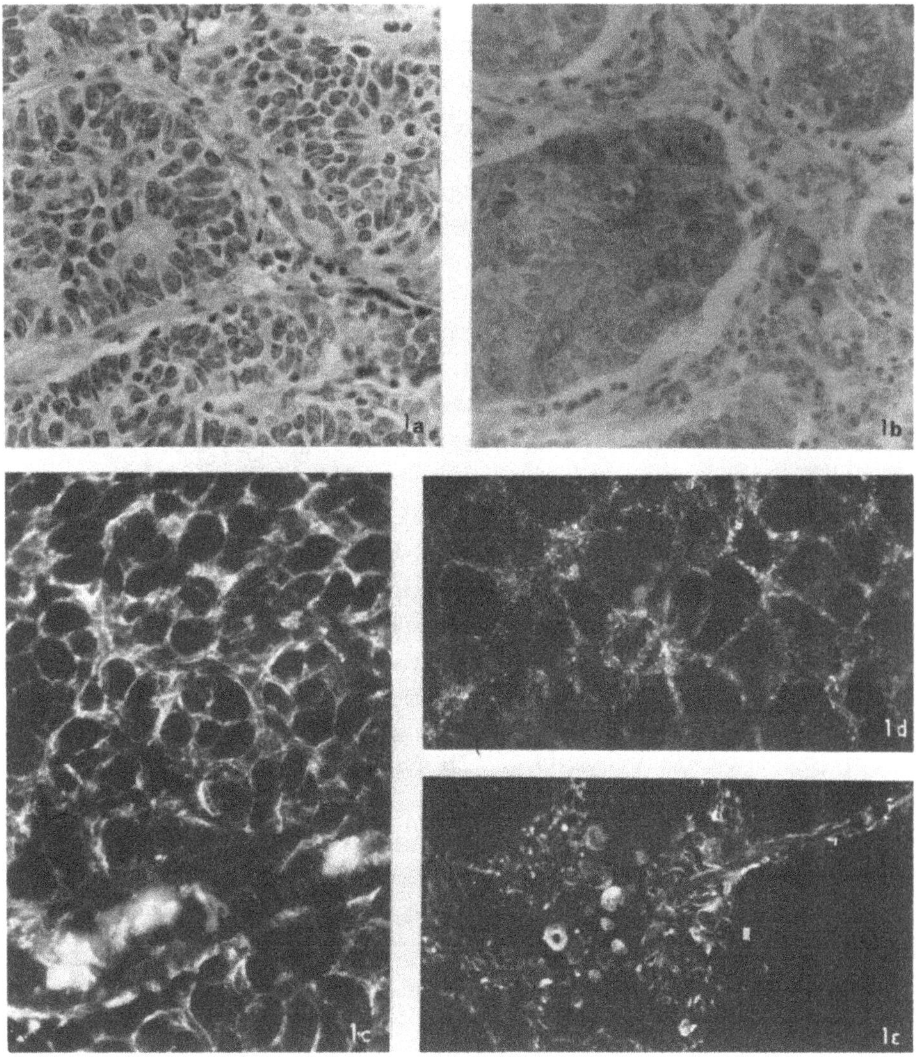

Figures 1a, b, c, d, e. Well-differentiated NE carcinoma of the bronchopulmonary tract. 1a. Note cellular pleomorphism and occasional mitoses; however the organoid pattern is retained, H&E, X380. 1b. Some neoplastic cells are strongly immunoreactive for NSE, PAP technique, X380. 1c Diffuse and strong immunoreactivity for cytokeratins #s 8 and 18, immunofluorescence on frozen section, X650. 1d. Immunofluorescence for desmoplakin; note small bright points indicating individual desmosomes, X750. 1e. Immunofluorescence for vimentin; connective tissue septa and blood vessels are positive, while the tumor is negative, X270.

confusing, mostly because the family of NE skin carcinomas encompasses a wide spectrum of entities reflected in multiple designations (for reviews see 12,13). Added to this confusion of taxonomy, is the frequently improper pathologic diagnoses of these neoplasms with widely diverse differential diagnoses such as lymphoma, neuroblastoma, or Ewing's sarcoma. Morphologic studies and clinical correlations have suggested that at least 3 distinct types of NE carcinoma of intermediate cell type, and NE skin carcinoma of small cell type.

NE skin carcinomas of trabecular cell type usually develop around the face. They seem to consistently arise in the dermis near the skin adnexal structures without connection to the overlying epidermis. The neoplastic cells are arranged in distinctly organoid clusters and trabeculae (Fig 2a). The clinical course is characterized by repeated recurrences followed and at times accompanied by regional lymph node metastases. All of our 7 cases survived longer than 4 years after presentation.

NE skin carcinomas of intermediate cell type appear to be the most frequent variant NE skin carcinoma. They also arise in the dermis. In the majority of cases, there is no connection between the tumor and the overlying epidermis. However, we have observed a case with a clear connection between it and a "pagetoid" change of the adjacent epidermis. These neoplasms are comprised of round, intermediate sized cells with poor cohesion. Focal necrosis is a consistent feature. Mitoses are abundant (Fig. 3a). This variant of NE skin carcinoma may mimick either lymphoma or Ewing's sarcoma. Primary sites of this variant are more diverse than in the trabecular variant. The clinical course is far more aggressive that the trabecular type.

NE skin carcinomas of small cell type may occur in "pure" form or admixed with intermediate cells. Morphologically this variant resembles neuroblastoma or small cell carcinomas of the lung or other sites. These tumors also develop in the dermis and are composed of solid sheets and clusters of small cells with hyperchromatic nuclei. Necrosis is relative abundant. There is frequent and characteristic crushing artifact. Cellular pleomorphism is conspicuous and the mitotic activity is brisk (Fig.4a). Clinically these neoplasms behave aggressively; regional and systemic metastases develop within 12-30 months subsequent to presentation.

Ultrastructurally the trabecular type has abundant neurosecretory granules, intermediate filaments, and cell junctions. The intermediate cell

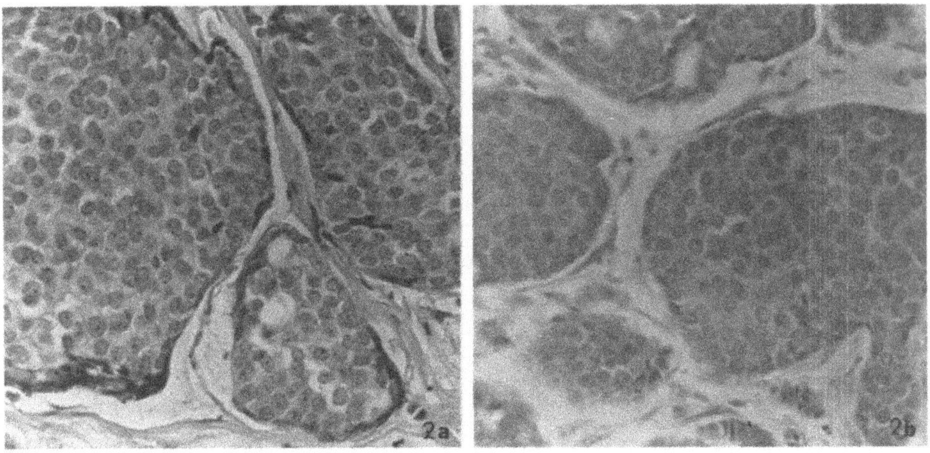

Figure 2a, b. NE skin carcinoma of trabecular type. 2a. Note clusters of relatively uniform cells with peripheral compression and gland-like cavities. H&E, X380. 2b. Neoplastic cells are moderately but diffusely immunostained for bombesin, PAP technique, X380

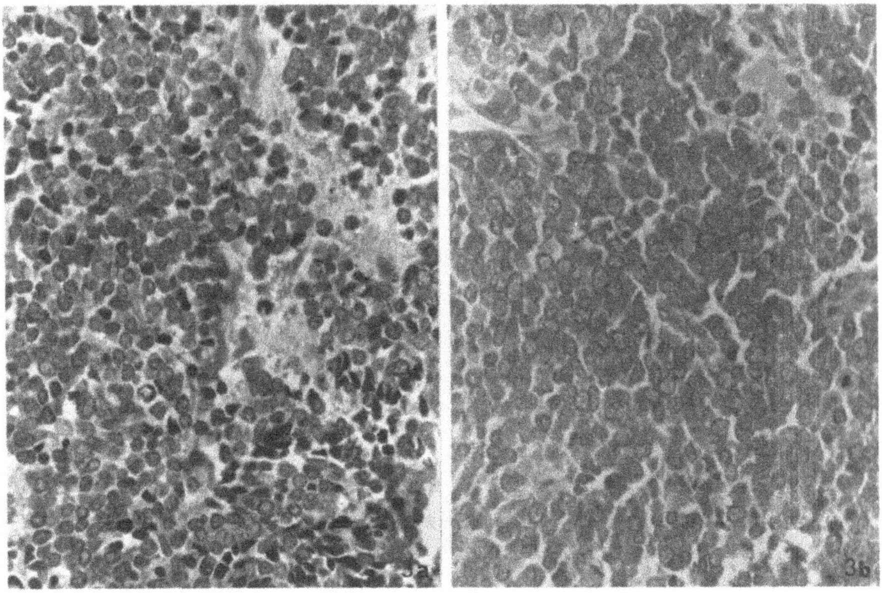

Figres 3a, b. NE skin carcinoma of intermediate cell type. 3a. Clusters of neoplastic cells lacking defined architectural pattern, note focal necrosis, poorly coferent round cells with frequent mitoses. H&E, X380. Neoplastic cells intensely immunostained for leu-enkephalin, PAP technique, X380.

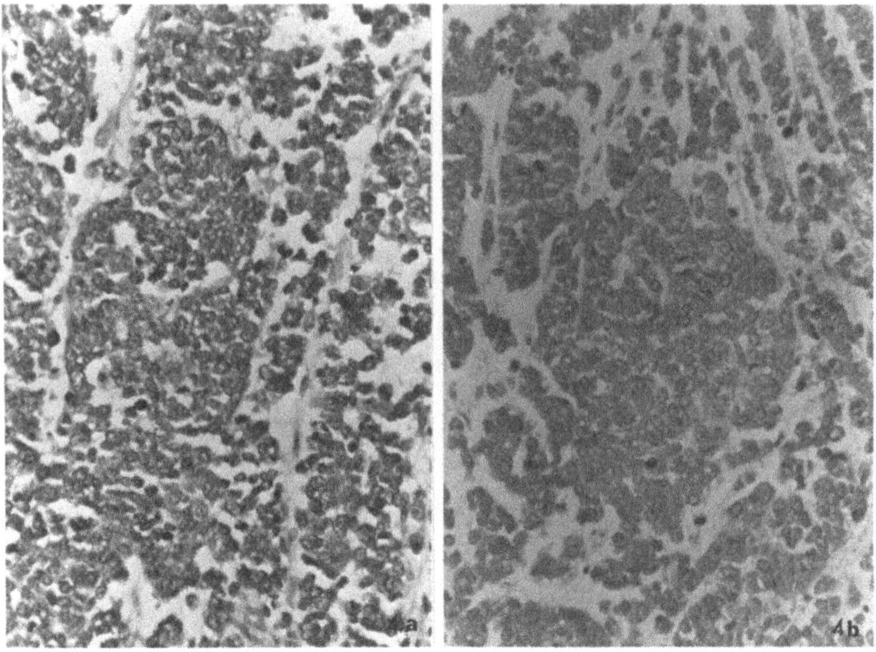

Figures 4a, b. NE skin carcinoma of small cell type. 4a. At identical magnification, the neoplastic cells are evidently smaller than those in the Fig.3a and 3b. Note scanty ill-defined cytoplasm, pleomorphic nuclei and numerous mitoses. H&E, X380. 4b. Neoplastic cells immunostained for NSE, PAP technique, X380.

variants show poorly developed junctions and are not richly granulated. In the small cell type, the neurosecretory granules are scanty and tend to aggregate in slender, dendrite-like processes.

Immunohistochemical analysis of NE markers has shown that NSE seems to be the most consistent and readily demonstrable marker in all types of NE skin carcinomas (14,15). We have observed also immunoreactivity for bombesin, leu-enkephalin, calcitonin, ACTH, and VIP (Figs.2b, 3b and 4b). This distribution of the immunoreactive cells is highly variable. Immunostaining for more than one neuropeptide is often demonstrable in a given tumor and also individual neoplastic cells (14).

Early reports indicated that NE skin carcinomas might exclusively express neurofilament protein (16) while subsequent investigations revealed that these tumors were capable of expressing cytokeratin (17). Initially, we studied the cytoskeletal chracteristics was demonstrated only in some carcinomas of trabecular and intermediate type.

We have examined frozen tissue samples of NE skin carcinomas by the double immunofluorescence technique (12). All these neoplasms expressed cytokeratins. One skin NE carcinomas of intermediate cell type displayed synchronous immunoreactivity for neurofilaments. Similar observations have been made by other investigators (18). Two dimensional gel electrophoresis revealed the presence of cytokeratin polypeptides 8,18 and small amounts of 19. In addition, a polypeptide in the position of the 68kD neurofilament protein was identified.

The expression of cytokeratin proteins of the simple epithelial type by NE skin carcinomas parallels findings in normal, developing Merkel cells (19), and in other NE carcinomas. However, as previously mentioned, this does not necessarily indicate that NE skin carcinomas are "derived" from Merkel cells. The finding of neurofilament protein immunoreactivity and the suggestive electrophoretic pattern are certainly indicative of the coexpression of neurofilaments and cytokeratin by at least some of these neoplasms. Although biochemical confirmation is required, this is an interesting finding because vimentin seems to be the usual addtional component, in cases of cells possessing more than one class of cytoskeletal protein (20).

REFERENCES

1. Gould VE, DeLellis RA: The neuroendocrine cell system: Its tumors, hyperplasias, and dysplasias. In Silverberg Sg (ed), Principles and Practice of Surgical Pathology. John Wiley & Sons, Inc. pp 1487-1501, 1983.
2. Gould VE, Linnoila I, Memoli VA, Warren WH: Neuroendocrine components of the bronchopulmonary tract: Hyperplasias, Dysplasias, and Neoplasms,. Lab Invest 49, (5); 519, 1983.
3. Gould VE, Linnoila RI, Memoli VA, Warren WH: Neuroendocrine cells and neuroendocrine neoplasms of the lung. Path Annu 18, (10; 287, 1983.
4. Warren WH, Memoli VA, Gould VE: Immunohistochemical and ultrastructural analyses of bronchopulmonary neuroendocrine neoplasms. I. carcinoids. Ultrastruct Pathol 6; 15, 1984.
5. Tstsumi Y, Osamura RY, Watanabe K, Yanaihara N: Immunohistochemical studies on gastrin-releasing peptide and adrenocorticotropic hormone-containing cells in the human lung. Lab Invest 48; 623, 1983.
6. Osborn M. Weber K: Tumor diagnosis by intermediate filament typing: A novel tool for surgical pathology. Lab Invest 48(4); 372, 1983.

7. Franek WW, Schmid E, Schiller DL, Witer S, Jarash E, Moll R, Denk H, Jackson BW, Illmensee K: Differentiation patterns of expression of proteins of intermediate-sized filaments in tissues and cultured cells. Cold Soring Harbor Symp Quant Biol 46; 413, 1982.
8. Moll R, Franke WW, Schiller DL, Geiger B, Krepler R: The catalog of human cytokeratin polypeptides: patterns of expression of specific cytokeratins in normal epithelia, tumors and cultured cells. Cell 31; 11-24.
9. Blobel G, Gould VE, Moll R, Lee I, Huszar M, Geiger B, Franke WW: Co-expression of neuroendocrine markers and epithelial cytoskeletal proteins in bronchopulmonary neuroendocrine neoplasms. Lab Invest, 1985 (In Press).
10. Lehto VP, Steman S, Miettinen M, Dahl D, Virtanen I: Expression of a neural type of intermediate filament as a distinguishing feature between oat cell carcinoma and other lung cancer. Am J Pathology 110; 113, 1983
11. Gazdar AF, Carney DN, Guccion JG, Baylin SB: Small cell carcinoma of the lung: cellular origin and relationship to other pulmonary tumors. In Small Cell Lung Cancer, Greco FA, Oldham RK, Bunn PA(eds), New York Grune & Stratton, 1981, pp 145-175.
12. Gould VE, Moll R, Moll I, Lee I, Franke WW: Neuroendocrine (Merkel) cells of the skin: Hyperplasias, Dysplasias and Neoplasms. Lab Invest, 1985 (In Press).
13. Silva EG, Mackay B, Goepfert H, Burgess MA, Fields RS: Endocrine carcinoma of the skin (merkel cell carcinoma). Pathol Annu 19(II)I; 1984.
14. Gould VE, Fodstad O, Memoil VA, Warren WH, Dardi LE, Johannessen JV: Neuroendocrine cells and associated neoplasms of the skin. In evolution and tumor pathology of the neuroendocrine system. Eds. Falkner S, Hakason, R, Sundler F. Elsevier Science Publishers, Amsterdam, pp 545-580, 1984.
15. Gu J, Polak JM, Tapia FJ, Pearse AGE: Neuron-specific enolase in the Merkel cells of mammalian skin. The use of specific antibody as a simple and reliable marker. Am J Pathol 104; 63, 1981.
16. Miettinen M, Lehto VP, Virtanen I, Asko-Seljavaara S, Pitkanen J: Neuroendocrine carcinoma of the skin (Merkel cell carcinoma): Ultrastructural and immunohistochemical demonstration of neurofilaments. Ultrastruct Pathol 4; 219, 1983.
17. Gree WR, Linnoila RI, Triche TJ: Neuroendocrine carcinoma of skin with simultaneous cytokeratin expression. Ultrastruct Pathol 6;141, 1984.
18. Hoefler H, Kerl H, Rauch HJ, Denk H: New immunohistochemical observations with diagnostic significance in cutaneous neuroendocrine carcinomas. Am J Dermatopathol (In press).
19. Moll R, Moll I, Franke WW: Indentification of Merkel cells in human skin by specific cytokeratin antibodies: Changes of cell density and distribution in fetal and adult plantar epidermis. Differentiation (In press).
20. Holthofer H, Miettinen A, Lehto VP, Lehtonen E, Virtanen I: Expression of vimentin and cytokeratin types of intermediate filament proteins in developing and adult human kidneys. Lab Invest 5; 552, 1984.

11

IMMUNOCYTOLOGY OF ENDOCRINE TUMORS

K. KOVACS

The introduction of immunocytologic techniques had a major impact on experimental and diagnostic histopathology. Whereas many previously applied staining procedures were nonspecific and yielded unreliable and irreproducible results, immunocytologic methods were capable of demonstrating various substances conclusively in the cells. The usefulness of immunocytology became especially apparent in the study of endocrine glands, since the products of hormone-secreting cells are antigenic and the generation of specific antisera poses no major problems. Another advantage of investigating endocrine glands is the fact that hormones are usually stored in large quantities in the cell cytoplasm, thus their localization is easier than that of other nonhormonal tissue antigens. In the last decade, numerous works have been published which dealt with immunocytologic findings related to endocrine glands. In these studies, various immunocytologic techniques were used and a deeper insight was obtained into structure-function relationships.

In the last few years, the application of immunocytologic procedures became popular among pathologists who realized that the immunocytologic approach has great potential in the better understanding of the pathogenesis of various lesions. The value of immunocytology is obvious in diagnostic tumor pathology. Tumors may have specific antigens, thus attempts can be made to distinguish between neoplastic and nonneoplastic cells. Since various tumor types may possess different antigenic markers, the primary site and cellular origin of the tumor may be established. Endocrine tumors may contain hormones in large concentrations facilitating the disclosure of their function and cytogenesis.

However, one must take into consideration that several factors may cause difficulties in the interpretation of findings. Some endocrine tumors release their hormones at an accelerated rate and the cells do not store the secretory products in sufficient amounts to permit their identification. Hormones produced by tumor cells may differ in antigenicity from those of normal cells; hence, no immunopositivity can be demonstrated by specific antisera raised against the hormonal products of normal cells. It may be that abnormal hormones are produced which cross react with some antisera, resulting in misleading conclusions.

It was regarded as a principal law in endocrinology that a hormone can only be synthesized by one single cell type and, furthermore, that a cell type is capable of producing only one hormone. Based on recent findings, this cornerstone of classic endocrinology requires revision. It became increasingly evident that a hormone can be produced by a variety of cell types, even under normal conditions and not only in tumors. Somatostatin is synthesized in the hypothalamus but also in normal and neoplastic pancreatic islets, certain carcinoid tumors, hypothalamic gangliocytomas and medullary carcinomas of the thyroid. It is well established that several tumors, such as pancreatic islet cell neoplasms, carcinoid tumors and pituitary adenomas are capable of synthesizing multiple hormones. Tumors arising in cells traditionally regarded as not belonging to the endocrine system can secrete hormones and cause clinical symptoms. In the last decade, much progress was made in achieving a deeper insight into the prevalence and diagnosis of ectopic hormone syndromes. Hence, great caution is advised when one wants to interpret immunocytologic findings and resolve the cytogenesis of a tumor.

There are two principal techniques which are used in immunocytologic studies: 1) immunofluorescence; 2) immunoperoxidase method. Although immunofluorescence techniques are widely applied, it appears that immunoperoxidase methods are gradually gaining ground and replacing previously favored immunofluroescence procedures. The immunoperoxidase techniques undoubtedly have advantages: formalin-fixed and paraffin-embedded tissue can be utilized; there is no need to make fresh frozen sections or to apply a fluorescence microscope. The sections are permanent and easier to store. Several modifications are described in the literature; currently the avidin-biotin-peroxidase complex (ABC) technique (1,2) is recommended. The immunoperoxidase methods can be applied at the electron microscopic level; immunoelectron microscopy is a time-consuming but sensitive technique for reliable identification of various hormones. Autopsy material is also suitable for immunocytologic investigation. Tissues fixed in formalin, embedded in paraffin and stored for several years can be immunostained; this approach opens considerable opportunities for retrospective pathologic studies. The technical details of various immunoperoxidase techniques will not be dealt with here.

The immunocytologic study of various endocrine tumors progressed so rapidly in the last few years that it is impossible to summarize the accumulated knowledge briefly in this chapter. Thus, only a short summary of recent findings will be given here, focusing mainly on diagnostic aspects which may be of interest in service pathology. There are a large number of excellent papers dealing with various areas of immunocytology of endocrine tumors. We cannot quote all of them; only a few pertinent review are included in the bibliography (3,4,5,6,7,8,9,10). This field is expanding and changing so rapidly that publications soon become obsolete.

This chapter is limited to human pathology and immunocytologic features of endocrine tumors of various animal species will not be dealt with here. Only tumors are included; no reference will be made to normal conditions or different non-neoplastic lesions. Hormone-producing tumors arise either in endocrine glands or in some special cases in non-endocrine organs. Hormone secretion in the former tumors is termed eutopic, whereas in the latter ones, ectopic. The distinction between eutopic and ectopic hormone secretion is not always clear and, to some extent, is arbitrary, since genetic information may be encoded, but repressed in normal cells and hormone production becomes manifest only after neoplastic transformation. A great variety of hormones can be produced ectopically and can be associated with diverse clinical symptoms and biochemical abnormalities. Neoplasms producing hormones ectopically are of great interest both theoretically and practically, since the hormones produced can be used as markers facilitating the correct diagnosis and the disclosure of the primary site and cellular origin of the tumor.

The following tumors are included in this chapter: 1) tumors of the hypothalamus; 2) tumors of the posterior pituitary; 3) tumors of the anterior pituitary; 4) tumors of the corpus pineale; 5) tumors of the thyroid; 6) tumors of the parathyroid; 7) tumors of the thymus; 8) tumors of the adrenal medulla; 9) tumors of the steroid-producing endocrine tissues; 10) tumors producing hormones ectopically; 11) tumors containing hormone receptors; 12) tumors containing hormone precursors or hormone fragments.

Tumors of the Hypothalamus.

Hamartomas or gangliocytomas, arising in the hypothalamus, can secrete various hypothalamic hormones and be associated with diverse clinical symptoms. Somatoliberin (GRF or GRH) producing hypothalamic gangliocytomas have been reported accompanied by growth hormone cell adenoma of the pituitary, excessive growth hormone secretion and acromegaly (11,12,13). Recently, somatoliberin has been demonstrated in these tumors by immunocytologic techniques (11). Gonadoliberin (GnRH or LRH) producing hypothalamic hamartomas are known to cause precocious puberty (14,15). The endocrine symptoms and biochemical abnormalities regress following surgical removal of the hypothalamic tumor (15). Immunocytologic studies of the tumors have revealed the presence of gonadoliberin in the cytoplasm of neoplastic nerve cells, underlining the pathogenetic role of this hypothalamic hormone in the causation of endocrine abnormalities (14,15). Corticoliberin (CRF or CRH) producing hypothalamic hamartomas have been found to be associated with Cushing's syndrome (16). It was suggested that corticoliberin released from neoplastic nerve cells results in increased pituitary ACTH secretion, corticotroph hyperplasia and cortisol excess (16). The presence of somatostatin has been detected by immunocytologic techniques in several cases of hypothalamic gangliocytoma (11,17). The endocrine significance of this intriguing finding has yet to be elucidated.

Tumors of the Posterior Pituitary.

Tumors arising from the posterior lobe are uncommon and, to our knowledge, have not been described in association with increased production of vasopressin, oxytocin, or any other hormone (18,19). Gliomas or granular cell tumors deriving from the neurohypophysis may contain nonhormonal markers, such as glial fibrillary acidic protein or S-100 protein (20); the discussion of these findings are beyond the scope of this review.

Tumors of the Anterior Pituitary.

Tumors originating in the adenohypophysis are not uncommon; they represent about 15% of intracranial neoplasms and can be detected in approximately 10-20% of unselected autopsy cases (21). Immunocytologic features of pituitary adenomas have been reported in detail recently (22,23,24,25,26,27), thus only a short summary of the main findings will be given here.

According to current knowledge, 5 distinct cell types can be demonstrated in the human adenohypophysis: 1) somatotrophs, 2) lactotrophs, 3) corticotrophs, 4) thyrotrophs and 5) gonadotrophs. All 5 cell types can give rise to adenoma. The immunoperoxidase technique is very useful in defining cellular composition, hormone production and, combined with ultrastructural studies, the cytogenesis of pituitary tumors.

Somatotroph adenomas contain growth hormone which can be demonstrated in the cell cytoplasm by immunocytologic techniques. Lactotroph adenomas contain prolactin, corticotroph adenomas ACTH and various fragments of the proopiomelanocortin molecule, thyrotroph adenomas TSH, and gonadotroph adenomas FSH and/or LH. Some clinically non-functioning adenomas mainly contain α-subunit.

Null cell adenomas are unassociated with clinical symptoms and laboratory alterations indicating hormone excess. They lack biochemical and morphologic markers; immunocytologic procedures show the absence of all known adenohypophysial hormones in the cytoplasm of adenoma cells. It is worth mentioning that, by electron microscopy, these tumors invariably contain secretory granules in their cytoplasm and possess all the cellular organelles required for hormone secretion. Thus, it is reasonable to assume that they produce certain peptides which are not recognized by the antibodies currently in use; they may be biologically inactive hormone fragments, precursors or unknown hormones.

Based on ultrastructural features, null cell adenomas can be divided into non-oncocytic and oncocytic tumors. The latter variety, called pituitary oncocytoma, is characterized by abundance of mitochondria. By immunocytology, oncocytomas contain no adenohypophysial hormones and are indistinguishable from non-oncocytic null cell adenomas.

In some non-oncocytic and oncocytic null cell adenomas, scattered individual adenoma cells or clusters of adenoma cells show immunopositivity for one or more adenohypophysial hormones, most frequently TSH, FSH, LH, α-subunit or prolactin. This finding is intriguing but difficult to interpret. It may be that hormone synthesis is a sign of functional maturation. These adenomas may originate in a precursor cell which differentiates into a hormone-producing cell line. Alternatively, it is possible, but less likely, that these adenomas arise in mature cells which undergo functional dedifferentiation and lose their capacity for hormone synthesis. According to the latter interpretation, they transform to null cells and discontinue to produce their immunocytologic markers; thus, by immunocytologic techniques, no hormones can be revealed in the cell cytoplasm.

Silent corticotroph adenomas contain ACTH and the related peptides, as shown by immunocytologic techniques, but are unassociated with clinical and biochemical evidence of increased ACTH release. The reason for the discrepancy between clinical and biochemical results and immunocytologic findings is obscure at present. It appears that silent corticotroph adenomas represent heterogeneous tumors which can be divided into various subtypes based on their electron microscopic appearance. Obviously, more work is needed to understand the cytogenesis of these unusual tumors, classify them properly and shed light on why they exhibit positive immunostaining for ACTH and other fragments of the proopiomelanocortin molecule by immunocytologic procedures without causing increased release of ACTH.

Plurihormonal pituitary adenomas produce two or more hormones which are different in chemical composition, immunoreactivity and biologic action. In monomorphous pituitary adenomas, two or more hormones can be demonstrated in the cytoplasm of the same cell type by the immunoperoxidase technique; whereas in plurimorphous pituitary adenomas, two or more separate cell types can be identified each of which contains one distinct immunoreactive hormone. Various combinations may occur, such as growth hormone and TSH - growth hormone, prolactin and TSH - growth hormone, prolactin and ACTH - growth hormone, prolactin and α-subunit, etc. The cellular derivation of these intriguing pituitary tumors is not clear and more investigation is required to obtain a deeper insight into their pathogenesis and secretory activity.

Pituitary carcinomas are exceptionally rare and are difficult to identify on the grounds of their histologic appearance. The diagnosis of pituitary carcinoma is justified only if the presence of distant metastases can be documented. They may produce growth hormone, prolactin or ACTH which can be demonstrated by immunocytologic techniques.

There are several tumors in the sella turcica which can cause clinical symptoms. Craniopharyngiomas, metastatic carcinomas, meningiomas, chordomas, malignant lymphomas and many other neoplasms may be found in the sella region. These tumors do not originate in nor are they composed of adenohypophysial cells; they neither produce nor contain adenohypophysial hormones. Thus, they are negative for all adenohypophysial hormones by immunocytologic techniques and their morphologic features will not be dealt with here. The immunostainings help in the differential diagnosis, since if the results are positive for one or more adenohypophysial hormones, it is evident that one is dealing with a tumor of adenohypophysial cell origin. However, if the tumor is negative, the diagnosis of pituitary adenoma cannot conclusively be excluded for it is known that pituitary null cell adenomas are negative for adenohypophysial hormones by the immunoperoxidase technique.

Tumors of the Corpus Pineale.

Tumors arising in the region of the pineal body are rare. They may be associated with precocious puberty (28,29). In some tumors, immunostaining for HCG may yield positive results (29,30).

Tumors of the Thyroid.

Immunocytology became increasingly valuable in the histopathologic differential diagnosis of various thyroid neoplasms. Many tumors, arising in the follicular epithelium, maintain their ability to produce thyroglobulin. Specific antisera are available against this protein molecule which can be conclusively revealed on formalin-fixed and paraffin-embedded sections (31,32,33,34,35). The demonstration of thyroglobulin is useful in cases of metastatic tumors, such as secondary carcinomas of lung, or bone if the primary site is unknown and thyroid derivation is suspected. The presence of thyroglobulin in these cases proves that the tumor arises in and consists of thyroid follicular cells. However, caution is required in the interpretation of immunocytologic results, since, some cases of thyroid carcinomas, especially the anaplastic ones, lose their capacity to synthesize thyroglobulin. Thus, negative immunohistologic findings do not exclude the possibility of thyroid follicular derivation of a neoplasm.

Medullary carcinomas of the thyroid produce calcitonin which can be conclusively disclosed in formalin-fixed, paraffin-embedded tissue sections (36,37,38,39,40,41). Calcitonin is produced by both non-neoplastic and neoplastic C cells and is a reliable marker of medullary carcinoma of the thyroid. Immunopositivity for calcitonin can confirm the diagnosis of medullary carcinoma of the thyroid, either at its primary site or in secondary deposits outside the thyroid gland. Immunocytologic techniques can distinguish between tumors of follicular cell origin, which are positive for thyroglobulin and negative for calcitonin and those of C cell origin, which are positive for calcitonin and negative for thyroglobulin. Recent results seem to indicate that certain tumors consist of a mixture of follicular cells and C cells (42,43,44,45). The cytogenesis of these tumors is not understood. It may be that they arise in a stem cell which can differentiate in two directions: one cell line producing thyroglobulin, the other, calcitonin. Caution is also advised in the differential diagnosis between medullary carcinomas of the thyroid and some extrathyroid tumors which may produce calcitonin, such as pheochromocytomas, pancreatic islet cell tumors or small cell carcinomas of the lung. Since some of these tumors may give distinct immunostaining for calcitonin, positive calcitonin immunoreactivity does not necessarily prove that the tumor has originated in C cells of the thyroid gland. Medullary carcinomas of the thyroid are often plurihormonal and produce several other hormones or proteins, such as ACTH, somatostatin, carcinoembryonic antigen, etc (39,41,46,47,48). These substances can also be used as markers and can be demonstrated by immunocytologic techniques. In contrast to tumors of follicular cell origin, medullary carcinomas of the thyroid show positive immunostaining for neuron specific enolase (41) and chromogranin (49,50) markers of various endocrine cells believed to belong to the APUD cell system.

Calcitonin immunostaining can be useful in the diagnosis of C cell hyperplasia (38,39,51,52,53). Accumulation of C cells in the nontumorous portion of the thyroid occurs in the familial form of medullary carcinoma and can be documented, in some cases in several members of the family, preceding the development of medullary carcinoma. Thus, the demonstration of C cell hyperplasia in the nontumorous thyroid, in patients with medullary carcinoma, should call attention to the fact that the disease may be familial. Identification of C cell hyperplasia may help to select patients in the family that may develop medullary carcinoma. Although the monitoring of these patients can be most effectively undertaken by measuring serum calcitonin levels, demonstration of C cell hyperplasia by immunocytologic methods has practical significance. However, one must be aware of the fact that C cell hyperplasia may develop in aging patients, in patients with long-standing hypercalcemia and hyperparathyroidism (38,54,55). Thus, demonstration of C cell hyperplasia does not necessarily mean a preneoplastic condition and does not prove that family members are prone to develop medullary carcinoma of the thyroid.

Recent studies seem to indicate that the immunoperoxidase technique can reveal the presence of thyroid hormones, thyroxine and triiodothyronine in follicular cell tumors of the human thyroid (56).

Tumors of the Parathyroid.

A few recent reports describe the immunocytochemical demonstration of various molecular forms of parathyroid hormone in tissue sections (57,58, 59). Immunopositivity can be disclosed in non-neoplastic, hyperplastic and adenomatous parathyroid cells; thus the application of immunostaining does not seem to be valuable in the differential diagnosis between hyperplasia and neoplasia. Immunocytologic methods can be useful in revealing the primary site of those secondary tumors which are suspected to originate in the parathyroid gland. In these rare cases, the demonstration of parathyroid hormone in the cytoplasm of tumor cells may prove the diagnosis of parathyroid carcinoma. Parathyroid adenoma cells exhibit positive immunostaining for chromogranin, a recently applied marker for a variety of endocrine cells (49,50).

Tumors of the Thymus.

Some of the endocrine tumors of the thymus may produce ACTH or other peptide hormones which can be demonstrated by immunostaining (60,61). Thymic carcinoids exhibit positive immunostaining for neuron specific enolase (60,62). However, the reliability of immunostaining for this enzyme has been questioned recently (63).

Tumors of the Adrenal Medulla.

Pheochromocytomas produce catecholamine hormones, such as epinephrine or adrenaline, and norepinephrine or noradrenaline. Recent evidence indicates that these tumors, in addition to catecholamines, may contain different peptides, which can be detected by immunocytologic methods. Calcitonin, vasoactive intestinal polypeptide, somatostatin, ACTH and other proopio-melanocortin-derived peptides have been identified in pheochromocytoma cells (64,65,66). However, their demonstration at present is primarily of academic significance and has little practical value. Nontumorous cells of the adrenal medulla and pheochromocytoma cells can be immunostained for chromogranin (49,50). More work is required to establish the value of this new immunocytologic marker in the diagnosis of pheochromocytomas.

Tumors of the Pancreatic Islets.

Like cells of the nontumorous islets of Langerhans (67) the substantial majority of pancreatic endocrine tumors produce insulin, glucagon, somatostatin or a combination of these 3 hormones which can be demonstrated conclusively by immunocytologic methods (68,69,70). Hence, the clinical and biochemical diagnosis of insulin, glucagon or somatostatin-producing tumors can be confirmed. The immunocytologic approach is useful in the presence of secondary tumors with unknown primary sites. The identification of insulin, glucagon or somatostatin confirms the diagnosis of an endocrine tumor, most probably originating in the pancreas. However, in cases of positive somatostatin immunostaining, the primary site cannot be proven unequivocally, since somatostatin can be synthesized by certain extrapancreatic neoplasms.

Several hormones can be produced ectopically by pancreatic islet cell tumors. The secretion of gastrin by pancreatic endocrine tumors and the Zollinger-Ellison syndrome, the clinical manifestations of gastrin excess are well known (68,71). A large number of other hormones, such as ACTH, calcitonin, vasoactive intestinal polypeptide, pancreatic polypeptide, growth hormone, somatoliberin, corticoliberin, thyroliberin, etc. can be produced by pancreatic islet cell tumors and demonstrated by immunocytologic techniques (68,72,73,74).

It appears that many islet cell tumors are plurihormonal; they are capable of producing several hormones (69). These tumors may arise in the epithelial cells of the ductules which serve as undifferentiated precursors of islets and, due to multidirectional differentiation, mature to islet cells. The various hormones can be revealed in one cell or in different cell types. In 1980 Asa et al. (72) reported a pancreatic islet cell carcinoma that produced gastrin, ACTH, β-endorphin, somatostatin and calcitonin. The cytogenesis of these plurihormonal pancreatic endocrine tumors is obscure.

Pancreatic islet cells and islet cell tumors have been shown to give positive immunostaining for neuron specific enolase (75,76,77) and it was proposed that the demonstration of this enzyme by immunocytology is valuable in distinguishing between neuron specific enolase positive endocrine tumors and neuron specific enolase negative non-endocrine tumors (75). However, it became evident that not all endocrine tumors are positive and some non-endocrine tumors may give positive immunostaining for this enzyme (63). Thus, the usefulness of neuron specific enolase in diagnostic histopathology is uncertain at present. Recent investigations show that chromogranin can be used as a marker for the endocrine tumors of the pancreas (49,50,77).

Tumors of the Steroid-producing Endocrine Tissues.

The adrenal cortex, the Leydig cell of the testis and the endocrine cells of the ovary produce various steroid hormones. The main classes are the various corticosteroids, such as cortisol and aldosterone, the sex steroids including androgens such as testosterone and dehydroepiandrosterone, estrogens such as estradiol, estrone and estriol as well as gestagens such as progesterone. Although immunocytologic techniques appear to be promising in the demonstration of these steroid hormones, several technical problems have to be resolved before they can gain wide acceptance in diagnostic pathology. Steroid hormones are not stored in large quantities in the cells; they are dissolved during the embedding procedure and can no longer be demonstrated by immunocytology. Recent evidence however, seems to indicate that various steroids can be localized in certain gonadal tumors (78,79,80,81,82). Although only a few studies have been reported so far, we predict that with further advances in methodology, this area will progress rapidly in the coming years and immunocytologic techniques will be of great value in the differential diagnosis of tumors capable of synthesizing various steroids.

Tumors Producing Hormones Ectopically.

The concept that hormones can only be synthesized in a specific cell type located in one single organ, has been challenged by the discovery of tumors secreting hormones ectopically (7,83,84,85,86,87,88,89). It became increasingly clear that the endocrine system is more complicated, and more widespread; tumor cells not regarded as deriving from the endocrine system can produce different hormones and endocrine cells assumed to synthesize one specific hormone may produce more than one hormone. There are several theories to explain ectopic hormone production, but they are beyond the scope of this review. Suffice it to say that various tumors, classified as non-endocrine neoplasms, can produce different hormones. Small cell arcinomas of the lung or prostate, medullary carcinomas of the thyroid, intestinal, bronchial, thymic carcinoids, etc. can produce ACTH and lead to rapidly progressing, severe hypercorticism. This syndrome, termed ectopic ACTH syndrome, is diagnosed with increasing frequency. Carcinoid tumors can produce a great variety of biologically active compounds, such as 5-hydroxytryptamine,

ACTH, somatoliberin, etc. Vasopressin excess or inappropriate ADH secretion or Schwartz-Bartter syndrome has been observed in association with various tumors, primarily carcinoma of the lung. Hypercalcemia, a not uncommon abnormality of cancer patients, has been attributed to the secretion of various hormones or peptides by tumor cells. Some tumors may produce several hormones ectopically, leading to unusual endocrine symptoms which are difficult to diagnose. Immunocytologic techniques have a fundamental role in exploring these intriguing tumors and conclusively demonstrating their products (7). It should be emphasized, however, that specific antibodies, appropriate tissue preservation and processing as well as rigorous control procedures are needed to achieve reliable results. One must keep in mind that without a critical attitude, erroneous conclusions can easily be drawn.

It is evident that many hormone-producing cells exist outside those endocrine organs which were traditionally classified as endocrine glands (3, 10,90,91,92,93) and were discussed above. These cells, located in the gastrointestinal tract, endometrium, lung, breast, prostate, ect. can synthesize different hormones and give rise to various neoplasms (3,9,10, 90). Tumors originating in these cells may retain their capability of hormone secretion leading to different endocrine symptoms. Immunocytology can be valuable in recognizing these tumors and unraveling their cytogenesis. Tissue stored for several years in formalin or embedded in paraffin can be used for hormone exploration. Such retrospective pathology will help to elucidate functional activity of those endocrine tumors which produce hormones unknown at present. Many pathology departments which have adequate funding to establish tissue banks collect tumors stored in paraffin for future testing. If a new antibody becomes available, the paraffin blocks can be retrieved, sections can be cut and immunostained for the newly discovered hormone.

Tumors Containing Hormone Receptors.

The demonstration of hormone receptors by immunocytology is a promising but controversial area of research at present (94,95,96) which will gain popularity. Various steroid receptors can be detected in different tissues and tumors by radioimmunoassay and immunocytochemistry (97,98,99,100,101, 102,103,104,105,106); their demonstration is valuable in predicting the prognosis and responsiveness of some tumors to different treatment modalities (103,104,105,107,108,109). The morphologic identification of hormone receptors is currently in an initial stage, but substantial advances can be expected in the coming years. Preliminary investigations have been made to localize protein and peptide hormone receptors and binding sites, such as somatostatin, FSH, LH, prolactin and dopamine receptors and binding sites by immunocytology (110,111,112,113,114))

Tumors Containing Hormone Precursors or Hormone Fragments.

With the generation of specific antisera against hormone precursors and fragments, one can foresee their immunocytologic demonstration. They include not only various hormone precursor molecules but also intermediary hormone metabolites. Future studies may shed light on multiple steps of hormone synthesis and degradation.

SUMMARY

This review briefly summarizes current knowledge related to immunocytology of endocrine tumors and stresses the usefulness and importance of immunocytologic methods in experimental and service pathology. With the wider availability of antibodies, the immunocytologic approach will expand rapidly and will contribute substantially to the diagnosis and the better understanding of cytogenesis of endocrine tumors.

The horizons of immunocytology are unlimited. We are convinced that it will continue to revolutionize experimental and service pathology and will provide new insights into the clinicopathologic correlations of tumors originating in hormone-producing cells.

ACKNOWLEDGEMENT

This work was supported in part by Grant MT-6349 of the Medical Research Council of Canada and the Physicians of Ontario through the P.S.I. Foundation. The author wishes to thank Dr. Eva Horvath, Mrs. Gezina Ilse and Mrs. Nancy Ryan for their invaluable contribution throughout this study, and Mrs. Wanda Wlodarski for excellent secretarial work.

References

1. Hsu SM, Raine L, Fanger H: A comparative study of the peroxidase-antiperoxidase method and an avidin-biotin complex method for studying polypeptide hormones with radioimmunoassay antibodies. Am J Clin Pathol(75): 734-738, 1981.

2. Hsu SM, Raine L, Fanger H: The use of antiavidin antibody and avidin-biotin-peroxidase complex in immunoperoxidase technics. Am J Clin Pathol(75): 816-821, 1981.
3. Welbourn RB: Current status of the apudomas. Ann Surg(185): 1-12, 1977.
4. DeLellis RA, Sternberger LA, Mann RB, Banks PM, Nakane PK: Immunoperoxidase technics in diagnostic pathology. Report of a workshop sponsored by the National Cancer Institute. Am J Clin Pathol(71): 483-488, 1979.
5. Mukai K, Rosai J: Applications of immunoperoxidase techniques in surgical pathology. Progr Surg Pathol(1): 15-49, 1980.
6. DeLellis RA: Diagnostic immunohistochemistry in tumor pathology: an overview. In: DeLellis RA (ed) Diagnostic immunohistochemistry. Masson, New York, 1981, pp 1-5.
7. Heitz PU, Kloppel G, Polak JM, Staub JJ: Ectopic hormone production by endocrine tumors: localization of hormones at the cellular level by immunocytochemistry. Cancer(48): 2029-2037, 1981.
8. Taylor CR, Kledzik G: Immunohistologic techniques in surgical pathology. A spectrum of "new" special stains. Human Pathol(12): 590-596, 1981.
9. Gould VE, DeLellis RA: The neuroendocrine cell system: its tumors, hyperplasias and dysplasias. In: Silverberg SG (ed) Principles and practice of surgical pathology. Wiley and Sons, New York, 1983, pp 1487-1501.
10. DeLellis RA, Tischler AS, Wolfe HJ: Multidirectional differentiation in neuroendocrine neoplasms. J Histochem Cytochem(32): 899-904, 1984.
11. Asa SL, Scheithauer BW, Bilbao JM, Horvath E, Ryan N, Kovacs K, Randall RV, Laws ERJr, Singer W, Linfoot JA, Thorner MO, Vale W: A case for hypothalamic acromegaly: a clinicopathological study of six patients with hypothalamic gangliocytomas producing growth hormone-releasing factor. J Clin Endocrinol Metab(58): 796-803, 1984.
12. Scheithauer BW, Kovacs K, Randall RV, Horvath E, Okazaki H, Laws ERJr: Hypothalamic neuronal hamartoma and adenohypophyseal neuronal choristoma: their association with growth hormone adenoma of the pituitary. J Neuropathol Exp Neurol(42): 648-663, 1983.
13. Asa SL, Bilbao JM, Kovacs K, Linfoot JA: Hypothalamic neuronal hamartoma associated with pituitary growth hormone cell adenoma and acromegaly. Acta Neuropathol(52): 231-234, 1980.
14. Judge DM, Kulin HE, Page R, Santen R, Trapukdi S: Hypothalamic hamartoma: a source of luteinizing hormone-releasing factor in precocious puberty. New Engl J Med(296): 7-10, 1977.
15. Price RA, Lee PA, Albright AL, Ronnekleiv OK, Gutai JP: Treatment of sexual precocity by removal of a luteinizing hormone-releasing hormone secreting hamartoma. J Am Med Ass(251): 2247-2249, 1984.
16. Asa SL, Kovacs K, Tindall GT, Barrow DL, Horvath E, Vecsei P: Cushing's disease associated with an intrasellar gangliocytoma producing corticotrophin-releasing factor. Ann Intern Med, in press.
17. Rhodes RH, Dusseau JJ, Boyd ASJr, Knigge KM: Intrasellar neural-adenohypophyseal choristoma: a morphological and immunocytochemical study. J Neuropathol Exp Neurol(41): 267-280, 1982.
18. Sheehan HL, Kovacs K: Neurohypophysis and hypothalamus. In: Bloodworth JMBJr (ed) Endocrine pathology. Williams and Wilkins, Baltimore, 1982, pp 45-99.
19. Kovacs K: Pathology of the neurohypophysis. In: Reichlin S (ed) The neurohypophysis. Physiological and clinical aspects. Plenum, New York, 1984, pp 95-113.

20. Bonnin JM, Rubinstein LJ: Immunohistochemistry of central nervous system tumors. Its contributions to neurosurgical diagnosis. J Neurosurg(60): 1121-1133, 1984.
21. McComb DJ, Ryan N, Horvath E, Kovacs K: Subclinical adenomas of the human pituitary. New light on old problems. Arch Pathol Lab Med(107): 488-491, 1983.
22. Horvath E, Kovacs K: Pathology of the pituitary gland. In: Ezrin C, Horvath E, Kaufman B, Kovacs K, Weiss MH (eds) Pituitary diseases. CRC Press, Boca Raton, 1980, pp 1-83.
23. Kovacs K, Horvath E, Ryan N: Immunocytology of the human pituitary. In: DeLellis RA (ed) Diagnostic immunohistochemistry. Masson, New York, 1981, pp 17-35.
24. Kovacs K, Horvath E: Pathology of pituitary adenomas. In: Givens JR (ed) Hormone secreting pituitary tumors. Yearbook Med Publ, Chicago, 1982, pp. 97-118.
25. Kovacs K, Horvath E: The pituitary. In: Silverberg SG (ed) Principles and practice of surgical pathology. Wiley and Sons, New York, 1983, pp 1393-1414.
26. Kovacs K, McComb DJ, Horvath E: Subcellular investigation of experimental and human pituitary adenomas. Neuroendocr Perspect(2): 251-291, 1983.
27. Scheithauer BW: Surgical pathology of the pituitary: the adenomas. Part I. Pathol Annu(19) Part I: 317-374, 1984.
28. Sklar CA, Conte FA, Kaplan SL, Grumbach MM: Human chorionic gonadotropin-secreting pineal tumor: relation to pathogenesis and sex limitation of sexual precocity. J Clin Endocrinol Metab(53): 656-660, 1981.
29. Laidler P, Pounder DJ: Pineal germinoma with syncytiotrophoblastic giant cells: a case with panhypopituitarism and isosexual pseudopuberty. Human Pathol(15): 285-287, 1984.
30. Sano K: Pineal region tumors: problems in pathology and treatment. Clin Neurosurg(30): 59-91, 1983.
31. Burt A, Goudie RB: Diagnosis of primary thyroid carcinoma by immunohistological demonstration of thyroglobulin. Histopathology(3):279-286,1979.
32. Böcker W, Dralle H, Hüsselmann H, Bay V, Brassow M: Immunohistochemical analysis of thyroglobulin synthesis in thyroid carcinomas. Virchows Arch Pathol Anat(385): 187-200, 1980.
33. Böcker W, Dralle H, Dorn G: Thyroglobulin: an immunohistochemical marker in thyroid disease. In: DeLellis RA (ed) Diagnostic immunohistochemistry Masson, New York, 1981, pp 37-59.
34. Permanetter W, Nathrath WBJ, Lohrs U: Immunohistochemical analysis of thyroglobulin and keratin in benign and malignant thyroid tumours. Virchows Arch Pathol Anat(398): 221-228, 1982.
35. Albores-Saavedra J, Nadji M, Civantos F, Morales AR: Thyroglobulin in carcinoma of the thyroid: an immunohistochemical study. Human Pathol(14): 62-66, 1983.
36. Kameda Y, Harada T, Ito K, Ikeda A: Immunohistochemical study of the medullary thyroid carcinoma with reference to C-thyroglobulin reaction of tumor cells. Cancer(44): 2071-2082, 1979.
37. Deftos LJ, Bone HG III, Parthemore JG: Immunohistological studies of medullary thyroid carcinoma and C cell hyperplasia. J Clin Endocrinol Metab(51): 857-862, 1980.
38. LiVolsi VA: Calcitonin: the hormone and its significance. Progr Surg Pathol(1): 71-103, 1980.
39. DeLellis RA, Wolfe HJ: Calcitonin immunohistochemistry. In: DeLellis RA

(ed) Diagnostic immunohistochemistry. Masson, New York, 1981, pp 61-74.
40. Charpin C, Andrac L, Monier-Faugere MC, Hassoun J, Cannoni M, Vagneur JP, Toga M: Calcitonin, somatostatin and ACTH immunoreactive cells in a case of familial bilateral thyroid medullary carcinoma. Cancer(50): 1806-1814, 1982.
41. Lloyd RV, Sisson JC, Marangos PJ: Calcitonin, carcinoembryonic antigen and neuron-specific enolase in medullary thyroid carcinoma. An immunohistochemical study. Cancer(51): 2234-2239, 1983.
42. Valenta LJ, Michel-Bechet M, Mattson JC, Singer FR: Microfollicular thyroid carcinoma with amyloid rich stroma, resembling the medullary carcinoma of the thyroid (MCT). Cancer(39): 1573-1586, 1977.
43. Hales M, Rosenau W, Okerlund MD, Galante M: Carcinoma of the thyroid with a mixed medullary and follicular pattern. Morphologic, immunohistochemical and clinical laboratory studies. Cancer(50): 1352-1359, 1982.
44. Ljungberg O, Ericsson U-B, Bondeson L, Thorell J: A compound follicular-parafollicular cell carcinoma of the thyroid: a new tumor entity? Cancer(52): 1053-1061, 1983.
45. Pfaltz M, Hedinger CE, Mühlethaler JP: Mixed medullary and follicular carcinoma of the thyroid. Virchows Arch Pathol Histol(400): 53-59,1983.
46. Kameya T, Shimosato Y, Adachi I, Abe K, Kasai N, Kimura K, Baba K: Immunohistochemical and ultrastructural analysis of medullary carcinoma of the thyroid in relation to hormone production. Am J Pathol(89): 555-574, 1977.
47. Sundler F, Alumets J, Hakanson R, Björklund L, Ljungberg O: Somatostatin-immunoreactive cells in medullary carcinoma of the thyroid. Am J Pathol(88): 381-386, 1977.
48. DeLellis RA, Rule AH, Spiler I, Nathanson L, Tashjian AHJr, Wolfe HJ: Calcitonin and carcinoembryonic antigen as tumor markers in medullary thyroid carcinoma. Am J Clin Pathol(70): 587-594, 1978.
49. Lloyd RV, Wilson BS: Specific endocrine marker defined by a monoclonal antibody. Science(222): 628-630, 1983.
50. Wilson BS, Lloyd RV: Detection of chromogranin in neuroendocrine cells with a monoclonal antibody. Am J Pathol(115): 458-468, 1984.
51. Graze K, Spiler IJ, Tashjian AHJr, Melvin KEW, Cervi-Skinner S, Gagel RF, Miller HH, Wolfe HJ, DeLellis RA, Leape L, Feldman ZT, Reichlin S: Natural history of familial medullary thyroid carcinoma. Effect of a program for early diagnosis. New Engl J Med(299): 980-985, 1978.
52. Mendelsohn G, Eggleston JC, Weisburger WR, Gann DS, Baylin SB: Calcitonin and histaminase in C-cell hyperplasia and medullary thyroid carinoma. A light microscopic and immunohistochemical study. Am J Pathol(92): 35-52, 1978.,
53. Gibson WGH, Peng TC, Croker BP: C-cell nodules in adult human thyroid. A common autopsy finding. Am J Clin Pathol(75): 347-350, 1981.
54. LiVolsi VA, Feind CR, LoGerfo P, Tashjian AHJr: Demonstration by immunoperoxidase staining of hyperplasia of parafollicular cells in the thyroid gland in hyperparathyroidism. J Clin Endocrinol Metab(37): 550-559, 1973.
55. Gibson WGH, Peng T-C, Croker BP: Age-associated C-cell hyperplasia in the human thyroid. Am J Pathol(106): 388-393, 1982.
56. Kawaoi A, Okano T, Nemoto N, Shiina Y, Shikata T: Simultaneous detection of thyroglobulin (Tg), thyroxine (T_4) and triiodothyronine (T_3) in nontoxic thyroid tumors by the immunoperoxidase method. Am J Pathol(108): 39-49, 1982.

57. Futrell JM, Roth SI, Su SPC, Habener JF, Segre GV, Potts JTJr: Immunocytochemical localization of parathyroid hormone in bovine parathyroid glands and human parathyroid adenomas. Am J Pathol(94): 615-622, 1979.
58. Ordonez NG, Ibanez MD, Mackay B, Samaan NA, Hickey RC: Functioning oxyphil cell adenomas in parathyroid gland: evidence of hormonal activity in oxyphil cells. Am J Clin Pathol(78): 681-689, 1982.
59. Ordonez NG, Ibanez ML, Samaan NA, Hickey RC: Immunoperoxidase study of uncommon parathyroid tumors. Report of two cases of nonfunctioning parathyroid carcinoma and one intrathyroid parathyroid tumor-producing amyloid. Am J Surg Pathol(7): 535-542, 1983.
60. Huntracoon M, Lin F, Heitz PU, Tomita T: Thymic carcinoid tumor with Cushing's syndrome. Report of a case with electron microscopic and immunoperoxidase studies for neuron-specific enolase and corticotropin. Arch Pathol Lab Med(108): 551-554, 1984.
61. Wick MR, Scheithauer BW: Thymic carcinoid. A histologic, immunohistochemical,and ultrastructural study of 12 cases. Cancer(53): 475-484, 1984.
62. Wick MR, Scheithauer BW, Kovacs K: Neuron-specific enolase in neuroendocrine tumors in the thymus, bronchus and skin. Am J Clin Pathol(79): 703-707, 1983.
63. Vinores SA, Bonnin JM, Rubinstein LJ, Marangos PJ: Immunohistochemical demonstration of neuron-specific enolase in neoplasms of the CNS and other tissues. Arch Pathol Lab Med(108): 536-540, 1984.
64. Sano T, Saito H, Inaba H, Hizawa K, Saito S, Yamanoi A, Mizunuma Y, Matsumura M, Yuasa M, Hiraishi K: Immunoreactive somatostatin and vasoactive intestinal polypeptide in adrenal pheochromocytoma. An immunochemical and ultrastructural study. Cancer(52): 282-289, 1983.
65. Hassoun J, Monges G, Giraud P, Henry JF, Charpin C, Payan H, Toga M: Immunohistochemical study of pheochromocytomas. An investigation of methionine-enkephalin, vasoactive intestinal peptide, somatostatin, corticotropin, β-endorphin, and calcitonin in 16 tumors. Am J Pathol(114): 56-63, 1984.
66. Lloyd RV, Shapiro B, Sisson JC, Kalff V, Thompson NW, Beierwaltes WA: An immunohistochemical study of pheochromocytomas. Arch Pathol Lab Med(108): 541-544, 1984.
67. Mukai K: Functional pathology of pancreatic islets: immunocytochemical exploration. Pathol Annu 18(part 2): 87-107, 1983.
68. Dayal Y, O'Briain DS: The pathology of the pancreatic endocrine cells. In: DeLellis RA (ed) Diagnostic immunohistochemistry. Masson, New York, 1981, pp 111-135.
69. Heitz PU, Kasper M, Polak JM, Kloppel G: Pancreatic endocrine tumors: immunocytochemical analysis of 125 tumors. Human Pathol(13): 263-271, 1982.
70. Mukai K, Grotting JC, Greider MH, Rosai J: Retrospective study of 77 pancreatic endocrine tumors using the immunoperoxidase method. Am J Surg Pathol(6): 387-399, 1982.
71. Solcia E, Capella C, Buffa R, Frigerio B, Fiocca R: Pathology of the Zollinger-Ellison syndrome. Progr Surg Pathol(1): 119-133, 1980.
72. Asa SL, Kovacs K, Killinger DW, Marcon N, Platts M: Pancreatic islet cell carcinoma producing gastrin, ACTH, β-endorphin, somatostatin and calcitonin. Am J Gastroenterol(74): 30-35, 1980.
73. Tomita T, Friesen SR, Kimmel JR, Doull V, Pollock HG: Pancreatic polypeptide-secreting islet-cell tumors. A study of three cases. Am J Pathol(113): 134-142, 1983.

74. Lyons DF, Eisen BR, Clark MR, Pysher TJ, Welsh JD, Kem DC: Concurrent Cushing's and Zollinger-Ellison syndromes in a patient with islet cell carcinoma. Case report and review of the literature. Am J Med(76): 729-733, 1984.
75. Tapia FJ, Polak JM, Barbosa AJA, Bloom SR, Marangos PJ, Dermody C, Pearse AGE: Neuron-specific enolase produced by neuroendocrine tumours. Lancet(1): 808-811, 1981.
76. Bishop AE, Polak JM, Facer P, Ferri GL, Marangos PJ, Pearse AGE: Neuron specific enolase: a common marker for the endocrine cells and innervation of the gut and pancreas. Gastroenterology(83): 902-915, 1982.
77. Lloyd RV, Mervak T, Schmidt K, Warner TFCS, Wilson BS: Immunohistochemical detection of chromogranin and neuron-specific enolase in pancreatic endocrine neoplasms. Am J Surg Pathol(8): 607-614, 1984.
78. Kurman RJ, Andrade D, Goebelsmann U, Taylor CR: An immunohistological study of steroid localization in Sertoli-Leydig tumors of the ovary and testis. Cancer(42): 1772-1783, 1978.
79. Taylor CR, Kurman RJ, Warner NE: The potential value of immunohistologic techniques in the classification of ovarian and testicular tumors. Human Pathol(9): 417-427, 1978.
80. Kurman RJ, Goebelsmann U, Taylor CR: Steroid localization in granulosa-theca tumors of the ovary. Cancer(43): 2377-2384, 1979.
81. Kurman RJ, Goebelsmann U, Taylor CR: Localization of steroid hormones in functional ovarian tumors. In: DeLellis RA (ed) Diagnostic immunohistochemistry. Masson, New York, 1981, pp. 137-164.
82. Gaffney EF, Majmudar B, Hertzler GL, Zane R, Furlong B, Breding E: Ovarian granulosa cell tumors - Immunohistochemical localization of estradiol and ultrastructure, with functional correlations. Obstet Gynecol(61): 311-319, 1983.
83. Rees LH, Radcliffe JG: Ectopic hormone production by non-endocrine tumours. Clin Endocrinol(3): 263-299, 1974.
84. Rees LH: The biosynthesis of hormones by non-endocrine tumours: a review. J Endocrinol(67): 143-175, 1975.
85. Baylin SB, Mendelsohn G: Ectopic (inappropriate) hormone production by tumors: mechanisms involved and the biological and clinical implications. Endocr Rev(1): 45-76, 1980.
86. Imura H: Ectopic hormone syndromes. Clin Endocrin Metab(9): 235-260, 1980.
87. Frohman LA: Ectopic hormone production. Am J Med(70): 995-997, 1981.
88. Sommers SC, Gould VE: Endocrine activities of tumors (ectopic hormones). In: Bloodworth JMBJr (ed) Endocrine pathology. Williams and Wilkins, Baltimore, 1982, pp. 221-243.
89. Frohman LA: Ectopic hormone production by tumors: growth hormone-releasing factor. Neuroendocr Perspect(3): 201-224, 1984.
90. Pearse AGE, Polak JM: Endocrine tumours of neural crest origin: neurolophomas, apudomas and the APUD concept. Med Biol(52): 3-18, 1974.
91. Pearse AGE: The APUD cell concept and its implications in pathology. Endocr Pathol Decennial 1966-1975. Sommers SC (ed) Appleton-Century-Crofts, New York, 1975, pp 147-163.
92. Pearse AGE, Takor Takor T: Embryology of the diffuse neuroendocrine system and its relationship to the common peptides. Fed Proc(38): 2288-2294, 1979.
93. Pearse AGE: The APUD concept and hormone production. Clin Endocrin Metab(9): 211-222, 1980.

94. Chamness GC, Mercer WD, McGuire WL: Are histochemical methods for estrogen receptor valid? J Histochem Cytochem(28): 792-798, 1980.
95. Chamness GC, McGuire WL: Questions about histochemical methods for steroid receptors. Arch Pathol Lab Med(106): 53-54, 1982.
96. Panko WB, Mattioli CA, Wheeler TM: Lack of correlation of a histochemical method for estrogen receptor analysis with the biochemical assay results. Cancer(49): 2148-2152, 1982.
97. Kurzon RM, Sternberger LA: Estrogen receptor immunocytochemistry. J Histochem Cytochem(26): 803-808, 1978.
98. Lee SH: Cancer cell estrogen receptor of human mammary carcinoma. Cancer(44): 1-12, 1979.
99. Lee SH: Cellular estrogen and progesterone receptors in mammary carcinoma. Am J Clin Pathol(73): 323-329, 1980.
100. Lee SH: Sex steroid hormone receptors in mammary carcinoma. In: DeLellis RA (ed) Diagnostic immunohistochemistry. Masson, New York, 1981, pp. 149-164.
101. Nenci I: Estrogen receptor cytochemistry in human breast cancer: status and prospects. Cancer(48): 2674-2686, 1981.
102. Taylor CR, Cooper CL: Kurman RJ, Goebelsmann U, Markland FSJr: Detection of estrogen receptor in breast and endometrial carcinoma by the immunoperoxidase technique. Cancer(47): 2634-2640, 1981.
103. Clark GM, McGuire WL: Progesterone receptors and human breast cancer. Breast Cancer Res Treat(3): 157-163, 1983.
104. Saez S, Cheix F, Asselain B: Prognostic value of estrogen and progesterone receptors in primary breast cancer. Breast Cancer Res Treat(3): 345-354, 1983.
105. LeDoussal V, Pichon MF, Pallud C, Hacene K, Gest J, Milgrom E: Relationship between ultrastructure and receptor content of human primary breast cancer. Histopathology(8): 89-103, 1984.
106. Press MF, Greene GL: An immunocytochemical method for demonstrating estrogen receptor in human uterus using monoclonal antibodies to human estrophilin. Lab Invest(50): 480-486, 1984.
107. Antoniades K, Spector H: Correlation of estrogen receptor levels with histology and cytomorphology in human mammary cancer. Am J Clin Pathol(71): 497-503, 1979.
108. Parl FF, Wagner RK: The histopathological evaluation of human breast cancers in correlation with estrogen receptor values. Cancer(46): 362-367, 1980.
109. Walker RA, Cove DH, Howell A: Histological detection of oestrogen receptor in human breast carcinomas. Lancet(1): 171-173, 1980.
110. Goldsmith PC, Cronin MJ, Weiner RI: Dopamine receptor sites in the anterior pituitary. J Histochem Cytochem(27): 1205-1207, 1979.
111. Witorsch RJ: The application of immunoperoxidase methodology for the visualization of prolactin binding sites in human prostate tissue. Human Pathol(10): 521-532, 1979.
112. Childs GV, Hutson JC, Bauer TW: Immunocytochemical detection of hormones at target binding sites. In: DeLellis RA (ed) Diagnostic immunohistochemistry. Masson, New York, 1981, pp. 165-177.
113. Cronin MJ: The role of direct measurement of the dopamine receptor(s) in the anterior pituitary. Neuroendocr Perspect(1): 169-210, 1982.
114. Wahlstrom T, Huhtaniemi I, Hovatta O, Seppala M: Localization of luteinizing hormone, follicle-stimulating hormone, prolactin, and their receptors in human and rat testis using immunohistochemistry and radioreceptor assay. J Clin Endocrinol Metab(57): 825-830, 1983.

12

IMMUNOCYTOCHEMICAL DEMONSTRATION OF CARDIONATRINS IN HUMAN ATRIAL MYOCARDIUM

M.L. de Bold and A.J. de Bold

The bulk of muscle cells of the mammalian heart atria contain elements found in endocrine cells. These elements include a highly developed Golgi complex, a relatively high proportion of rough endoplasmic reticulum and membrane-bound granules referred to as specific atrial granules. Morphologically as well as histochemically these granules resemble storage granules known to store polypeptide hormones (1,2).

It is now known that the presence of atrial granules is due to the fact that the atria of the mammalian heart synthetizes and stores polypeptides - cardionatrins (3,4) - which are powerful diuretic and vasoactive agents. Cardionatrins are synthetized by atrial muscle as a prepropeptide which contains about 150 aminoacids (5,6,7). The exact processing pathway for this peptide is not known but its carboxyl terminal portion which contains a 17-member disulfide loop is essential for biological activity. Several fragments of the prepropeptide have been isolated to date. We first isolated and sequenced (4) a 28 amino acid peptide from rat atria and named it cardionatrin 1 (Fig. 1).

H-Ser-Leu-Arg-Arg-Ser-Ser-Cys-Phe-Gly-Gly-Arg-Ile-Asp-Arg-Ile-

S-S

Gly-Ala-Gln-Ser-Gly-Leu-Gly-Cys-Asn-Ser-Phe-Arg-Tyr-OH

Figure 1. Primary structure of cardionatrin I

The human sequence proved remarkably similar to rat cardionatrin I (8); differing from the latter by only a single amino acid replacement. In the rat prepropeptide, cardionatrin I comprises residues 123 to 150.

We have raised antibodies in rabbits against synthetic rat cardionatrin I coupled to keyhole limpet hemocyanin using carbodiimide as the coupling agent. For the studies presented here human atrial appendages obtained from patients undergoing coronary bypass were fixed in 3% glutaraldehyde. The tissues were dehydrated through graded alcohols and embedded in Epon. Pale gold sections were mounted on nickel grids annd incubated on a drop of half saturated solution of metabisulfite for 5 min. The grids were then washed in the distilled water and treated with 3% hydrogen peroxide for 30 min. After a rapid rinse with water, incubation in 10% normal goat serum for 5 min followed. The grids were then placed for 60 min directly on a drop of rat cardionatrin I antiserum diluted 1:100 to 1:1000 in phosphate buffered saline (PBS) containing 10% normal goat serum. The grids were then washed with PBS, transfered to a drop of 10% normal goat serum for 5 min. and incubated for 60 min in colloidal gold (10 nm)-goat anti-rabbit IgG diluted 1:4 in PBS containing 1% normal goat serum. After thoroughly washing the grids in PBS and water, they were dried, stained with uranyl acetate and lead citrate. The specificity of the immunostain was assessed by omitting the primary antiserum and application of immunogold complex.

As shown in Figs. 2 and 3, immunogold complexes were found mainly in association with specific granules. At higher magnification (Fig. 3) some Golgi complexes showed associated gold complexes indicating that the antibody recognizes granules early in their formation. It is apparent the the antiserum obtained against rat cardionatrin is satisfactory to demonstrate human cardionatrin. In fact, the antiserum used in the present studies demonstrates specific granules on a large variety of both mammalian and non-mammalian species suggesting that the cardionatrin molecule is a highly conserved one from the evolutionary point of view.

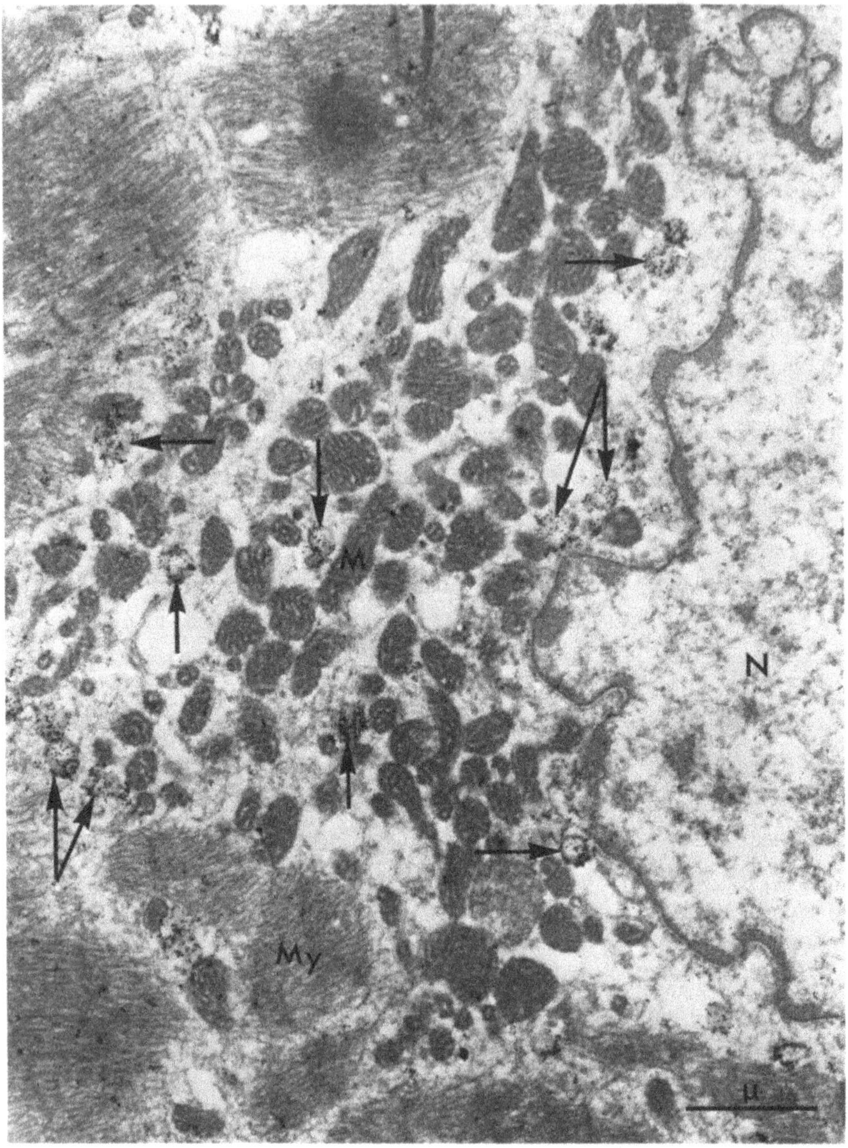

Figure 2. Human atrial cardiocyte. Immunochemical staining with cardionatrin I antiserum. A large number of immunogold complexes are present over the specific atrial granules (arrows). N: nucleus. My: myofibrils. M: mitochondria.

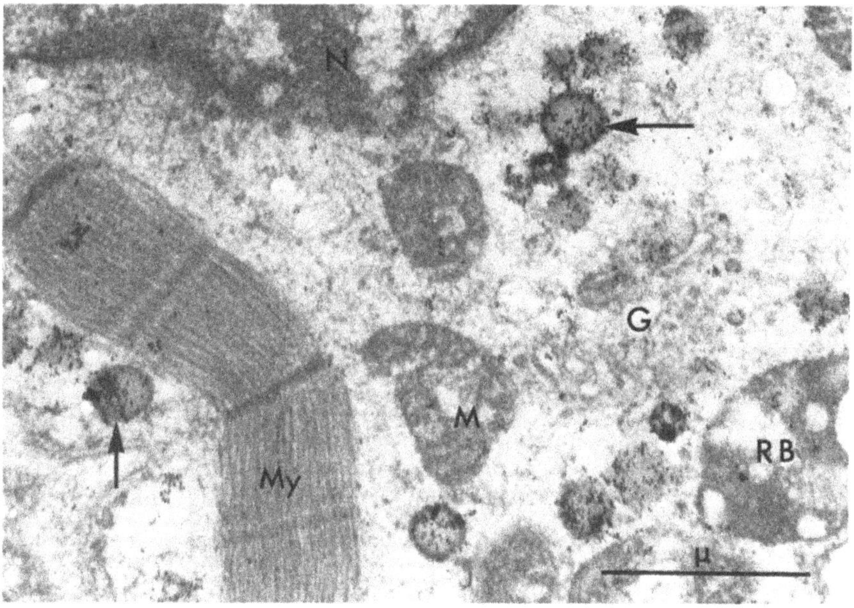

Figure 3. Human Atrial cardiocyte. Immunochemical staining with cardionatrin I antiserum. High magnification of immunogold complexes associated with atrial granules (arrows). Some of these complexes are seen associated with a Golgi complex (G). RB: residual body. M: mitochondria. N: nucleus. My: myofibril. G: Golgi complex.

Although no pathology has been associated as yet with the cardionatrins, their biological actions make them likely of involvement in major clincal entities associated with disturbances in water and electrolyte balance. In addition to their powerful natriuretic (diuretic) and vasodilatory actions, the atrial peptides are potent inhibitors of aldosterone and renin release (9,10). In some experimental animal models such as in the cardiomyopathic hamster (11) and in the spontaneously hypertensive rat (12) significant alteration in tissue levels of the atrial peptides are found.

1. Jamison JD and Palade GE: Specific granules in atrial muscle cells. J. Cell Biol. (23):151-172, 1964.
2. de Bold AJ, Raymond J, Bencosme SA: Atrial specific granules of the rat heart. Light microscopic staining and histochemical reactions. J. Histochem. (26): 1094-1102, 1978.
3. de Bold AJ, and Flynn TG: Cardionatrin I. A novel heart peptide with potent diuretic and natriuretic properties. Life Sciences (33):297-302, 1983.
4. Flynn TG, de Bold ML, de Bold AJ: The amino acid sequence of an atrial peptide with potent diuretic and natriuretic properties. Biochem. Biophys. Res. Commun. (117):859-865, 1983.
5. Kennedy BP, Marsden JJ, Flynn TG, de Bold AJ, Davies PL: Isolation and nucleotide sequence of a cloned cardionatrin cDNA. Biochem. Biophys. Res. Commun. (122):1076-1082, 1984
6. Yamanada M, Greenberg B, Johnson L, Seilhammer J, Friedemann T, Miller J, Atlas S, Laragh J, Lewicki J, Fiddes J: Cloning and sequence analysis of the cDNA for the rat atrial natriuretic factor precursor. Nature (309):724-726, 1984.
7. Oikawa S, Imai M, Veno A, Tanaka S, Noguchi T, Nakazato H, Kangawa K, Fukuola A, Matsuo H: Cloning and sequence analysis of cDNA encoding a precursor for human atrial natriuretic polypeptide. Nature (309):724-726, 1984.
8. Kangawa K, and Matsuo H: Purification and complete amino acid sequence of α-human atrial natriuretic polypeptide (α hANP). Biochem. Biophys. Res. Commun. (118):131-139, 1984.
9. Goodfriend TL, Elliott ME, Atlas SA: Actions of synthetic atrial natriuretic factor on bovine adrenal glomerulosa. Life Sciences (35):1675-1682, 1984.
10. Freeman RH, Davis IO, Vari RC, Sweat WD: The anti-renin/ anti-aldosterone actions of synthetic atrial natriuretic factor in concious dogs with canal constriction and ascites. 17th Annual meeting Amer. Soc. Nephrol., Washington D.C., U.S.A. Dec. 9-12 Abstr. 28, 1 984.
11. Chimoskey JE, Spielman WS, Brandt MA, Heidemann SR: Cardiac atria of Bio 14.6 hamsters are deficient in natriuretic factor. Science (233):820-821, 1984.
12. Sonnenberg H, Milojevic S, Chong CK, Veress AT: Atrial natriuretic factor: reduced cardiac content in spontaneously hypertensive rats. Hypertension (5):672-675, 1984.

13

IMMUNOCYTOCHEMICAL MARKERS IN BREAST CANCER

JOSE RUSSO, M.D.

1. INTRODUCTION

Tumor associated antigens (TAA) are presently used widely as markers of neoplasia and as a help in the evaluation and prognosis of the disease; such is the case with carcinoembryonic antigens (2,3) and alpha fetoprotein (3,5). However, these particular TAA are not specific markers for a given type of cancer, because they can be detected in different kinds of tumors, such as lung carcinoma (1), mucinous ovarian carcinoma (7), as well as in breast carcinomas (9). At the present time, however, no TAA can be considered breast specific. What is needed is a set of immunocytochemical markers that allows us: a) to determine the breast epithelial nature of neoplastic tissues, b) to define the neoplastic characteristics, c) be of prognostic significance and, (d) have therapeutic application. In this review, I will concentrate my attention on the three first topics. The use of monoclonal antibodies as a therapeutic tool has been reviewed by other authors (9-11).

2. HISTOCHEMICAL MARKERS OF BREAST EPITHELIUM

The mammary gland of humans and mammals is composed of two main cell types, epithelial and myoepithelial cells, the latter lying on a basement membrane (12). In Table 1 are depicted the antibodies available against the different components of the breast. Myoepithelial cells are characterized by the presence of filaments of actin and myosin, and present reactivity against these two components (13-15). Bussolati has done extensive studies on the distribution of actin in normal as well as in neoplastic breast tissue. Myoepithelial cells are absent from the lining epithelium of cysts, whereas they are abundant in sclerosing adenosis (16). Their identification using antiactin allows their precise location when entrapped in the sclerosed stroma (17). In the lobular carcinoma in situ the disappearance of myoepithelial cells observed when the process turns invasive is detected using antiactin and myosin (15, 18). Antiactin has been shown to be a reliable criterion for differentiating tubular carcinoma from sclerosing adenosis (19). Another use of this marker is in the cases in which hyperplasia must be differentiated from carcinoma in situ. In the former, there is abundant proliferation of myoepithelial cells with a rich reaction for actin (18).

Table 1. Histochemical Markers of Human or Animal Breast Tissue

	Cell Type or Structure	Antibody	Reference
a.	Myoepithelial Cells	Anti-Myosin	13
		Anti-Actin	14,15
b.	Epithelial Cells	Anti-Keratin	20-29
		Anti-Fat Globule Membrane	31-39
		Anti-Breast Tissue	40-41
		Anti-Epithelial Membrane	9-12,41
		Anti-Casein	49-50
		Anti-Alpha Lactalbumin	42-48
		Anti-lactoferrin	51-54
c.	Basement Membrane	Anti-Collagen IV	11,55,56
		Anti-Laminin	11,56
		Anti-Elastin	58

The epithelial cells of the mammary gland, at difference of the myoepithelial cells, have a large variety of cell markers that can be identified in the normal as well as in the neoplastic process. In Table 1 are outlined the different kinds of antibodies raised against specific components of the gland. Keratin is positive in breast epithelium (20). Keratin or cytokeratin stain intermediate-sized filaments, which represent a family of proteins ranging from 40,000 to 70,000 in molecular weight (21). Both monoclonal and polyclonal antibodies have been obtained and are very useful in staining a variety of epithelial cells including breast (Figs. 1 and 2). Antibodies to cytokeratins are extremely useful as markers of epithelial differentiation in carcinomas of various sites (22-25). Ductal and lobular carcinomas of the breast are strongly positive for keratin, however they present a great variation from area to area within the same tumor, or a "patch work" configuration (Figs.3-5).

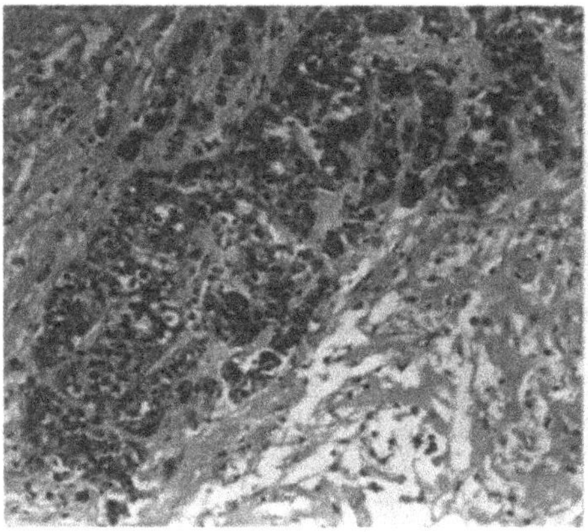

Figure 1. Infiltrating ductal carcinoma immunoperoxidase reaction for keratin, X100.

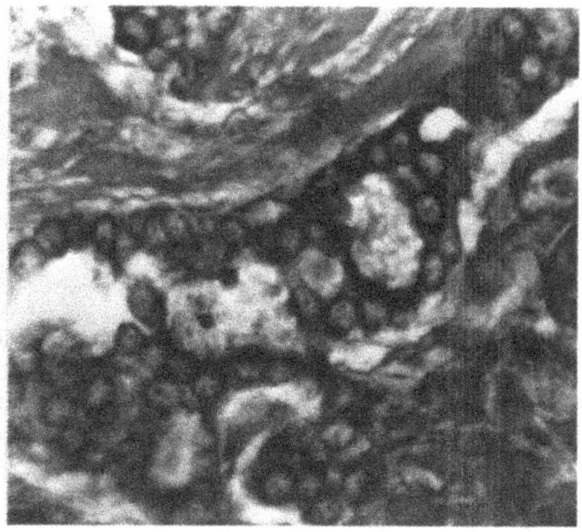

Figure 2. Higher magnification of the epithelial component of the ductal carcinoma stained for keratin, X400.

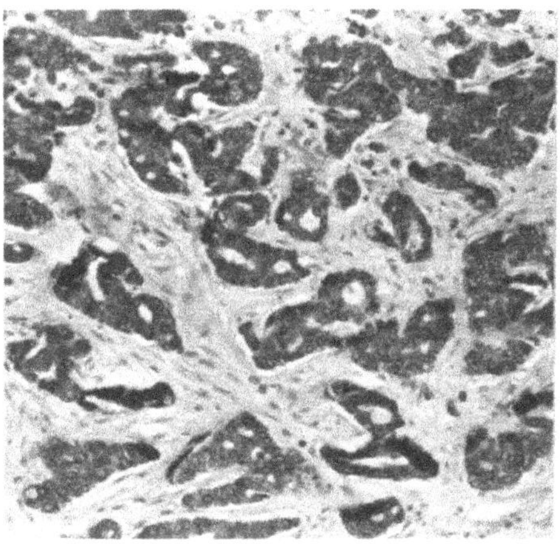

Figure 3. Patch work pattern of keratin stain in moderately differentiated carcinoma, X160.

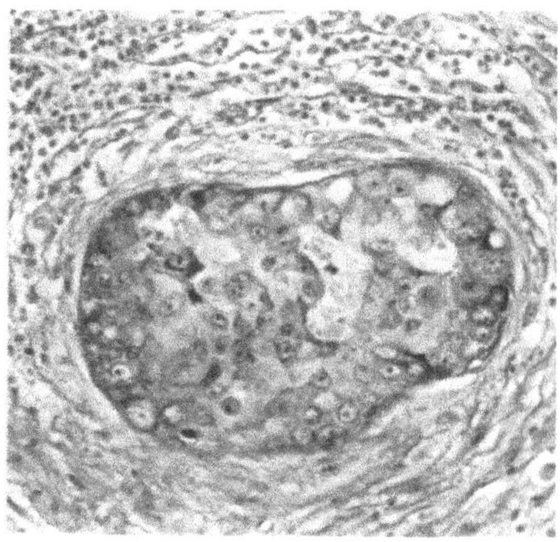

Figure 4. Intraductal carcinoma showing few cells positive for keratin X160.

Keratin is negative in spindle-shaped cells of cystosarcoma phylloides and in fibroadenomas (26,27). In our series of cases, keratin was expressed in 81% of the breast carcinomas, 14% were negative and 5% presented a borderline reaction (Table 5).

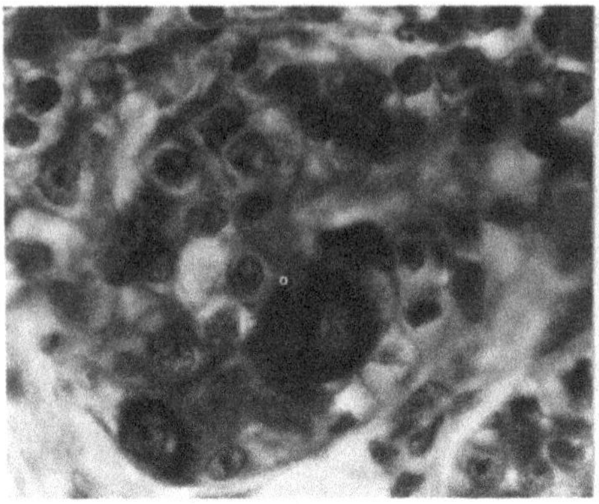

Figure 5. Observe the difference in reaction for keratin intensity among the epithelial cells of the infiltrating ductal carcinoma, X400.

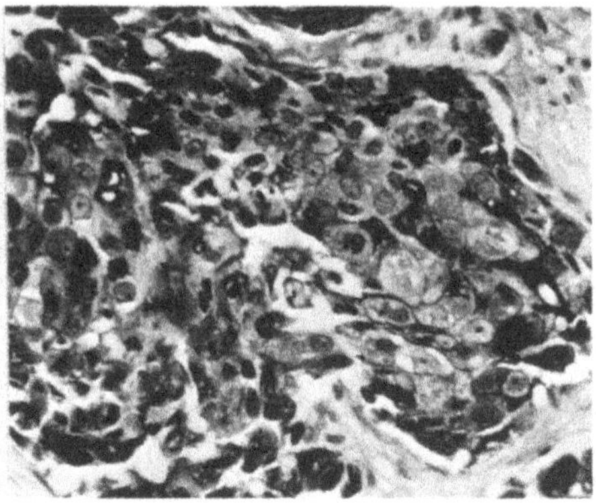

Figure 6. Infiltrating ductal carcinoma reacted with MC5. The heterogeneity in the expression of the of the antigen is evident, X160.

Table 2. Antigens Associated With Breast Epithelium

Antibody	Source of Antigen	References
1 - 14-A-3	Milk Fat Globule Membranes	32,33
2 - 1-10-F3	Milk Fat Globule Membranes	32,33
3 - MFGH-gP70	Milk Fat Globule Membranes	31
4 - HME	Milk Fat Globule Membranes	34
5 - HMFG-(MC-5)	400,000 Dalton Protein (MFGM)	35
6 - EMA	Defatted Human Milk	40,41
7 - LICR-LON-M8	Breast Epithelium	13,38,39
8 - LICR-LON-M18	Breast Epithelium	13,38,39

By determining reactivity with two keratins (28,29) one that reacts with tonofilament-associated prekeratin and the other with a 49,000 molecular weight keratin, more than one cell type has been identified in the mammary epithelium (27). In our series, keratin was always negative in myoepithelial cells, although keratin has been reported to react positively with myoepithelial cells by other authors (30).

In Table 2 are depicted the different monoclonal and polyclonal antibodies obtained from the breast epithelial membrane. An available source is the macromolecules from plasma membranes of mammary epithelial cells obtained from the milk fat globule. The cream portion of milk consists of fat droplets stabilized by an external membrane. The antibody against milk fat globule membrane (MFGM) obtained by Tokes and his group is a glycoprotein of 70,000 molecular weight (31). It is a heterologous antibody that reacts with the antigen that is preserved in buffered formalin fixed tissue embedded in paraffin. This antibody reacts with normal breast tissue, mainly lactating gland, giving a positive reaction in the luminal surface. It is not detected in myoepithelial cells, fat, fibroblasts or other tissue of the breast. It presents cross reactivity with columnar epithelium of colon, collecting tubules of kidney, salivary gland, stomach, eccrine sweat and sebaceous glands. This antibody reacts with morphologically well-differentiated tumors in the luminal border and less intensely in the less differentiated tumors.

Using the same source of antigen, milk fat globule membranes, other antibodies have been obtained, like 1-4A3, 1-10F3 (32,33), human fat globule membrane antibody (34) and human milk fat globule membrane monoclonal antibody (MC-5)(35). The antigen identified by MC5 is a mucin-like glycoprotein with an apparent molecular weight of 400,000 (36). However, this antigen is not unique to breast epithelial cells, since it is found in some other secretory cells or other tissues (33). Using the avidin biotinylated peroxidase, we have found that the luminal material and the luminal border of ductal and lobular epithelial cells of normal breast and the lobular epithelium, react specifically with MC5. In breast carcinomas, independently of tumor type, we found MC5 positivity in 95% of the tumors studied (Table 5). Only in 3% of the case the reaction was weak and considered borderline. In intraductal carcinomas, as well as in lobular carcinomas in situ, the reaction occurs in the cytoplasm and/or in the free surface. Not all of the cells react with this antibody, and a "patchwork" pattern is often found in different areas of the same tumor. In invasive, both ductal and lobular carcinomas, there is a consistent positive reaction that goes from very strong in all the tumor cells to a "patchwork" pattern in others (Figs. 6-8). Four tumors show only isolated positive cells (Fig.9). Besides the high percentage of reactivity of this monoclonal antibody with human breast cancer cells in paraffin embedded tissues, its use is also advantageous in cytospin preparations of cytologic specimens. A further advantage of the antigen detected by MC5 is that it is also present in the circulation and can be detected by sensitive radioimmunoassay. The levels of antigen are useful in detecting relapse of breast tumors or for monitoring the effectiveness of therapy. Dr. Ceriani has demonstrated that mixtures of these antibodies can inhibit the growth of human breast tumors implanted in nude mice, whereas other human epithelial tumors are not affected (37). Other monoclonal antibodies have been developed like LICR-LON-M8 and LICR-LON-M18. The monoclonal LICR-LON-M8 (antibreast) is positive in the luminal border of ductal epithelial cells, however, not all the littoral cells express the epitope. The monoclonal LICR-LON-M18 stains positively the luminal material and the cytoplasmic component. This has been interpreted as a segmental distribution of some antigens, so that they are present in some ducts and absent from others (39).

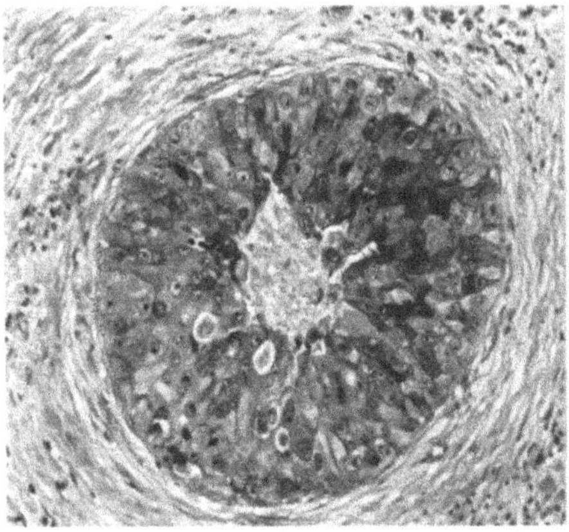

Figure 7. Intraductal carcinoma reacted with MC5, X160.

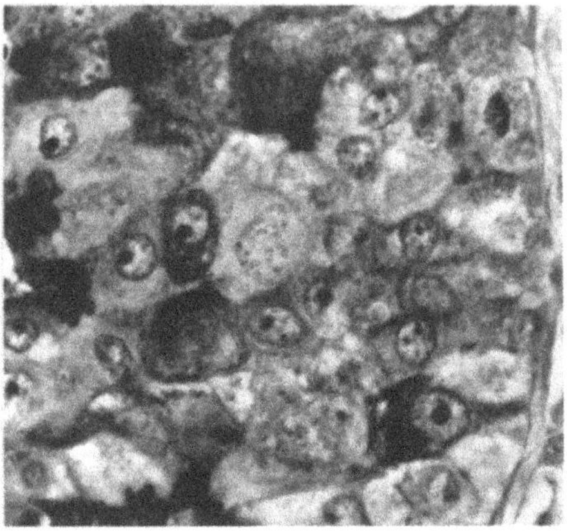

Figure 8. Intraductal carcinoma reacted with MC5. Only epithelial cells are positive showing different degrees of reactivity, X400.

Another antibody obtained against defatted human milk (EMA) (Table 2) has been observed to react with breast epithelium, but also with squamous epithelium and urothelium (40). EMA has been useful to a certain extent in the detection of breast cancer metastases in bone in 50% of the cases when a biopsy aspiration was done. However, it is not reliable in detection of breast carcinoma in other sites (41).

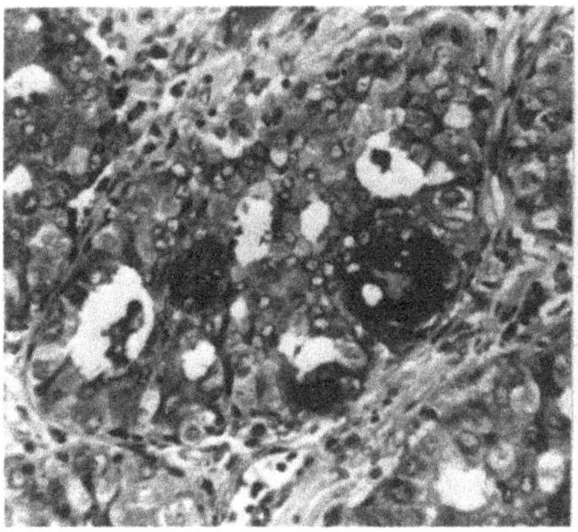

Figure 9. Infiltrating ductal carcinoma in which only one cluster of cells presented reactivity with MC5

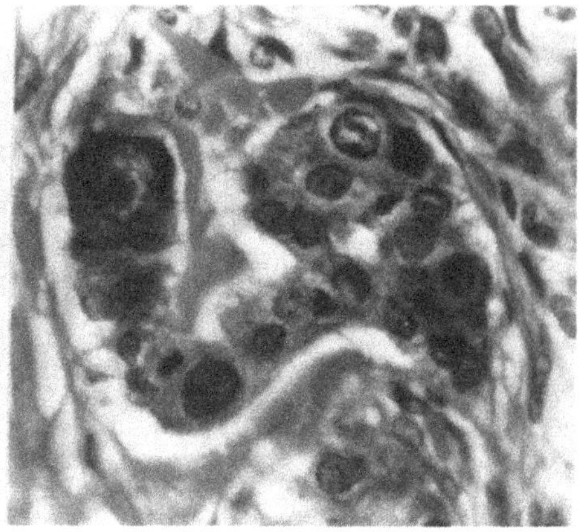

Figure 10. Cluster of neoplastic cells showing dense reaction in cytoplasm with B6:2 monoclonal antibody, X400.

Putting in perspective our own results, as well as those obtained by others and reported in the literature, the monoclonal antibody MC5, raised against human fat globule membrane, has the highest reactivity with breast epithelium in normal and malignant conditions.

In Table 1 are also described additional antibodies that react with specific gene products of breast epithelium. They are alpha lactalbumin, casein, and lactoferrin. Alpha lactalbumin is the beta protein of lactose synthetase secreted by the differentiated mammary epithelium (41). The localization of alpha lactalbumin using immunocytochemical techniques has been reported by different researchers (43-47). Unfortunately, the fixation procedures and the immunohistochemical techniques used differ from one author to another. In normal breast as well as in benign lesions, such as fibrocystic disease, sclerosing adenosis and epithelial hyperplasia, the range of reactivity varies from series to series (43, 46, 47). The major discrepancy is in breast carcinoma, that goes from 0% for Bailey (43) to 70% for Bussolati, et al. (45). When tumor type is considered, infiltrating ductal carcinoma presents reactivity in 54% (47),

63% (44) and 77% (20) of the cases depending on the series studied. The discrepancy is even larger for infiltrating lobular carcinoma, ranging from 7% (44) to 42% (46). No correlation has been found between degree of histological differentiation and the reactivity to alpha-lactalbumin (46,47). The expression of alpha-lactalbumin has not been found to correlate with prognosis of the disease (47), or with the presence of estrogen receptor or level of prolactin in serum (44). Even though alpha-lactalbumin has been found in the seminiferous epithelium and in epididymus (48) it must still be considered as a specific gene product of differentiated mammary epithelium.

Casein is a protein specific to the mammary epithelial cells and has been considered a marker of differentiation of human cells in dysplastic and neoplastic lesions of the breast. Studies done by Bussolati et al (49), using immunofluorescence and an anti-human casein, showed that casein reactivity was located in the lining surface or filling the cavity of dilated alveoli and in the apical portion of the acinar border but negative in atrophic and prepuberal glands. Minute positive reaction has been observed in all cases of mammary dysplasia, but negative in carcinoma of the breast. In well differentiated carcinomas casein has been localized in the inner border of gland-like structures. Even though casein is a breast epithelial product, the polyclonal antibody against human casein obtained by Bussolati (49) has been shown to react also with non-breast tissues like sebaceous and sweat glands of the skin, bronchial epithelium, exocrine pancreas, endometrium in proliferative phase and ductal collecting tubules of the kidney (50). The obtention of monoclonal antibody against casein may help to obtain a more specific marker of breast epithelium and still be usable as a differentiation associated product.

Lactoferrin, an iron-binding protein, found in milk and other human secretions (51), has not been consistently used in diagnostic pathology as a marker of differentiation in mammary epithelium of normal, dysplastic and neoplastic breast (52-54).

Recognition of the basement membrane of the mammary gland has been done using reagents against laminin and collagen type IV, which are their main components (55,56). Early recognition of the invasive process can be achieved by using monoclonal antibodies against these two components.

Elastosis has been indicated to play a role in the prognosis of human breast cancer (57). An adequate and specific immunocytochemical reaction using an antibody against alpha elastin has been developed (58). However, more studies are needed before it can be considered for practical use in diagnostic pathology over the usual procedure of elastin stain.

3. MARKERS ASSOCIATED WITH HUMAN MAMMARY TUMORS

Numerous works have been published with regards to the existence and detection of antigens associated with human mammary tumors. Table 3 summarizes the main findings in this area (59,69).

In the present work we will discuss three sets of histochemical markers in human breast cancer: a) monoclonal antibodies against cell membrane components of cancer cells; b) markers considered to be present in different types of cancer cells including breast carcinoma and c) pregnancy related products that have been shown to be present in breast cancer tissue as well as in the patient's serum.

3.1 Monoclonal Antibodies Against Cell Membrane Components of Cancer Cells

In the work of Schlom and associates (70,71) they used human metastatic tumor cells as immunogens in an attempt to generate and characterize monoclonal antibodies reactive with determinants that would be maintained on metastatic as well as primary human mammary carcinoma cells. Membrane enriched cell extracts were prepared from breast tumor metastases to the liver and using hybridoma technique 11 monoclonal antibodies were prepared. From these 11, we have had access to three of them B1:1, B72:3 and B6:2 that were directly supplied by Dr. Schlom. Table 4 summarizes the main characteristics of these monoclonal antibodies. The reactivity of B1:1, due to its cross reactivity with different epitopes of CEA glycoprotein molecules, will be discussed in the next section.

In Table 5 are tabulated results of our study of 35 primary breast cancers that were reacted with monoclonal B72:3 and B6:2, using the avidin-biotin-peroxidase complex (Vectastain ABC Kit, Vector Laboratories). B72:3 resulted to be the most reactive of both monoclonals; 86% of the tumors reacted positively and 11% presented a $\pm$ or borderline reactivity. Only 3% of the tumors were negative. B6:2 presented a lower

Table 3. Markers Associated With Human Mammary Tumors

Source	Reactivity	References
1- Crude membrane extracts of breast cancer	Delay hypersensitivity in skin of breast cancer patient	59
2- Peripheral lymphocytes of patients with fibrocystic disease (FCD)	Cytotoxic to breast adeno - carcinoma cells. They are blocked using serum of patients free of FCD or fibroadenomas.	60
3- GP-52 (52,000 dalton glycoprotein of mouse mammary tumor virus)	39 to 63% of breast cancer of various histologic types react positively. There is negative reaction in normal and benign lesions.	61,66,67
4- Autologous breast cancer serum	Window test to measure cell mediated immunity. 86% Stage 0; 57% Invasive carcinoma with 5-year-survival. 27% in patients with recurrent breast cancer 4 year post-surgery.	62
5- Human mammary glycoprotein (MTGP) purified from breast cancer	Soluble MTGP is negative in normal tissue. 76.5% (+) in all breast cancer (It is independent of histological pattern of ductal carcinoma; degree of anaplasia or nuclear atypia; histological features of host response.)	63
6- Presence of tumor associated antigen in human serum (TAA)	PAP reaction shows positive binding of TAA in breast cancer but not in normal tissue.	64, 65
7- Monoclonal antibody against a membrane preparation of MCF.7 cells (MBRI) (A neutral glycolipid).	It reacts with mammary gland epithelium, and primary metastatic carcinoma.	68, 69

reactivity, only 50% of the tumors were positive, 26% were borderline and 24% negative. Interestingly enough, we observed that the pattern of reactivity was very heterogeneous from tumor to tumor. Some tumors (Fig.10) presented a focal staining, with a dense reaction in the cytoplasm, whereas others showed a more diffuse cytoplasmic staining (Fig.11) or membrane staining in the apical portion of the cells (Fig.12). Other authors have also observed the same phenomenon (70,71)

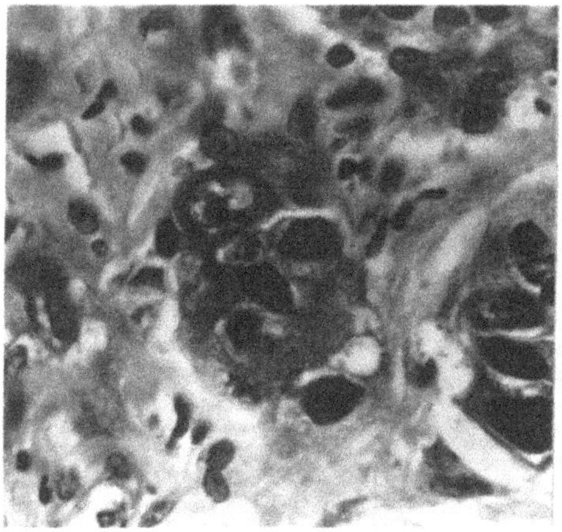

Figure 11. Diffuse staining reaction for B72:3 monoclonal antibody in an infiltrating ductal carcinoma, X400.

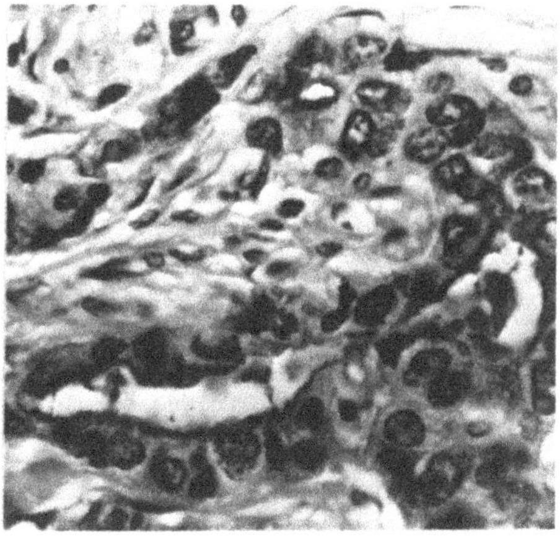

Figure 12. Apical localization of B72:3 in an infiltrating ductal carcinoma, X400.

which has been called "patchwork" pattern, because of the presence of one group of tumor cells expressing the specific antigen adjacent to tumor cells that are negative for the same antigen (Fig.13). Intraluminal variation in reactivity was detected for both monoclonal antibodies (B72:3 and B6:2). In addition, intertumoral variation was observed. For example, one tumor showed reactivity with one monoclonal and not with the other. In Table 7 is a crucigram in which it is easily appreciated the diversity in reactivity from tumor to tumor. These wide ranges of antigenic phenotypes expressed in human mammary tumors are interpreted as manifestations of tumor heterogeneity in a single cell type, being at different stages of functional cell membrane composition due to variation in the stages of the cell cycle, or to post-translational cellular events that are controlling the reactivity of the peptide side chains to the antibody (72). Heterogeneity in the expression of those TAA have been observed using MCF-7 clones (70); similar finding has also been reported within normal and neoplastic mammary epithelium using a non-breast specific monoclonal antibody raised to the human milk fat globule membrane (38,39). This variability in the antigenic expression is not unique to breast cancer cells and has been shown in other human and rodent tumors (73-75).

Table 4. Mammary Carcinoma Antigens

Monoclonal Ab	Biochemical Characteristics
- B72:3	Binds to a high molecular weight protein (Mr 200,000 complex)
- B6:2	Reacts with a Mr 90,000 component Mr 180,000 CEA glycoprotein
- B1:1	Binds to different epitopes of the Mr 180,000 CEA glycoprotein

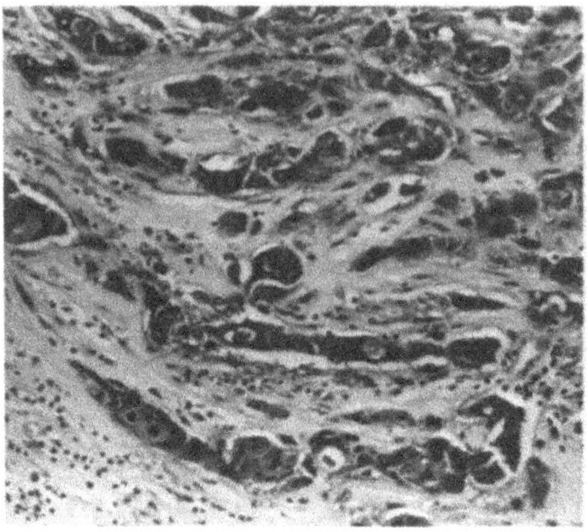

Figure 13. Infiltrating ductal carcinoma with few patches of cells reacting with B72:3, X100.

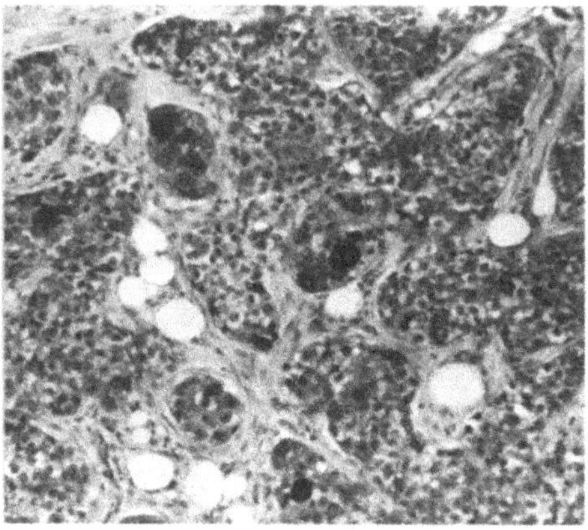

Figure 14. Reactivity of ductal carcinoma to polyclonal antibody against CEA, X100.

We found that B72:3 displayed a higher range of reactivity with breast carcinomas than B6:2, an observation also reported by Nuti et al. (71), although the percentage of tumors reacting with B72:3 reported by those authors was lower than those in our series. The monoclonal B72:3 has shown some reactivity with few colon and lung carcinomas, but cross reactivity with CEA has been excluded (71).

Regarding the monoclonal antibody B6:2, we obtained 50% strongly positive and 26% $\pm$ reactivity in the primary breast carcinomas studied (Table 5). In a study done by Colcher et al (76), they found 74%

reactivity in primary breast carcinomas, but in their report the intensity of the reaction in the section was not considered. B6:2 has been found to be negative in normal mammary ductal tissue and other normal tissues (76). One of the advantages of B6:2 is its use in the radiolocalization of human mammary tumors in athymic mice (86) and therefore its potential application in human radiodiagnosis.

Table 5. Expression of Various Cell Markers in Human Breast Carcinoma.

			Positive		Negative		Borderline	
Marker of	Antibody	#Cases	#	%	#	%	#	%
Epithelial	MC5	36	35	97	0	0	1	3
Cells	Keratin	36	29	81	5	14	2	5
Breast	B72:3	35	30	86	1	3	4	11
Cancer Cell	B6:2	34	17	50	8	24	9	26
Membranes								
Neoplastic	CEA	36	21	58	11	31	4	11
Cells	B1:1	28	19	68	6	21	3	11
Pregnancy	hCG	25	1	4	23	92	1	4
Related	BhCG	35	14	40	12	34	9	26
Products	SP1	38	23	60	12	32	3	8

3.2 Reactivity of Breast Carcinoma Usings Markers Common to Other Neoplasias

Under this subset we will discuss the distribution of CEA and B1:1. The latter is a monoclonal antibody developed by the Schlom's group (70) that binds to different epitopes of Mr 180,000 CEA glycoprotein. CEA has been established as a useful marker in patients with breast cancer (77-79). However, conflicting results have been reported with regards to immunocytochemical localization in tissue sections, the value of positivity ranging from 1.6 to 83% of the breast cancers studied (80-85). In our study (Table 5) CEA was found to be positive in 58% of breast carcinomas, and borderline in 11%. Thirty-one percent of breast carcinomas were negative. In the tumors in which positive reaction was

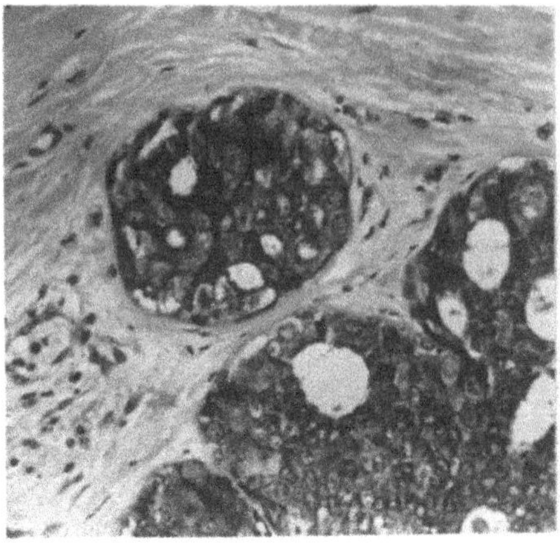

Figure 15. Reactivity of CEA in the cell membrane, X160.

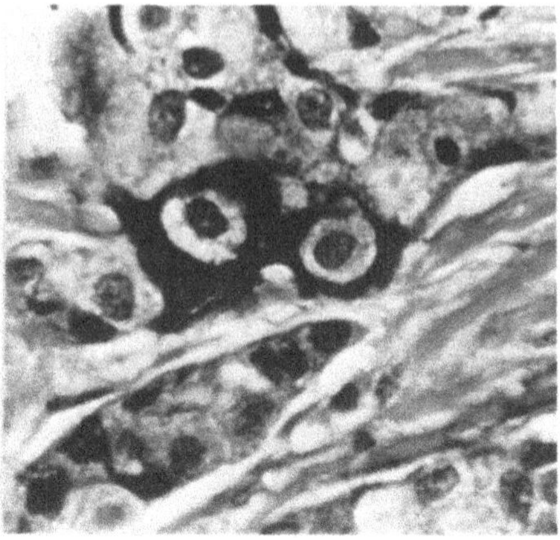

Figure 16. Infiltrating ductal carcinoma showing intense reaction to CEA adjacent to negative areas in the same cluster, X400.

detected there was no difference in the subtypes studied. Positive staining was predominantly cytoplasmic with a diffuse intracytoplasmic distribution; in some cases, however prominent staining of cell membranes occurred (Fig.15). These cytologic differences in CEA staining did not correlate with histologic pattern or type of tumor. Heterogeneity was a notable feature of CEA staining in all in situ and infiltrating carcinomas, with variability from patient to patient and from one area of the tumor to the next. In many cases, like that shown in Figure 16, areas showing strong 3+ CEA positivity were immediately adjacent to or admixed with negative areas. Cellular debris in areas of tumor necrosis were frequently detected as CEA+, even in tumors with weak or minimal CEA+. Some normal areas of breast tissue adjacent to the tumor may show a weak positive reaction in the apical border of the cells.

The reactivity of mammary carcinomas to monoclonal B1:1, that has a direct reactivity against CEA, was in our series 68% positive, and 11% borderline. Twenty-one percent were negative (Table 5). In the series of Horan Hand et al (70) 25 out of 39 breast cancers reacted with B1:1, that is approximately 64% of the tumors reacted. The distribution pattern is similar to that described for CEA.

3.3 Pregnancy Related Products

Pregnancy related products are represented by placental hormones the main one being chorionic gonadotropin, whose production as native hCG and as free subunits has been identified in extracts of tumor tissues, as well as circulating in peripheral blood of patients harboring gonadotropin-secreting tumors (90). The secretion of human chorionic gonadotropin (hCG) by non-trophoblastic tumors is well recognized (87). The presence of placenta-specific hormones such as hCG and pregnancy specific protein (SP1) in breast tumors could represent the expression of developmental hormonal genes that are repressed in the more differentiated condition. Elevated serum levels of choriogonadotropin-like polypeptides have been reported to be present in the serum of up to 49-50% of patients with breast carcinoma (87,88), the incidence increasing to 60% when there is one metastatic organ site of involvement (88). The synthesis of choriogonadotropin-like material have been demonstrated in tissue sections and cell cultures of the R3230 AC rat mammary adenocarcinoma using immunocytochemical, radioimmunoassay and bioassay methods (89). Breast adenocarcinomas, either cell lines derived from breast tumors or primary breast cancers have been shown to stain positively for hCG using immunoperoxidase techniques. It is of interest to note that the profile of hCG and its subunits in serum varies with the degree of anaplasia of the tumors and correlates with their response to chemotherapy (90). The neoplasms of patients who readily respond to conventional chemotherapy synthesize and secrete native hCG, but not its free subunits, whereas the tumors of those women with widely metastatic cancer resistant to intensive chemotherapy, secrete almost exclusively free subunits of hCG (90).

The study of the immunocytochemical distribution of hCG and its subunit beta hCG in paraffin sections of 36 formalin-fixed primary breast carcinomas revealed that hCG is present in a very small percentage of tumors (4%) whereas the beta subunit is manifested more frequently, with 40% of the primary tumors strongly positive, 26% are borderline positive, and 34% negative (Table 5). The pattern of reactivity is also variable; whereas some tumors present a homogeneous reactivity in all the neoplastic cells, others present only focal clusters of isolated positive cells (Figs. 17 and 18).

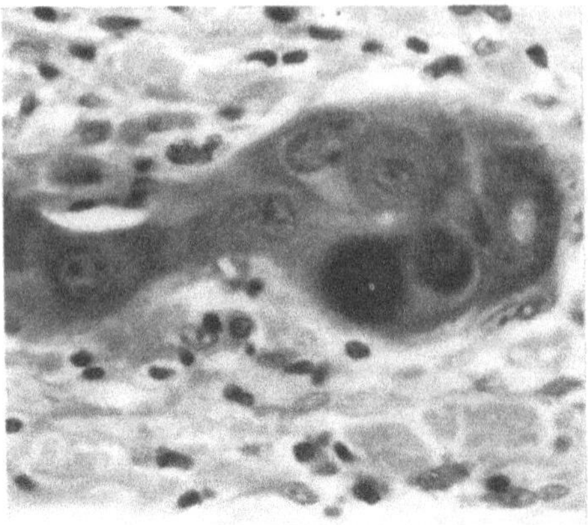

Figure 17. Cluster of cells with two cells showing positive reactivity for hCG, X400.

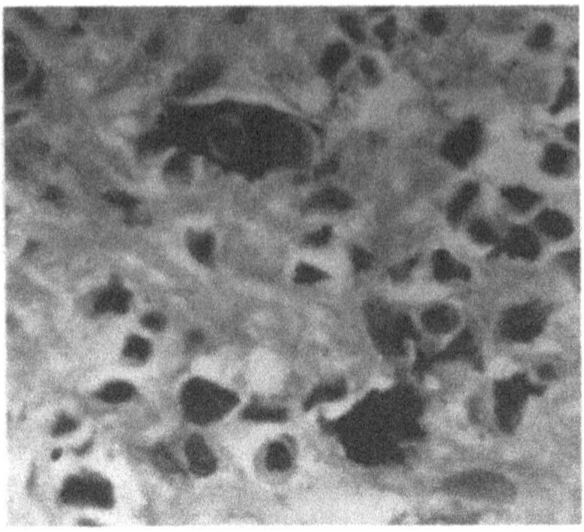

Figure 18. Isolated cells in an infiltrating ductal carcinoma with reactivity to hCG, X400.

Another placental hormone, pregnancy specific glycoprotein (SP1), is a product of the syncytiotrophoblast. By a variety of techniques it has been shown to be the inappropriate product of nontrophoblastic tumors, including breast cancer (60%) and gastrointestinal cancers (50%) (93). Horne et al, (91) in retrospective studies using immunoperoxidase techniques claim that tumors that stained positively for SP1 had a poorer prognosis than those that were negative. Wurz (92) found that SP1 levels detected by radioimmunoassay in the serum of patients bearing various malignant epithelial tumors fell rapidly following surgical removal of the tumor. The immunocytochemical detection of SP1 shows reactivity in breast carcinoma in 60% of the cases, and only 8% show a borderline reactivity (Table 5). The distribution in paraffin embedded, formalin-fixed sections is very heterogeneous. Some areas are strongly positive, whereas other areas are negative. In Figures 19 and 20 a common pattern of SP1 distribution is shown.

3.4 Prognostic Significance of Immunocytochemical Markers in Breast Carcinoma.

We have shown that mitotic grade alone or in combination with lymph node status at the time of surgery for primary breast carcinoma have a significant discriminant power to predict recurrence of the disease (93). It was of interest to correlate parameters like lymph node status, mitotic

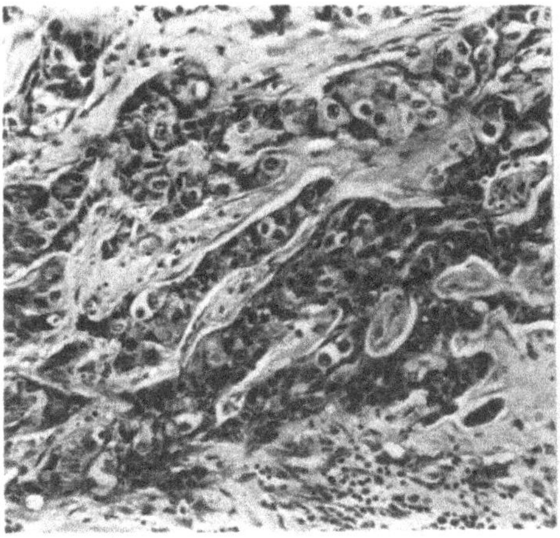

Figure 19. Pattern of reactivity for SP1, X100.

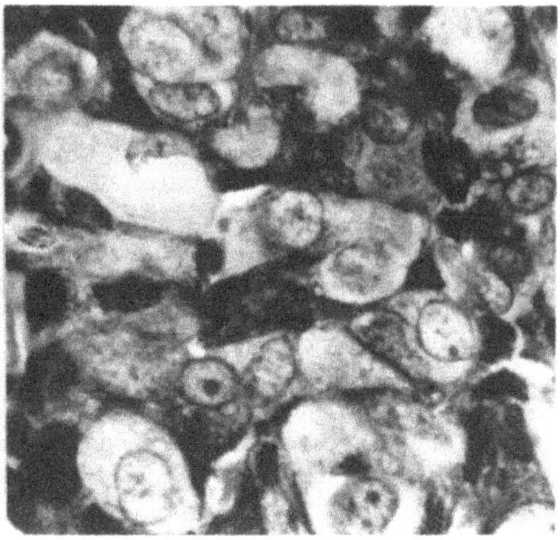

Figure 20. Higher magnification of of Figure 19, showing the heterogeneous pattern of reactivity of SP1, X400.

grade and estrogen receptors with the presence of immunocytochemical markers in primary breast tumors in order to determine whether they were associated with recurrence of the disease or mortality after five years followup. Table 6 summarizes the correlation between the markers studied in primary breast tumors and the other parameters above mentioned.

MC5 and keratin were positive in 100% and 86% of the tumors respectively; there was equal distribution between those that were lymph node positive, 56% and 50% respectively. The same distribution was observed when estrogen receptor content was considered. There was a slightly lower percentage of tumors mitotic grade(MG) 2-3 in those that were positive for MC5 and keratin. Recurrence occurred in 50% of MC5 and 44% keratin positive tumors. The survival rate was the same in both MC5 and keratin positive tumors and no different than that shown for other specific breast cancer markers, like B72:3 and B6:2. The reactivity of B72:3 and B6:2 in breast carcinomas was equally distributed among lymph node positive and lymph node negative tumors. There was a slightly higher number of E2R estrogen receptor negative in those tumors that presented these two antigens. The percentage of tumors with low mitotic grade was slightly higher and recurrence was lower in those B6:2 positive tumors than in B72:3 positive tumors, and both markers were associated with lower

Table 6. Correlation Between TAA and Cell Markers With Prognostic Factors In Breast Cancer

Markers	No. Positive/ No. Cases	%+	LN+	E2R+	MG (2-3)	Recur-rence	Mor-tality
MC5	36/36	100	20(56%)	18(50%)	15(42%)	18(50%)	12(33%)
Keratin	31/36	86	18(50%)	17(47%)	14(39%)	16(44%)	11(31%)
B72:3	34/35	97	19(54%)	16(46%)	16(46%)	17(49%)	11(31%)
B6:2	26/34	76	16(47%)	14(41%)	15(44%)	13(38%)	10(29%)
CEA	25/36	69	15(42%)	14(39%)	10(28%)	14(39%)	10(28%)
B1:1	22/28	79	14(50%)	12(43%)	11(39%)	13(46%)	9(32%)
hCG	2/25	8	1(4%)	2(8%)	1(4%)	0(0%)	0(0%)
BhCG	23/35	66	12(34%)	12(34%)	10(29%)	10(29%)	7(20%)
SP1	26/38	68	15(39%)	15(39%)	10(26%)	15(39%)	9(24%)

recurrence than those with keratin and MC5 positive reaction. The survival rate however, was no different. The expression of CEA has been shown to correlate with the presence of lymph node metastases (81) and it has been demonstrated that patients with CEA negative tumors have significantly higher 5 to 10 year-survival rates (94). On the other hand, Walker (82) failed to find a correlation between CEA positive and lymph node metastases or recurrence within two years of the discovery of the primary disease. In our results (Table 6) 69% of the tumors were CEA positive, and 42% were lymph node positive, 39% were estrogen receptor positive and 28% had MG(2-3). A five-year follow up showed that 39% of the tumors with CEA positive tumors presented recurrence with lower mortality rate. Interestingly enough, B1:1, the monoclonal antibody that reacts with one of the epitopes of CEA, shows approximately the same behavior that those CEA positive tumors. There is a positive correlation between B1:1 and CEA (X^2=6.26 p=0.01).

The presence of pregnancy related markers in breast cancer showed that hCG was expressed in 8% of the tumors and seemed to be associated with better prognosis (Table 6) No recurrence or mortality has been found in those cases that hCG reacted positively in the tumor. All breast cancers positive for hCG were also positive for estrogen receptor (X^2=2.95 p=0.08). Beta hCG and SP1 behaved both in the same fashion (Table 6) when compared with other markers like MC5, B72:3, B6:2, B1:1 and CEA.

Table 7. Relationship Between Recurrence, Mortality and Presence of Tumors Cells Markers

Patient I.D.	Recur- rence.	LN	E2R	MG	MC5	Kera- tin	B72:3	B6:2	CEA	B1:1	hCG	BhCG	SP1
62	+	+	-	2-3	++	+	+	++	±	+	ND	-	-
75	+	+	-	2-3	++	+	++	±	ND	ND	ND	+	-
110	+	-	-	2-3	++	-	+	±	-	-	-	+	-
220	+	+	-	2-3	ND	ND	ND	ND	ND	ND	ND	++	±
260	+	+	-	2-3	++	++	++	+++	++	++	++	-	ND
336	+	-	-	1	++	++	-	-	-	-	-	++	++
472	+	+	+	1	++	+	+	±	+	++	-	++	++
489	+	-	+	2-3	++	++	ND	±	++	±	ND	-	++
492	+	+	+	2-3	+	++	++	-	-	-	ND	-	++
597	+	+	-	2-3	+	+	++	++++	++	+++	-	-	++
605	+	+	+	2-3	++	+	++	±	++	++	ND	±	+
609	+	+	-	1	++	++	+++	+	+++	+	ND	-	++
662	+	-	+	1	+	-	+	±	+++	-	-	-	++
813	+	+	+	2-3	+	±	±	++	+++	+++	-	+	++

However, SP1 was associated with higher recurrence and slightly lower survival rate beta hCG at five years followup. Table 7 lists all the patients that died as a consequence of the disease and had recurrence; It can be observed that there is a markedly heterogeneous expression of the TAA in these tumors. Whereas in some of them the reactivity is very strong, and in others it is very weak; and even in the same tumor different degrees of reactivity for different TAA are observed.

5. CONCLUSIONS

a - MC5 a monoclonal antibody against milk fat globule, is positively expressed in 100% of all types of breast cancer studied.

b - Keratin is an epithelial cell marker and is expressed in 86% of the tumors studied.

c - B72:3, a monoclonal Ab raised against breast cancer cells is present in 97% of the tumors, whereas B6:2 is only found in 76% of the breast cancer studied.

d - The use of general antibodies against TAA like CEA and B1:1 showed that they are present in 69 and 79% of the breast cancer studied.

e - Pregnancy related products like hCG, Beta hCG and SP1 are expressed in 8%, 66% and 68% of breast cancer respectively.

f - It seems that the most reliable marker for breast cancer is MC5, that determines the epithelial breast origin, and B72:3 that determines the neoplastic nature of the cells.

g - The presence of MC5 and keratin does not indicate advantage in the prediction of recurrence or mortality and they seem to be equally distributed among LN+ or LN-, E2R+ or E2R- or high and low mitotic grade.

h- The presence of the breast cancer cell markers B72:3 and B6:2 does not differ significantly in their predicting capability from markers like MC5 and keratin. They are approximately equally distributed among LN+ or LN-, E2R+ or E2R- or high and low mitotic grade patients.

i - Similar conclusions reached in (7) and (8) can be obtained when general neoplastic markers as CEA or B1:1 are used. However, CEA positive tumors have a trend to have a lower mitotic grade.

j - Those tumors that are hCG positive (8%) do not show recurrence or mortality.

k - The use of beta hCG is more discriminative than hCG; however, the percentage of patients with LN+, E2R+, high mitotic grade, recurrence and mortality are lower than those detected for other markers indicated in (7), (8) and (9).

l - SP1 reactivity is associated with higher rate of recurrence, 39%, when compared with recurrence in Beta hCG and hCG positive tumors.

References

1. McCluskey RT and Bhan, AK: Cell-mediated reactions in vivo. In: Green I, Cohen S, and McCluskey RT (eds), Mechanisms of Tumor Immunity. John Wiley and Sons, New York, 1977, pp 1-25.
2. Kupchik HK: Antibodies to alphafetoprotein and carcinoembryonic antigen produced by somatic cell fusion. In Hurrel JG (ed). Monoclonal Hybridoma Antibodies: Techniques and Applications. CRC Press Inc. Boca Raton, Florida, 1981, pp 81-89.
3. Primus FJ, Clark CA and Goldenberg DM: Immunohistochemical detection of carcinoembryonic antigen. In: DeLellis RA (ed). Diagnostic Immunohistochemistry, Masson Publishing, USA 1981, pp 263-276.
4. Prat J, Bhan AK, Dickersin GR, Robboy SJ and Scully RE: Hepatoid yolk tumor of the ovary (endodermal sinus tumor with hepatoid differentiation); A light microscopic, ultrastructural and immunohistochemical study of seven cases. Cancer (50):2355-2368, 1982.
5. Waldman TA and McIntire RR: The use of radioimmunoassay for alphafetoprotein in the diagnosis of malignancy. Cancer (34): 1510-1515, 1974.
6. Carson JM and Pinkus GS: Mesothelioma: Profile of keratin proteins and carcinoembryonic antigen. An immunoperoxidase study of 20 cases and comparison with pulmonary adenocarcinomas. Am J Pathol (108):80-88, 1982.
7. Carpin C, Phan AK, Zurwski JR, Jr. and Scully RE: Carcinoembryonic antigen (CEA) and carbohydrate determinant 19-9(CA19-9) localization in 2 primary and metastatic ovarian tumors. An immunohistochemical study with the use of monoclonal antibodies. Int J Gynecol. Pathology (1):231-245, 1982.
8. Kuhada FP, Offutt LE, Mendelsohn G: The distribution of carcinoembryonic antigen in breast carcinoma. Diagnostic and Prognostic Implications. Cancer (52): 1257-1264, 1983.
9. Gilliland DG, Steplewski, Z, Collie RJ, Mitchell KF, Chang TH and Koprowski H: Antibody directed cytotoxic agents: Use of monoclonal antibody to direct the action of toxin. A chain to colorectal carcinoma cells. Proc Natl Acad Sci USA (77): 4539-4573, 1980.
10. Miller RA and Levey R: Response of cutaneous T-cell lymphoma to therapy with hybridoma monoclonal antibody. Lancet (2):226-230, 1981.
11. Nadler LM, Stashenko P, Hardy R, Kaplan WD, Button LN, Kufe DW, Antman, KH and Schlossman SF: Serotherapy of a patient with a monoclonal antibody directed against a human lymphoma associated antigen. Cancer Res (40): 3147-3154, 1980.
12. Russo J, Tay LK, and Russo, IH: differentiation of the mammary gland and susceptibility to carcinogenesis. Breast Cancer Res and Treatment (2):5-73, 1982.
13. Neville M, Foster CS, Moshkis V and Gore M: Monoclonal antibodies and Human Tumor Pathology. Human Pathology (13):1067-1081, 1982.
14. Bussolati G, Gugliotta P and Fulcheri E: Immunohistochemistry of actin in normal and neoplastic tissues. In DeLellis, RA (ed) Advances in immunohistochemistry, pp 325-341, 1981.
15. Ozello L: Ultrastructures of the human mammary gland. Pathol Ann (6):1-79, 1971.
16. Bussolati G, Botta G and Gugliotta P: Histology and histochemistry of cystic breast disease. In: Angeli A, Bradlow HL and Dogliotti L (eds). Endocrinology of cystic breast disease. Raven Press, New York, pp 7-18, 1983.

17. Bussolati G, Alfani V, Weber K, and Osborn M: Immunocytochemical detection of actin of fixed and embedded tissues: Its potential use in routine pathology. J Histochem Cytochem (28):169-173, 1980.
18. Bussolati G, Botta G, and Gugliotta P: Actin-rich (myoepithelial cells in ductal carcinoma in situ of the breast. Virchows Arch (Cell Pathol) (34):252-259,1980.
19. Eusebi V, Betts, CM and Bussolati G: Tubular carcinoma: A variant of secretory breast carcinoma. Histopathology (3):407-419, 1979.
20. Heyderman E, Steele K, Ormerad, MG: A new antigen on the epithelial membrane: Its immunoperoxidase localization in normal and neoplastic tissue. J Clin Pathol (32):35-39,1975.
21. Moll R, Franke WW, Schiller DL, Geiger B and Krepler R: The catalog of human cytokeratins: Patterns of expression in normal epithelia, tumors and cultured cells. Cell 31:11-24, 1982.
22. Battifora H, Sun TT, Bahu RM and Rao S: The use of antikeratin antiserum as a diagnostic tool: Thymoma versus lymphoma. Hum Pathol (11):635-240, 1980.
23. Espinoza CG, and Azar HA: Immunocytochemical localization of keratin-type proteins in epithelial neoplasms. Am J Clin Pathol (78):500-507, 1982.
24. Gabbiani G, Kapanci Y, Barazzana P and Franke WW: Immunochemical identification of intermediate-sized filaments in human neoplastic cells: A diagnostic aid for the surgical pathologist. Am J Pathol (104):206-216, 1981.
25. Ramaekers FCS, Putts JJG, Kant A, Moestker O, Jap PHK, and Voojis GP: Antibodies to intermediate filaments as a tool in tumor diagnosis. Cell Biol Int Rep (6):652, 1982.
26. Almannsberger M, Osborn M, Holscher A, Schauer A, and Weber K: The distribution of keratin type intermediate filaments in human breast cancer: An immunohistological study. Virchows Arch (Cell Pathol) (37):277-284, 1981.
27. Krepler R, Denk H, Weirich E, Schmid E and Franke WW: Keratin-like proteins in normal and neoplastic cells of human and rat mammary gland as revealed by immunofluorescence microscopy. Differentiation (20):242-252, 1981.
28. Franke WW, Denk H, Kalt R and Schmid E: Biochemical and immunological identification of cytokeratin proteins present in hepatocytes of mammalian liver tissue. Exp Cell Res (131):299-318, 1981.
29. Asch BB, Burstein NA, Vidrich A and Sun TT: Identification of mouse mammary epithelial cells by immunofluorescence with rabbit and guinea pig antikeratin antiserum. Proc Natl Acad Sci, USA (78):5643-5647, 1981.
30. Franke WW, Schmid E, Freudenstein C, Apellhans B, Osborn M, Weber K and Keeman TW: Intermediate filaments of the prekeratin type in myoepithelial cells. J Cell Biol (84):633-654, 1980.
31. Iman A, Taylor CR, Tokes ZA: Immunohistochemical study of the expression of human milk fat globule membrane glycoprotein 70. Cancer Research (44):2016-2022, 1984.
32. Taylor-Papadimitriaou J, Peterson JA, Arklie J, Burchell J, Ceriani R and Badner WI: Monoclonal antibodies to epithelium specific components of the human milk fat globule membrane. Production and reaction with cells in culture. Int J Cancer (28):17-21, 1981.
33. Arklie J, Taylor-Papadimitriaou J, Badner W, Egan M and Millis R: Differentiation antigens expressed by epithelial cells in the lactating breast are also detectable in breast cancers. Int J Cancer (28):23-29, 1981.

34. Ceriani RL, Thompson K, Peterson JA, Abraham S: Surface differentiation antigens on human mammary epithelial cells carried on the human milk fat globules. Proc Natl Acad Sci, USA (14):582-586, 1977.
35. Ceriani RL, Peterson JA and Blank E: Variability in surface antigen expression of human breast epithelial cells cultured from normal breast normal tissue peripheral to breast carcinomas and breast carcinomas. Cancer Research (44): 3033-3039, 1984.
36. Ceriani RL, Peterson JA, Lee JY, Moncada R and Blank EW: Characterization of cell surface antigens of normal human mammary epithelial cells with monoclonal antibodies. Somatic Cell Genet (9):415-427, 1983.
37. Henson DE: New Methods for the early detection and diagnosis of breast cancer. JNCI (73):549-552, 1984.
38. Foster CS, Edwards PAW, Dinsdale E: Monoclonal antibodies for the human mammary gland I. Distribution of determinants in non-neoplastic mammary and extra mammary tissues. Virchows Arch (Pathol Anat) (94):279-293, 1982.
39. Foster CS, Dinsdale EA, Edwards, PAW: Monoclonal antibodies for the human mammary gland II. Distribution of determinants in breast carcinomas. Virchows Arch (Pathol Anat) (394):295-305, 1982.
40. Sloane JP, Ormerod MG, Carter RL, Gusterson BA and Foster CS: An immunocytochemical study of the distribution of epithelial membrane antigen in normal and disordered squamous epithelium. Diagnostic Histopathol (5):11-17, 1982.
41. Heyderman E, Steele K, Ormerod MG: A new antigen on the epithelial membrane: Its immunoperoxidase localization in normal and neoplastic tissue. J. Clin Pathol (32):35-39, 1979.
42. Fitzgerald DK, Bradbeck V, Kiyosawa I, Marval R, Calvin B and Ebner KE: Alpha lactalbumin and the lactose synthetase reaction. J Biol Chem (245): 2103-2108, 1970.
43. Bailey AJ, Sloane JP, Trickey BS and Ormerod, MG: An immunocytochemical study of alpha lactalbumin in human breast tissue. J Pathology (137):13-23, 1982.
44. Bahu RM, Mangkormkonok-Mark M, Albertson D, Fors E, Molteni A, and Battifora H: Detection of alpha lactalbumin in breast lesions and relationship to estrogen receptor and serum prolactin. Cancer (46):1775-1780, 1980.
45. Bussolati G, Ghiringhello B, Carlo FD, Aimone V and Voglino GF: Lactalbumin synthesis in breast cancer tissue. Lancet (2):252, 1977.
46. Clayton F, Ordonez NG Hanssen GM, and Hanssen H: Immunoperoxidase localization of lactalbumin in malignant breast neoplasms. Arch Pathol Lab Med (106):268-270, 1982.
47. Walker RA: The demonstration of alpha lactalbumin in human breast carcinomas. J Pathol (129):37-42, 1979.
48. Byers SW, Qasba PK, Poulson HL, and Dym M: Immunocytochemical localization of alpha lactalbumin in the male reproductive tract. Biology of Reproduction (30):171-178, 1984.
49. Bussolati G, Pich A, Alfani V: Immunofluorescence detection of casein in human mammary dysplastic and neoplastic tissues. Virchows Arch A Path and Histol (365):15-21, 1973.
50. Pich A, Bussolati G and Carbonara A: Immunocytochemical detection of casein and casein-like proteins in human tissues. J of Histochem Cytochem (24):940-947, 1976.
51. Masson PL and Heremans JF: Studies on lactoferrin: The iron-binding protein of secretions. Prot Biol fluids (14):115-124, 1966.

52. Hurlimann J, Lichaa M and Ozello L: In vitro synthesis of immunoglobulins and other proteins by dysplastic and neoplastic human mammary tissues. Cancer Res (36):1284-1292, 1975.
53. Masson OY and Taylor CR: Distribution of transferrin in human tissues. J Clin Pathol (31):316-327, 1978.
54. Rumke PH, Bisser D, Kwa HG and Hart AAH: Radioimmunoassay of actoferrin in blood plasma of breast cancer patients: lactating and normal women. Folia Med Neerl (14):156-168, 1971.
55. Siegal GP, Barsky SM, Teranova VP: Stages of neoplastic transformation of human breast tissue as monitored by dissection of basement membrane components an immunoperoxidase study. Invasion Metastasis (14):54-59, 1981.
56. Warburton HJ, Fern SA, Rudland PS: Enhanced synthesis of basement membrane during differentiation of rat mammary tumor epithelial cells into myoepithelial-like cells in vitro. Exp Cell Res (137):373-380, 1982.
57. Shivas AA, Douglas JG: The prognostic significance of elastosis in breast carcinoma. Royal College of Surgeons of Edimburgh Journal (17):315-320, 1972.
58. Davies JD, Barnard K and Young EW: Immunoreactive elastin in benign breast tissues. An immunoperoxidase study, Virchows Arch (Pathol Anat) (398):109-117, 1982.
59. Hollinshead AC, Jaffurs WT, Albert LK, Harris JE and Herberman RB: Isolation and identification of soluble skin-reactive membrane antigens of malignant and normal human breast cells. Cancer Res (34):2961-2968, 1974.
60. Avis F, Avis I, Newsome JF and Haughton G: Antigenic cross reactivity between adenocarcinoma of the breast and fibrocystic disease of the breast. J Natl Cancer Inst (56):17-25, 1976.
61. Mesa Tejada R, Keydar I, Ramanarayan M, Ohno T, Fenoglio C and Spiegelman S: Detection in human breast carcinomas of an antigen immunologically related to group-specific antigen of mouse mammary tumor virus. Proc Natl Acad of Sci, USA (75):1529-1530, 1978.
62. Black MM, Sachrau RE, Shore B, Dion A and Leis HP: Cellular immunity to autologous breast cancer and RIII - Murine Mammary Tumor Virus Preparation Cancer Res (38):2008-2078, 1978.
63. Leung JP, Bordin GM, Nakamura RM, Dotlear D, and Edington TS: Frequency of association of mammary tumor glycoprotein antigen and other markers with human breast tumors. Cancer Research (39):2057-2061, 1979.
64. Howard DR, Taylor CR: Amethod for distinguishing benign from malignant breast lesions utilizing antibody present in normal human sera. Cancer (43):2279-2287, 1979.
65. Springer GF, Desai PR and Scanlon EF: Blood group MN precursors as human breast carcinoma associated antigens and "naturally" occurring human cytotoxin against them. Cancer (37):169-176, 1976.
66. Yang NS, McGrath CM, Furmanski P: Presence of a mouse mammary tumor virus-related antigen in human breast carcinoma cells and its absence from normal mammary epithelial cells. J Natl Cancer Inst (61):1205-1205, 1978.
67. Keydar I, Selzer G, Chaitchek S, Hareuveni M, Karby S and Hizi A: A viral antigen as a marker of human breast cancer. Eur J. Cancer Clin Oncol (18):1321-1328, 1982.
68. Menard S, Talgiabue E, Canevari S, Fossati G, Colnaghi MI: Generation of monoclonal antibodies reacting with normal and cancer cells of human breast. Cancer Res (43):1295-1300,1983.

69. Canevari S, Fossati G, Balsari A, Sonnine S, and Colnaghi MI: Immunochemical analysis of the determinant recognized by a monoclonal antibody (MBrl) which specifically binds to human mammary epithelial cells. Cancer Research (43):1301-1305, 1983.
70. Horan Hand PM, Nuti M, Colcher D, and Schlom J: Definition of antigenic heterogeneity among human mammary carcinoma cell population using monoclonal antibodies to tumor associated antigens. Cancer Res (43): 728-735, 1983.
71. Nuti M, Teramoto YA, Mariani-Constantini R, Horan Hand P, Colcher D and Schlom J: A monoclonal antibody (B72:3) defines patterns of distribution of a novel tumor associated antigen in human mammary carcinoma cell populations. Int J Cancer (29):539-545, 1982.
72. Neville MA, Foster CS, Moshakis V and Gore M: Monoclonal antibodies and human tumor pathology. Human Pathology (13):1067-1081, 1982.
73. Byers VS, and Johnston JO: Antigenic differences among antigenic sarcoma tumor cells taken from different location in human tumors. Cancer Res (37):3173-3183, 1977.
74. Fogel M, Gorelik E, Segal S and Feldman M: Differences in cell surface antigens of tumor metastases and those of the local tumor. J Natl Cancer Inst (62):585-588, 1979.
75. Pimm NV, Baldwin RW: Antigenic differences between primary methylcholanthrene-induced rat sarcomas and post surgical recurrences. Int J Cancer 20:37-43, 1977.
76. Colcher D, Horan Hand P, Nuti M and Schlom J: A spectum of monoclonal antibodies reactive with human mammary tumors cells. Proc Natl Acad Sci, USA (78):3199-3203, 1981.
77. Tormey DC, Waalkes, TP, Snyder, JJ, Simon, RM: Biological markers in breast carcinoma: III Clinical correlation with carcinoembryonic antigen. Cancer (39):2397-2404, 1977.
78. Haagensen DE, Kister SJ, Panick J, Giannola J, Hansen, HJ and Wells SA: Comparative evaluation of carcinoembryonic antigen and gross cystic disease fluid protein as plasma markers for human breast carcinoma. Cancer (42):1512-1519, 1978.
79. Steward AM, Dixson D, Xamcheck N, Aisenberg A: Carcinoembryonic antigen in breast cancer patients: Serum levels and disease progress. Cancer (33):1245-1251, 1974.
80. Goldenberg DM, Sharkey RM, Primus FJ: Immunocytochemical detection of carcinoembryonic antigen in conventional histopathology specimens. Cancer (42):1526-1533, 1972.
81. Shousha S, Lyssiotis, T: Correlation of carcinoembryonic antigens in tissue sections with spread of mammary carcinomas. Histopathology (2):433-447, 1978.
82. Walker RA: Demonstration of carcinoembryonic antigen in human breast carcinomas by the immunoperoxidase technique. J Clin Pathol (33):356-366, 1980.
83. Wahren B, Lidbrink E, Willgren A, Eneroth P, Zajicek J: Carcinoembryonic antigen and other tumor markers in tissue and serum or plasma of patients with primary mammary carcinoma. Cancer (42):1870-1878, 1978.
84. Walter SA, Fuaker LD, Dupont WD, Mitchell WM: Carcinoembryonic antigen and patient survival in stage II. Carcinoma of the breast. Lab Invest (44):26a, 1981.
85. Heyderman E, Neville MB: A shorter immunoperoxidase technique for the demonstration of carcinoembryonic antigen and other cell products. J Clin Pathol (30:138-140, 1977.

86. Colcher D. Zalutsky, M, Kaplan W, Kufe D, Austin F, Schlom, J: Radiolocalization of human mammary tumors in athymic mice by a monoclonal antibody. Cancer Res (43):736-742, 1983.
87. Braunstein GD, Vaitukaitis JL, Carbone PP and Ross GT: Ectopic production of human chorionic gonadotropin by neoplasms. Ann Intern Med. (78):39-45, 1973.
88. Tormey DC, Waalken TP and Simon RM: Biological markers in breast carcinoma II clinical correlations with human chorionic gonadotropin. Cancer (39):2391-2396, 1977.
89. Kellen JA, Malkin A, Teodorczyk-Injeyan JA: Gonadotropin-like peptides and their subunits in an experimental mammary adenocarcinoma of the rat. Proc Am Assoc. Cancer Res (21):4, 1980.
90. Vaitukaitis JR and Ebersole ER: Evidence for altered synthesis of human chorionic gonadotropin in gestational trophoblastic tumors. J Clin Endocrinol Metab (42):1048-1052, 1976.
91. Horne CHN, Reid IN and Milne GD: Prognostic significance of inappropriate production of pregnancy proteins by breast cancer. Lancet II, 279, 1976.
92. Wurz H: Serum concentrations of SP1 (pregnancy specific B-glycoprotein) in healthy, nonpregnant individuals, and in patients with nontrophoblastic malignant neoplasm. Arch Gynecol (227):1-5, 1979.
93. Russo J, Fine G, Husain M, Krickstein H, Robbins T, Rosenberg B, Miller J, Ownby H, Roi L, Brooks S, Furmanski P, Rich MA, and Brennan MJ: Tumor grade, estrogen receptor and lymph node status as predictors of early recurrence of breast tumors. Proc Am Assoc. Cancer Research (22):577a, 1981.
94. Shousha S, Lyssiotis, L. Godfrey, VM, Schever, PJ: Carcinoembryonic antigen in breast cancer tissue; A useful prognostic indicator. Br Med J (1):777-779, 1979.

ACKNOWLEDGEMENTS:
This work was supported by the Ida Faigle Charitable Foundation and an Institutional Grant from the United Foundation of Greater Detroit.

The author thanks the secretarial assistance of Kalem Amin Hasan for his meticulous and conscientious work.

14

IMMUNOHISTOCHEMICAL STUDIES IN BREAST CANCER USING MONOCLONAL ANTIBODIES AGAINST BREAST EPITHELIAL CELL COMPONENTS AND WITH LECTINS

CERIANI, R.L. , D.L. HILL , L. OSVALDO , C. KANDELL AND E.W. BLANK

INTRODUCTION

We initially described anti-human mammary epithelial heterologous polyclonal antibodies (1)(anti-HME) that identified normal differentiation antigens of breast epithelial cells. These antigens were present in normal breast epithelial cells at any state of development (2,3), in the human milk fat globule (1), as well as in fibroadenomas, fibrocystic disease and every breast cancer investigated (3). Antigens expressed in high prevalence on human breast epithelial cells and not in other epithelial cells or fibroblasts and recognized by anti-HME are called human mammary epithelial antigens (HME-Ags). Specificity was conferred to anti-HME by repeated absorptions against different human epithelial cells (1).

An important quality of HME-Ags has been the persistence of their expression both after progression and metastatic dissemination (4), prolonged transplantation of human breast tumors in nude mice (5), prolonged *in vitro* culture (3) and cell line passage (6). These HME-Ags have been identified as glycoproteins with molecular weights of 150,000, 70,000 and 46,000 daltons (7). Once identified, these antigens were also found in the plasma of breast cancer patients and not in other patients (8), a fact that again testifies to their specificity and value. In addition, anti-HME Fab fragments labelled with radioiodine were used successfully to image simulated metastases of human breast tumors in nude mice (9). Thus, these cell surface antigens we discovered in breast epithelial cells can be used as markers for this cell type and its specific components, and alterations in expression of these antigens could represent changes of relative significance in cellular metabolism. In the precise case of breast cancer, it is conceivable that absences, increases, or diminutions in HME-Ags synthesis could correlate with breast neoplastic cells' important characteristics, such as invasiveness, response to therapy, de-differentiative potentiality, etc.

With all of the above in mind, and in view of the fact that monocolonal antibodies, above all, represent stable and possibly inexhaustible reagents, we initiated their preparation and successfully created several of them (10). These antibodies, as opposed to other monoclonal antibodies created against the surface of breast epithelial cell lines, were prepared against bona fide normal components, since the immunizing antigens came from the human milk fat globule membrane (10). Later a new series of monoclonal antibodies against milk fat globule were prepared and identified both by intra- and inter-species hybridizations (11).

In earlier studies we were the first to establish that breast epithelial cell populations, either normal or neoplastic, were heterogeneous in terms of their cell surface antigenic expression on a cell-per-cell basis (12). A significant corresponding finding was that, when histological sections were stained by immunoperoxidase techniques using these monoclonal antibodies, a heterogeneous pattern of expression was obtained at the cellular level. There were breast epithelial cells stained at different levels of intensity, and there were cells not stained at all. In view of this, using techniques for breast neoplastic cell-cloning we had previously developed (13), we prepared clonal colonies from normal breast epithelial tissue, from neoplastic breast epithelial tissue, from normal tissue surrounding breast tumors, and from human breast epithelial cell lines. In every instance cellular heterogeneity of antigen expression was proven to be a true phenomenon and not the result of fixation or tissue processing (14, 15). Clonal colonies were obtained where breast epithelial antigens were expressed at different levels, and even negative colonies were found. Confident that cell heterogeneity detected by the antibodies in the histological sections was the representation of the antigenic distribution in the breast tumor, many human breast tumors were stained by immunoperoxidase to determine their antigenic content as evidenced by the binding by monoclonal antibodies. This was done in an attempt to subclassify the several histologic types in which breast cancers are divided. Thus, there could be ductal carcinomas positive or negative for a given monoclonal antibody, or with a certain percentage of positive cells, or with a given per cell content of the antigen under study. This subclassification eventually could be correlated with the natural history of the tumor and possibly valuable prognostic implications could be discerned from it.

An important advantage of using normal cell surface antigens of the breast epithelial cells that are very prevalent, as those under study, is that localization images obtained are always intense and also histological staining very stong, facilitating the measurement of quantitative changes. This is the case for the monoclonal antibodies we created, where screening in their preparation was developed to select antibodies detecting very prevalent cell surface antigens (11).

In the course of these studies one item became evident: the monoclonal antibodies used were breast epithelial membrane-directed and thus they highlighted cell membranous organelles in histological preparations far above what could normally be detected with standard histological techniques, and made structures hitherto seen only with the electron microscope clearly visible. Such was the case with intracytoplasmic lumina (16). These membrane patterns are more abundant in transformed cells, and in some cases exclusive of neoplastic cells. Detection of specialized differentiative organelles is easily accomplished with our monoclonal antibodies, and could perhaps give deeper insight into the membranous differentiation ability of a given breast epithelial cell (or for a whole tumor for the case). Previously, in attempts by other investigators, only levels of expression of the antigens were taken into consideration, but now we propose their study at the levels of membranous organelles, and hope that their correlation with clinical findings could alert us regarding intrinsic characteristics of breast tumors.

In summary, there are increasing expectations that information regarding cell surface antigen expression of breast epithelial cells could be used to help predict clinical outcome or provide indications toward therapeutic choices. Increasing information using straight-forward approaches as to antigen content on the cells will now have to be upgraded to more refined histochemical and structural approaches, wherever possible quantitative, that will give further insight into cellular membrane differentiative processes.

MATERIALS AND METHODS

Paraffin-embedded material from 104 separate cancer cases (78 infiltrating ductal carcinoma, 11 colloid carcinoma, 5 micro-papillary carcinoma, 3 Paget's Disease of the nipple, and 7 carcinoma *in situ*) were sectioned at 5-8 microns and stored at room temperature until needed. Sections were de-paraffinized and rehydrated just prior to labelling and staining. All 104 tumors in the study were classified to type and grade by the same pathologist (L. O.). Estrogen receptor status of each tumor was determined in the Hormone Receptor Laboratory of the University of California, San Francisco School of Medicine.

Three murine monoclonal antibodies [Mc1, Mc5, (11) anti-Fatty Acid Synthetase] and two plant lectins, Concanavalin A and peanut agglutinin, were used to localize cytoplasmic and membrane determinants on tumor cells. Monoclonals Mc1 and Mc5 recognize two distinct antigens found on normal and malignant human mammary epithelial cells (11). Purified rat fatty acid synthetase was a gift from Dr. Stuart Smith. Murine monoclonal antibodies to FAS were developed in accordance to reported techniques (11). The plant lectins were a commercial preparation (E. Y. Laboratories, San Mateo, CA).

Visualization of labelled cells was done using peroxidase-diaminobenzidine in an avidin-biotin system ("Vectastain" from

Vector Laboratories, Inc.). All sections were counterstained with either hematoxylin or methylene blue prior to dehydration, mounting under coverslips (Permount) and examination.

Subjective data were obtained by microscopic evaluation of each slide, and scores representing average density of labelling on each of three possible cellular domains: apical region, membranous or cytoplasmic. A membrane staining surrounding a lumen or lumen-like structure (pseudo-lumen) was designated as apical. A membrane stain not surrounding a lumen or lumen-like structure but present on the cell membrane, either opposed to the basement membrane and/or another cell or structure was designated membranous. A score of 0-4 was given for each domain labelled by Mc1, Mc5 or anti-FAS. Only cytoplasmic scoring was recorded for labelling with plant lectins.

Microspectrum Analyzer (MSA) Determinations were obtained through use of a Farrand Spectrum Analyzer apparatus attached to a Leitz optical microscope. The instrument was "zeroed" either on an unstained tumor cell or, if no negative cells were present, on adjacent connective tissue. Fifty random readings of tumor cell cytoplasm were recorded per slide, and the mean (x), standard deviation (S.D.) and coefficient of variation (C.V. = S.D./$\bar{x}$) calculated for each specimen.

RESULTS

In infiltrating ductal carcinoma, the largest group of tumors examined, the degree of differentiation and estrogen receptor status of each tumor was compared to the binding pattern of Mc1 and Mc5 monoclonal antibodies to the tumor cells. A significantly greater percentage of tumors having some type (i.e., apical, membranous or both) of membrane-associated staining were estrogen receptor-positive (76-82%) compared to tumors staining exclusively in the cytoplasm (56-57%). This was noted regardless of the degree of tumor differentiation (Graphs A & B).

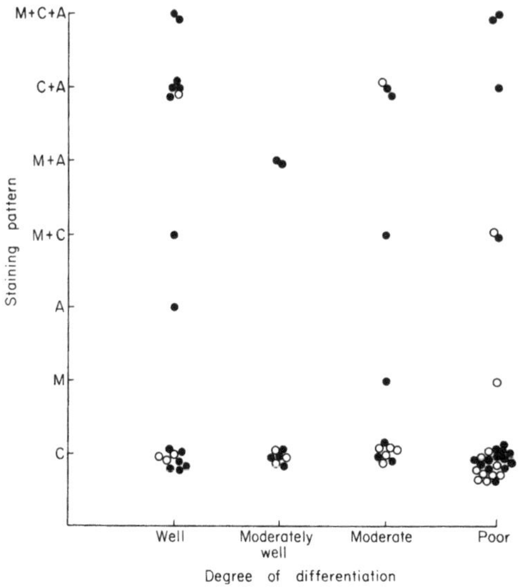

GRAPH A
Comparison of degree of differentiation, estrogen receptor status and staining pattern with breast-specific monoclonal antibodies (Mc1) in infiltrating ductal carcinomas. Percentage of tumors with membranous and/or apical staining with Mc1 that are estrogen-receptor positive = 76%. Percentage of tumors with only cytoplasmic staining with Mc1 that are estrogen receptor-positive = 57%.

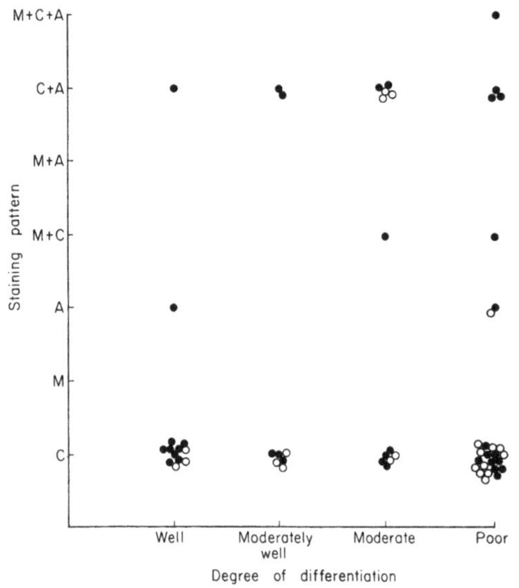

GRAPH B
Comparison of degree of differentiation, estrogen receptor status and staining pattern with breast-specific monoclonal antibodies (Mc5) in infiltrating ductal carcinomas. Percentage of tumors with membranous and/or apical staining with Mc5 that are estrogen-receptor positive = 82%. Percentage of tumors with only cytoplasmic staining with Mc5 that are estrogen receptor-positive = 56%.

M = membranous staining
C = cytoplasmic staining
A = apical staining
O = estrogen receptor negative
● = estrogen receptor positive

The percentage of tumors positive for estrogen receptors (see below) was developed for each degree of histological differentiation (Table I.). The greatest percentage of cells with estrogen receptors were in well-differentiated tumors, decreasing in frequency in a linear fashion as the degree of differentiation worsened.

Eye-scoring data for mean intensity of monoclonal antibody labelling (cytoplasmic) as it related to the degree of differentiation may be seen in Table II. It is clear that all three monoclonals stained the cytoplasm of cells in all four differentiation categories to approximately the same level. A comparison of the fifteen scores from Table II gives an overall average of 2.50 on a 0-4 intensity scale, the latter the most intense.

Table I. Estrogen Receptor Status of Infiltrating Ductal Carcinoma:

Differentiation	Percent ER-Positive Tumors
Well	78.9 (15/19)
Moderately well	75.0 (6/8)
Moderate	61.5 (8/13)
Poor	58.6 (17/29)

Table II. Relative levels (eye-scoring data) of cytoplasmic staining with breast-specific monoclonal antibodies (Mcl, Mc5) and anti-FAS monoclonal antibodies of infiltrating ductal carcinomas with respect to degree of differentiation.

Differentiation	Mcl	Mc5	Anti-FAS
Well	2.42 (13)	2.88 (16)	2.33 (15)
E-R(+)	2.35 (14)	2.91 (14)	2.15 (14)
E-R(-)	2.31 (4)	2.88 (4)	2.15.(4)
Mod. Well	2.52 (10)	2.76 (10)	2.11 (9)
Moderate	2.56 (13)	2.53 (14)	2.27 (11)
Poor	2.48 (27)	2.77 (29)	2.37.(24)

SCALE OF 0-4

Table III shows a breakdown of the numbers of estrogen-positive tumors that also had positive apical staining for each degree of histological differentiation. Data was analyzed for Mc1 and Mc5 binding only.

Anti-FAS stained apically only 8 of 104 tumors (not shown). This size sample group was considered inappropriate to show a meaningful breakdown of staining patterns with respect to differentiation. However, all eight that did apically stain with anti-FAS were either well or moderately well differentiated. Out of the 78 tumors in the infiltrating ductal carcinoma category, only 2 of the Mc1 and 4 of the Mc5 - labelled tumors that stained apically were estrogen receptor negative.

Mc1

Table III. Percentage of breast tumors estrogen receptor positive or negative that had apical-type staining.

Degree of Differentiation	% E-R (+)	% E-R (-)
Well	13 (2/15)	0 (0/4)
Moderately Well	33 (2/6)	0 (0/2)
Moderate	25 (2/8)	80 (4/5)
Poor	29 (5/17)	8 (1/12)

Mc5

Degree of Differentiation	% E-R (+)	% E-R (-)
Well	40 (6/15)	25 (1/4)
Moderately Well	33 (2/6)	0 (0/2)
Moderate	12 (1/8)	20 (1/5)
Poor	17 (3/17)	0 (0/12)

Table IV shows monoclonal antibody and lectin binding to different mammary carcinomas, expressed as the percentage of total tumors per category that positively stained with each reagent. This table demonstrates binding of monoclonal anti-breast antibodies and anti-FAS, as well as the two plant lectins tested to tumor cells, regardless of histopathologic classification.

Table IV. Monoclonal antibody and lectin binding to different mammary carcinomas, expressed as the percentage positively stained with each reagent.

Classification	Mc1	Mc5	anti-FAS	PNA	ConA
Infiltrating Ductal	90(70/78)	98(77/78)	83(65/78)	87(68/78)	78(61/78)
Micropap- illary	100 (5/5)	100 (5/5)	100 (5/5)	100 (5/5)	80 (4/5)
Paget's Dis. (Nipple)	100 (3/3)	100 (3/3)	100 (3/3)	33 (1/3)	66 (2/3)
Colloid Carcinoma	91(10/11)	100(11/11)	91(10/11)	36 (4/11)	91(10/11)
Carcinoma in situ	100 (7/7)	100 (7/7)	100 (7/7)	66 (4/6)	100 (6/6)

Tables V and VI demonstrate lectin binding patterns compared to estrogen receptor status in infiltrating ductal carcinoma for Concanavalin A and peanut agglutinin, respectively. Both of these tables show a greater likelihood of tumors that were well to moderately well differentiated to be positive for both lectin and estrogen binding than being positive only for a lectin. More poorly differentiated tumors, on the other hand, had a high frequency of lectin-positive, estrogen-negative results.

Table V. Concanavalin A binding patterns compared to estrogen receptor status in infiltrating ductal carcinoma.

Differentiation	% total ConA (+)	% ConA(+), E-R(+)	% ConA(+), E-R(-)
Well	88 (15/17)	76 (13/17)	17 (9/25)
Moderately Well	71 (5/7)	71 (5/7)	0 (0/7)
Moderate	60 (6/10)	20 (2/10)	50 (5/10)
Poor	88 (22/25)	52 (13/25)	36 (9/25)

Table VI. Peanut agglutinin binding patterns compared to estrogen receptor status in infiltrating ductal carcinoma.

Differentiation	% total PNA()	%PNA(+), E-R(+)	%PNA(+), E-R(-)
Well	71 (12/17)	52 (9/17)	18 (3/17)
Moderately Well	100 (5/5)	100 (5/5)	0 (0/5)
Moderate	63 (7/11)	45 (5/11)	18 (2/11)
Poor	60 (13/22)	36 (8/22)	22 (5/22)

A result similar to the lectin data shown in Tables V and VI held for anti-FAS monoclonal binding patterns compared to estrogen receptor status in infiltrating ductal carcinoma, shown in Table VII. Again, more well-differentiated tumors were about twice as likely to have positive binding in both parameters than their less well-differentiated counterparts.

One pattern that did emerge was the correlation between positive estrogen receptor status and binding of plant lectins or anti-FAS in infiltrating ductal carcinoma. A tumor positive for estrogen receptor was nearly twice as likely to stain positively for either plant lectin or anti-FAS. This finding, coupled with data showing a positive correlation in tumor cell membrane staining and estrogen receptor status, suggests that both availability of the estrogen receptor and that of cell membrane and cytoplasmic (FAS) antigens are all in some way related to the state of cellular differentiation.

Due to sample size, statistical data was not performed on Paget's Disease cases. Of three cases of Paget's Disease, all stained at least cytoplasmically with Mcl, Mc5 and anti-FAS.

MSA studies were performed on several cases of infiltrating ductal carcinoma, stained with murine monoclonals Mcl and Mc5. Each symbol represents a tumor from which 50 single-cell readings were recorded to calculate mean and coefficient of variation for each tumor. Graphs C and D compare three different parameters for each tumor examined.

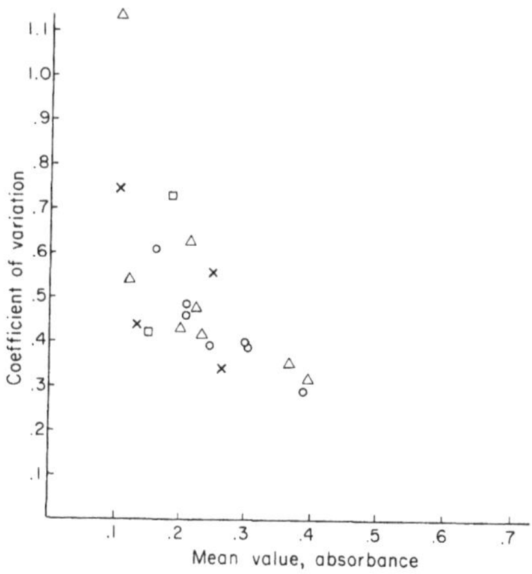

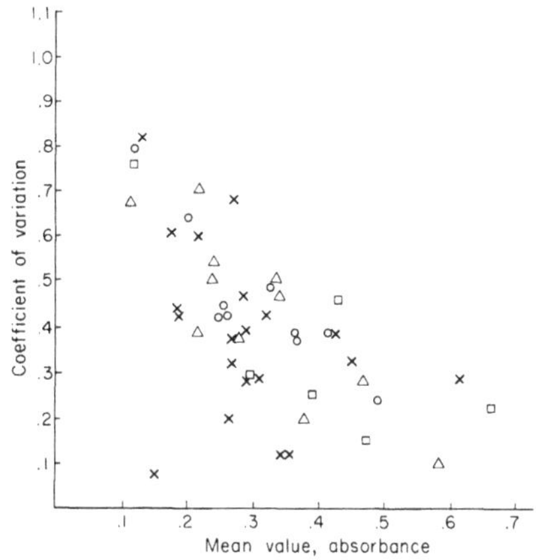

Graph C. Range of variation in mean values and coefficients of variation in binding of anti-HMFG monoclonal antibodies (Mc1) to single tumor cells in infiltrating ductal carcinomas. Each character represents a tumor from which 50 single-cell readings were recorded to calculate mean and coefficient of variation for each tumor.

Graph D. Range of variation in mean values and coefficients of variation in binding of anti-HMFG monoclonal antibodies (Mc5) to single tumor cells in infiltrating ductal carcinomas. Each character represents a tumor from which 50 single-cell readings were recorded to calculate mean and coefficient of variation for each tumor.

△ = well-differentiated
▢ = moderately well-differentiated
O = moderately differentiated
X = poorly differentiated

By examining these graphs it is possible to see that cytoplasmically-located, Mc1 or Mc5-defined HMFG antigen found in each differentiation category of tumor was variable in amount. Moreover, well-differentiated tumors did not, for example, cluster about a particular value of absorbance, but instead were spread through a range of absorbance values.

What these graphs also show is that, regardless of the level of differentiation, low mean absorbance seemed to correlate with greater values for coefficient of variation ($C.V. = S.D./\overline{x}$). Plotting the mean absorbance vs. the coefficient of variation for each individual tumor allows one to see the variability in absorbance values for each tumor, or differentiation grouping of tumors. In a previous study (12), the quantity of HME antigen found in breast tumors was generally lower than that found in normal mammary glands. What may be inferred from the data shown in graphs C and D is a furtherance of this finding to show how tumors containing the least amount of antigen (and hence most diverse from normal) may also be the most variable in their expression of antigen, thus having the greatest amount of phenotypic heterogeneity within a given tumor.

In this paper, we describe quantitative aspects of anti-breast epithelial antibody binding to breast tumors of different histopathological types, with reference to their degree of differentiation and steroid receptor content. In addition, we describe new cellular membrane differentiative patterns that are readily detectable by our monoclonal antibodies, and that appear to be, in some cases, privative of the aberrant cellular differentiation patterns of breast tumor cells.

Anti-breast epithelial monoclonal antibodies can also be very successful in identifying different membranous structures of breast epithelial cells. These structures can be highlighted by the use of these monoclonal antibodies far above their almost subliminal appearance in H & E staining. To this effect two monoclonal antibodies that we created, Mc1 and Mc5, that bind to a surface component with high prevalence on the breast epithelium were used (11).

After immunoperoxidase staining of breast carcinomas with Mc1 and Mc5, the cell membranes limiting lumina were usually strongly positive as were also the apical membranes of normal breast epithelial cells. In these carcinomas it was also clearly noticeable that the cytoplasm of many of their cells stained to various degrees in most tumors. In total, we reviewed 29 cases for this section of the study of in situ and infiltrating carcinomas that included solid, comedo and micropapillary cribriform patterns. Upon reviewing the different cases at the cytological levels, the patterns identified by the immunoperoxidase staining highlighted four distinctive cytological images : i) Intracytoplasmic lumina (ICL), ii) potential or pseudo-lumina (PL), iii) marginal labelling (staining)(ML), and iv) polar bodies (PB).

i.) ICL's

Close inspection of the immunoperoxidase-stained sections showed the ease with which ICL's (16) can be identified by this method using monoclonal antibodies Mc1 and Mc5. These membrane-directed monoclonal antibodies clearly detected these organelles wherever they existed. ICL's were seen in all cases of breast carcinoma as round bodies (1-2 microns in diameter), showing no particular association with apical or basilar portions of the cell. A barely visible central space was sometimes seen, but only distension of the lumina displayed the typical aggregates of tiny microvilli (Fig. 1, 2).

The emerging central space was sometimes partially filled with a secretory-like material, creating then the so-called target structure, showing a similar positive reaction (Fig. 1, 3). The remarkable increase in size of ICL's was secondary to dilation of their lumen (Fig. 1). They were always easy to recognize because they remained as sharply circumscribed spherical spaces outlined by thick, smooth membranes (Fig. 1, 2, 3, 4). The degree of enlargement of ICL's was variable, but sometimes the lumen was so ample that with the H & E sections

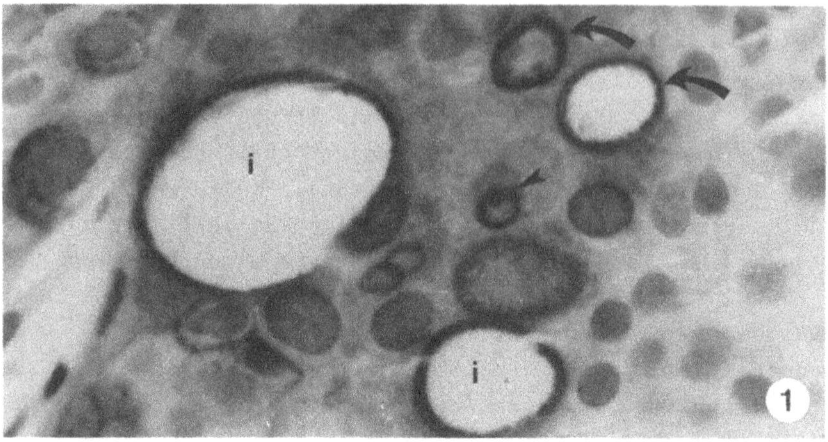

Figure 1. Immunoperoxidase staining with MC5 monoclonal antibody of intraductal carcinoma of the breast. There is a variable degree of dilatation of ICL. The fuzzy inner portion made up of microvilli - (long arrows) contrasts with microvilli cut tangentially (short arrow). A small ICL contains a positive eccentric deposit (arrowhead) and the membranes of two neighboring ICL overlap. Large ICL (i) show focal interruption of the thick membrane, X400.

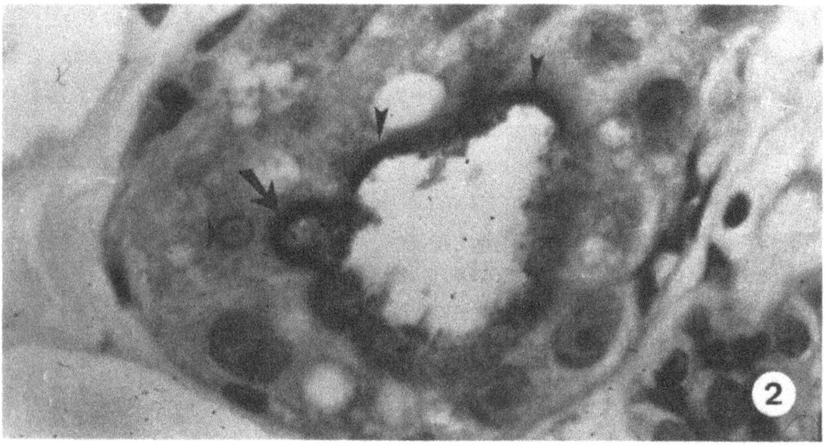

Figure 2. Immunoperoxidase staining with MC5 monoclonal antibody of ductal carcinoma of the breast. One ICL (long arrow) and two curved segments of ICL membrane (long arrownheads), together with microvilli and cell surface material outline a space. A small ICL is noted (short arrowhead). The cellular cluster mimics a gland, X400.

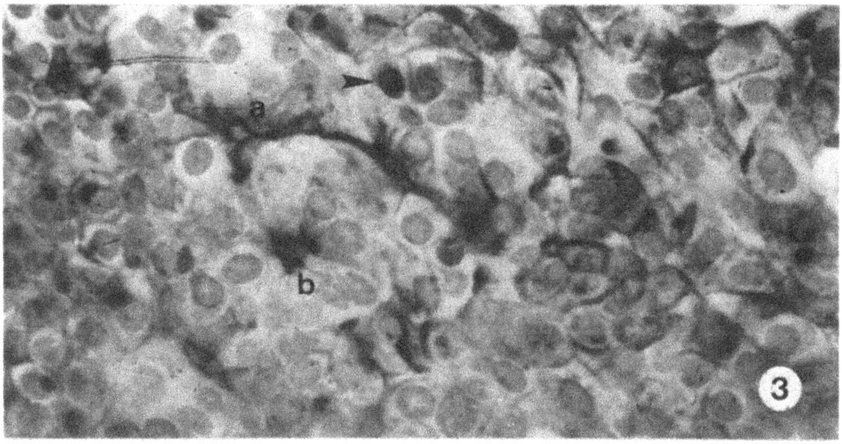

Figure 3. Immunoperoxidase staining with MC5 monoclonal antibody of ductal carcinoma with heterogeneous pattern of staining. There are many ICL and one (arrowhead) shows incipient dilatation. At the bottom of the figure, there is an ICL with target structure. Strongly stained membranes delineate two potential lumina in longitudinal (a) and cross sections (b) (See also Fig.5), X250.

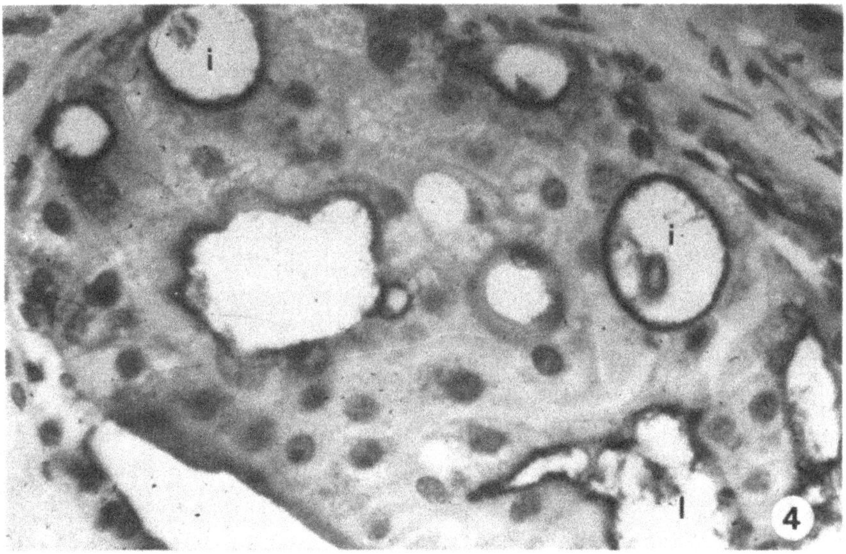

Figure 4. Immunoperoxidase staining with MC5 monoclonal antibody of ductal carcinoma of the breast with apocrine differentiation. There are several dilated ICL and microcystic transformations. Positive material is present in the spaces of two ICL (i) and a large lumina (l). A rigid membranous fragment (long arrow) lies free close to the basement membrane, X250.

they were visualized as "microcystic" spaces within a solid tumor mass (Fig. 4). Microvilli remained attached to the thick membrane with no obvious increase in length (Fig. 1, 2, 3). Microvilli formed a fuzzy, darkly-stained band, and their characteristic shape was sometimes discerned at high magnification. In sections tangential to the wall of the lumina, microvilli cut at different angles filled the entire space (Fig. 1). The apparent fusion of several ICL's produce a cloverleaf-like or scalloped contour (Fig. 2, 4). It was not certain that all "microcysts" were secondary to fusion of ICL's. It is quite likely that many of them originated from a single, gradually enlarging vacuole. Thus, morphological patterns can be established for breast tumors whereby increased dilation of ICL's can produce focal or diffuse microcystic transformation (as the result of dilation of one ICL)(Fig. 1); or, alternatively, formation of gland-like structures (Fig. 2) could result from the confluence of several ICL's. Both these variants can hypothetically be linked to an effort toward glandular differentiation by the neoplastic breast cells.

Previous authors (16, 17, 18) have described ICL's in some detail, but with the use of such sensitive and suitable methods as the one proposed, it can be established that ICL's exist both in normal breast epithelium and any type of breast tumor that we happened to inspect, thus making it a much more prevalent phenomenon than previously thought (23).

ii) PL

Another membranous structure characteristic of ductal breast carcinomas are PL's, which also are clearly detected at the light microscopic level by the use of Mc1 and Mc5 (Fig. 3, 5). The appearance of pseudo-lumina or potential lumina can also be viewed as an effort toward differentiation by the breast carcinoma, and again its clear visualization by the methods proposed could aid in establishing the differentiative level of a given breast tumor.

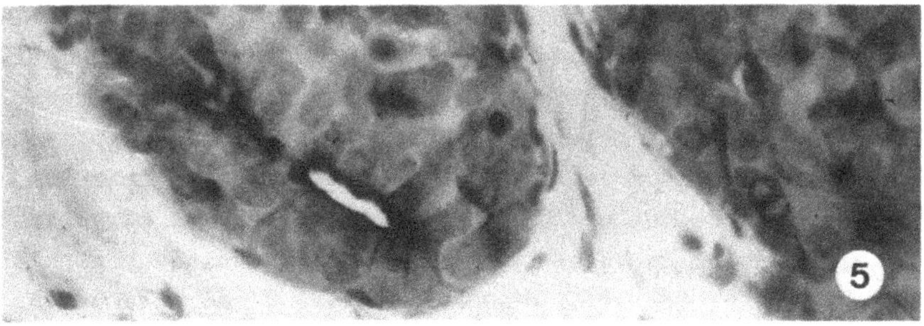

Figure 5. Immunoperoxidase staining with Mc5 monoclonal antibody of ductal carcinoma of the breast. A slit-like potential lumen shows positive labeling of apical membrane of cells and underlying cytoplasm. Many small underlying ICL are seen, X250.

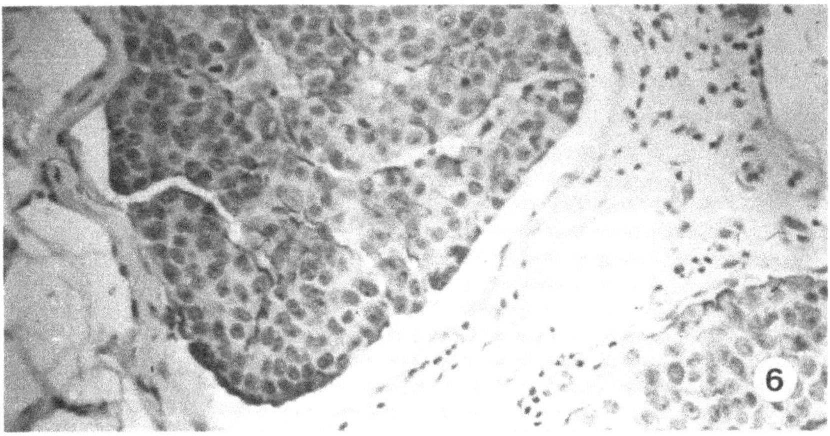

Figure 6. Immunoperoxidase staining with Mc5 monoclonal antibody of ductal carcinoma of the breast shows a tumor embolus with marginal labeling of cells segregated into cluster, X100.

These PL's are seen as malignant cells showing strong positive staining of a segment of the surface membrane usually associated with a similar pattern in opposing and/or adjacent cells (Fig. 3). The underlying cytoplasm revealed equally strong reactivity. Groups of cells showing this polarized reaction of membrane and cytoplasm were arranged in a linear or slightly curved fashion, or converged toward a darkly stained center (Fig. 3). In other carcinomas, PL's were minimal gland-like lumina, surrounded by orderly arranged cells with positive apical membranes (Fig. 5). These slits, devoid of any secretion, were different from the "punched out" spaces produced by dilation of ICL, although ICL may be present in cells showing a polarized segmental reaction. The spatial relationship of ICL, positive cell membrane reaction, and the appearance of pseudolumina is likely to be clarified only at the ultrastructural level. We draw attention to this pattern of membrane reaction because it was also present in solid nests of infiltrative ductal carcinomas. The minimally opened or virtual lumina were remarkably delineated by Mc1 and Mc5 and are easily missed in H & E sections.

iii) ML

The use of immunoperoxidase staining with Mc1 and Mc5 allowed for detection of yet another distinctive accumulation and polarization of membrane material. This pattern of membrane reactivity constituted the ML's that could only be identified by histochemistry as cell clusters surrounded by a thin, strongly reactive membrane following the contour of peripheral cells in each cluster. This image was clearly seen on tumor emboli in veins and lymphatics (Fig. 6). In addition, ML's were identified in solid masses of cells in intraductal tumors. In some carcinomas, groups of cells within the solid intraductal mass were segregated into clusters. Single or layered membranes were admixed with necrotic debris, and lined the positively stained, basement membranes of the ducts.

Another variation of the pattern of marginal labeling not uncommon in invasive ductal carcinomas is shown in Figure 7. Solid nests of tumor cells were surrounded by strongly positive membranes that wrapped around each nest; only some peripheral epithelial cells in each cluster had positive staining of the lateral cell membrane.

iv) PB

Finally, there was a membrane differentiative pattern that appeared with some regularity which we have provisionally designated as "polar body." It is possible that it corresponds to the "villous polarity" studied by Eusebi et al. (19, 20). Polar bodies are sharply circumscribed, angular areas of the cell surface strongly stained by Mc1 and Mc5 (Fig. 8). The tiny projection was seen mostly in contact with the stroma, but it was easily obscured when the entire cytoplasm or surface membrane reacted strongly with monoclonal antibodies. We believed the designation of polar body was adequate since we cannot discern the microvilli recognized at the ultrastructural level. We have recognized polar bodies in the cells of three intraductal carcinomas, and all of them contained many such bodies in the invasive component.

As a summary, all these four membranous structures that are evidenced by the use of breast epithelial cell membrane antigens are now being evaluated for their ability to designate differentiation stages of breast epithelium. Their clear-cut appearance allows for easy recognition and quantitation at low magnification, as can be done for mitoses, thus increasing their potential value if they were to be found to possess prognostic significance.

DISCUSSION

In this paper we have described a series of immunohistochemical studies on 104 cases of breast tumors, wherein quantitative and qualitative aspects of monoclonal

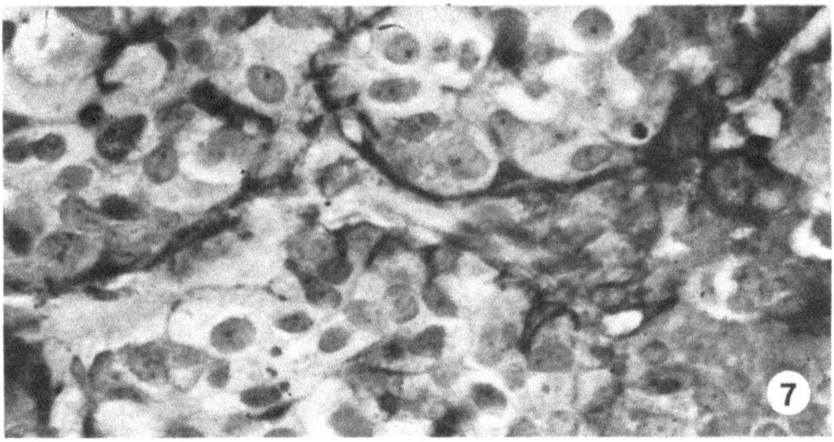

Figure 7. Immunoperoxidase staining with Mc5 monoclonal antibody of invasive poorly differentiated carcinoma shows segregation of cells into clusters by labeling of periphery of cell membranes. Heterogeneous staining of tumor is demonstrated, X400.

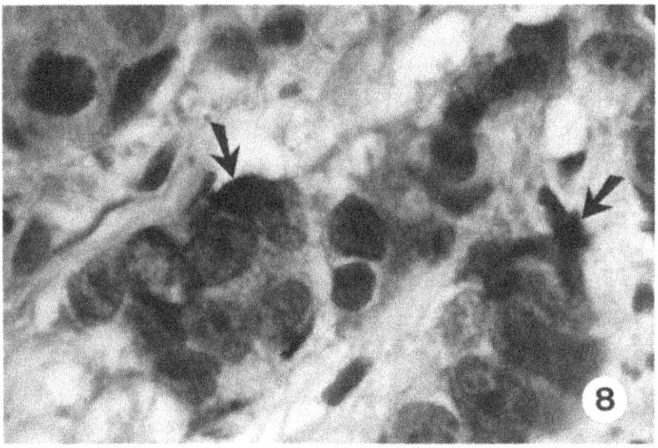

Figure 8. Immunoperoxidase staining with Mc5 monoclonal antibody of ductal carcinoma. Two polar bodies are demonstrated (arrows), X400.

antibody and lectin binding patterns are correllated with estrogen receptor status, histopathological classification and differentiation parameters of breast tumors. Comparisons were made not only between different histological tumor classifications, but also to their degree of differentiation. In addition, efforts were made to define subgroups within the standard breast tumor types as identified by the markers used. The findings in Table 1 corroborate previous findings of a direct positive relationship in estrogen receptor status to how well a tumor is differentiated. Results of monoclonal antibody to human breast epithelial cell differentiation antigens and lectin binding studies provide a means additional to classical histopathological diagnosis and estrogen binding assays for assessing a tumor's prognosis. Regardless of the degree of differentiation or estrogen receptor status, infiltrating ductal carcinomas had significant (2.5) on 0-4 density scale) cytoplasmic labelling by the three monoclonals tested. Cytoplasmic deposition of antigens normally found on the plasma membrane is a well-documented phenomenon, and such is apparently the case with the antigen defined by the monoclonals Mc1 and Mc5. The presence and density of FAS in tumor cells was unaffected by differentiation status, and differed little from results obtained from normal tissue.

Analysis of the infiltrating ductal carcinomas that had significant apical-type staining and were also estrogen receptor positive revealed a high percentage of poorly differentiated tumors having positive apical staining when being estrogen receptor positive as well. These findings appear at first to be a contradiction in terms. To categorize a tumor as being poorly differentiated indicates (among other parameters) a general lack of cellular polarity, essentially no "attempt" by the cancer cells to mimic normal glandular architecture. Staining with monoclonal antibodies of the tumor cells as was done here has a significant enhancing effect on visualization of cell membranes that contain Mc1 and Mc5 defined antigen, allowing for a degree of definition of cellular orientation and intercellular patterns not possible with conventional hematoxylin and eosin staining. While these more differentiated foci of tumor cells comprise a small percentage of the tumor section, they show a definite trend of the tumor as a whole towards a higher state of differentiation. Their presence intermingled with the more prevalent population of undifferentiated tumor cells may lend further evidence for phenotypic heterogeneity existing within the same neoplasm, even in regards to multicellular differentiation.

Breast tumors, when taken as a whole, showed a high overall degree of binding of both monoclonal antibodies and plant lectins. However, differences in morphology of these lesions that allowed for traditional histological categorization into distinct tumor classifications were not reflected into significantly different labelling profiles. All five of the ligands tested for were apparently conserved irrespective of tumor classification. Retention of monoclonal antibody-defined cell surface antigens by breast tumors of histopathological classification similar to our study have been reported (21) with staining patterns ranging from purely membranous to cytoplasmic. Together these findings indicate that differences between tumors placed in different histopathological types do not reflect differences on tumor cell surfaces detected by any known anti-breast, or anti-breast tumor-associated antibody.

Lectin binding studies on different grades of infiltrating ductal carcinoma compared to estrogen receptor status of the respective grades revealed a direct correlation found not only in the binding patterns of the two plant lectins but also in the binding of anti-FAS antibody. The reason for why tumor cells positive for estrogen receptors were also twice as likely to be positive for Con-A, PNA or anti-FAS may reflect a shift in either expression of antigenicity or accessibility of these ligands. An understanding of how multiple cellular constituents can be simultaneously affected to result in phenotypic alteration is under continuing investigation. A clearer understanding of this phenomenon of antigenic modulation may eventually allow for more effective immunotherapy of breast and other cancers with monoclonal antibodies.

In addition, detailed examination of the breast tissue sections stained with the monoclonal antibodies revealed unique cellular and tissue features, which could only be detected with this approach. Anti-normal breast epithelial cell membrane antibodies here used have to their advantage a high level of expression of their corresponding antigens. This high level of expression on cell membrane structures and organelles allows for their accurate recognition whenever they are present. An example of the latter is the clear identification at the light microscope level of ICL's. These organelles are of uncertain function in, the cell. Although found in normal tissue (22, 23), they are also found (usually in increased numbers) in breast carcinomas. They have usually been ascribed to lobular carcinomas (22), since in them they retain their usual pattern. In contrast, in ductal carcinomas they acquire an inflated look and punch-hole appearance and are often filled with secretory products. It is in ductal carcinoma, and not in the lobular ones, where coalescence of ICL's seems to occur; so much as to lead the authors to propose that those lacunar, punched-out, cloverleaf-like lumina found in ductal carcinomas could have as their origin ICL's. These lumina have to be distinguished from those slit-like structures we call PL's which, even when they form patent lumina, remain slit-like, and in further contrast to the lacunar type which in fact may be created by ICL's but are never seen to contain secretory material.

The strong staining obtained with monoclonal antibodies shows distinctively in solid ductal carcinoma the presence of slits that correspond to pseudo-lumina, a differentiative characteristic of these cells. Thus we postulate that the presence of such PL indicates a higher state of differentiation for a given tumor than does their absence. In fact, in our series of estrogen receptor positive, poorly differentiated ductal carcinomas, five out of six cases had PLs' as detected by monoclonal antibody Mc5 (Graph B). This finding could have definite prognostic significance. The creation of PL's comes as the result of accumulation of breast epithelial antigens in a polarized fashion, but very often with organized interaction with surrounding cells. This cell-to-cell interaction suggests that cells in the breast tumor are in fact interacting and communicating with each other so to generate membrane organized conditions that are common to several or many of them. This retained social behavior of the cell population can be ascribed to a higher level of tissue differentiation.

In another instance, this accumulation of breast epithelial antigens in certain segments of cells adjacent to each other takes a different look. Marginally staining breast carcinoma cells form aggregates, where only the portion of membrane of the cells in contact with the outside of the aggregate expresses the antigen. The area of membrane participating in intercellular contact within the aggregate does not express the antigen (fig. 6). Patterns of this kind found in venous and lymphatic emboli and in the infiltrating cell nests of invasive ductal carcinomas point to a possible relation between this pattern and an aggressive, disseminative behavior in the tumoral cells.

Thus the use of these immunohistochemical procedures highlights patterns of membrane specialization without having to resort to ultrastructural techniques in studies requiring the screening of a large population of cells or many fields in each histological section. In this regard, microvilli formation has been a common attribute of breast epithelial cells, and they have also been described to appear in a polarized, aberrant fashion in the midst of a sheet of breast carcinoma cells. As we have already noticed (unpublished observation), breast epithelial cell surface components concentrate in areas of largest membrane activity like pseudopodia and on microvilli in cultured cells. In those clusters of microvilli that were described by Azzopardi, et al. (20), we also found distinctive accumulation of cell surface antigen, and we called them thus polar bodies (PB). Polar bodies, a microvillous structure possibly associated with highly pleomorphic carcinomas (20), are easy to spot and could become, with the other pattern described, further aids in establishing the level of differentiation of a breast tumor.

In summary, with the power conferred to membrane antigen detection by histochemistry, we can define several cell membrane patterns that we believe represent efforts, albeit aberrant, toward differentiation of breast carcinoma cells. Intracytoplasmatic lumina are more abundant and coalescing in breast carcinoma as opposed to normal. Although their genesis seems obscure at the moment, their presence in normal tissue, especially in midpregnant tissues, could indicate a higher state of cell membrane production and assemblage by the cell. The other cellular patterns described, found only in carcinoma, seem to be a parody of cell membrane polarization and intercellular tissue arrangement as seen in normal breast epithelium, where the apical membrane of the many cells bordering a lumen stain strongly. The formation of pseudo-lumina speaks of a concerted effort of several adjacent breast epithelial cells to form a lumen and to acquire a "normal" state of differentiation, where concerted social behavior of adjacent cells exists. In this same line the marginal staining phenomenon (Mc5) shows again cell-to-cell interaction in a larger scale among few or many cells to create a boundary laden with cell surface antigens facing non-epithelial tissue or support material. All these patterns have in common a reliance for their recognition on the sensitivity provided by use of monoclonal antibodies against very prevalent normal differentiative components of the breast cell membrane.

The use of immunohistochemical procedures plus monoclonal antibodies and lectins both directed to cell membrane components of breast epithelial cells provide immense possibilities for the study of breast carcinomas. First, it is possible to quantitate their presence either for the whole tumor and on a cell-per-cell basis, recording the percent of positive or negative cells a tumor has and even to quantitate the level of antigen cell-per-cell. Second, as the antigens recognized by the monoclonal antibodies are associated with cell membrane differentiation (they are found in high levels in the milk fat globule) an accurate study of cell membrane differentiation of the breast tumor cell can be accomplished. Normal cellular membrane patterns can be shown that mimic possibly in an asynchronous way the abnormal pathway of differentiation taken by breast tumor cells. These cell membrane patterns could correspond to different stages in the final differentiation of the breast epithelial cell and therefore represent markers for given levels. Their presence can then be interpreted as indicating the level of arrest in differentiation of the clonal cell population composing the breast tumor. The differentiation autigens of the breast epithlial cells can also be used in cell lineage studies, as in the case of Paget's disease of the breast.

Different views have been expressed regarding the origins of the cells of Paget's disease of the breast. As it was originally described, carcinomatous infiltration of the nipple and areola in Paget's disease of the breast are accompanied by intraglandular carcinoma of similar histologic or cytologic appearance. We have studied three cases of Paget's disease of the breast, two of them with physical or radiological evidence of both nipple and intraglandular disease, and the last one with only nipple evidence of disease. Paraffin-embedded sections of many blocks of both nipple and the corresponding breast were stained with monoclonal antibodies Mc1, Mc5 and anti-fatty acid synthetase, using immunoperoxidase staining.

The typical light, large and round Paget cells in the epidermis stained intensely with the three antisera (Fig. 9). In the case of Mc1 and Mc5, the staining, which occurred in most Paget cells, was mainly membranous; however, the cytoplasm stained at times lighter in most cells. The rest of the cells of the epidermis and dermis were negative. With anti-fatty acid synthetase both Paget and normal skin epidermal cells were stained. However, the skin cells stained in a fine, granular pattern, while the Paget cells stained in a clumped and sometimes vacuolar (with deeply stained edges) pattern.

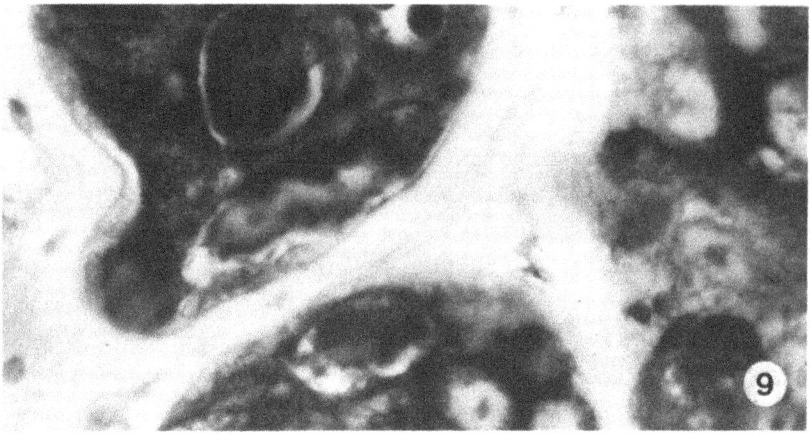

Figure 9. Immunoperoxidase staining with Mc5 monoclonal antibody of Paget cells infiltrating the epidermis. There is strong and heterogeneous labeling of membranes and cytoplasm equal to the cells of the underlying breast carcinoma. Some cells show only a remnant of surface membrane and empty cytoplasm, (section counterstained with methylene blue), X400.

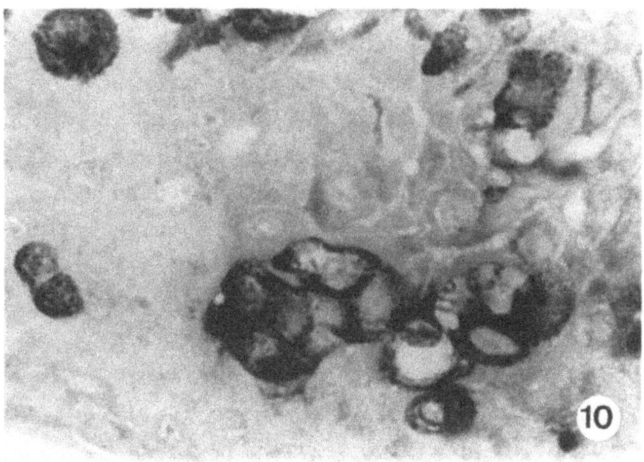

Figure 10. Immunoperoxidase staining with Mc5 monoclonal antibody of Paget cells invading a duct. There is strong cytoplasmic staining in most breast tumor cells, (section counterstained with metylene blue), X400.

In the first two cases, intraductal carcinomatous growth was deeply stained by both Mc1 and Mc5 (Fig. 10); the pattern of cellular staining and overall appearance was in no way different from the way the Paget cells of the nipple stained. In addition, the staining pattern with anti-fatty acid synthetase in intraductal carcinoma cells was coarse and vacuolar as that of Paget cells in the epidermis.

The third case is worth noting since it was the one without breast gland clinical manifestation of the disease. There were only nipple manifestations in this case. Paget cells of the epidermis were stained and resembled closely those of the previous case with the three monoclonal antibodies and tumor cells found only in larger galactophores a short distance from the nipple orifice. These cells also were as deeply stained with the antibodies as the previous two intraductal carcinomas were. This case shows conspicuously two points. First, both nipple and intraglandular cells are again identical, but also that at a very early stage of putative cancerization of ducts and alveoli the cells correspond to those of a full-blown case of Paget's disease, according to the immunohistological pattern.

In addition, a new membrane maturation marker (easily detected by monoclonal antibodies Mc1 and Mc5), the intracytoplasmic lumina, ICL's were also observed. ICL's are plasma membrane-related organelles that have been clearly seen in secretory epithelial cells, and not in skin cells. Close inspection at high magnification revealed ICL's in cancer cells both in the nipple and in the intraductal components of all three cases of Paget's disease of the breast under study. Therefore, on three confirmatory lines we can base our contention that both the nipple and ductal components belong to similar strains of carcinoma cells, namely: a) All epidermal and intraductal Paget cells stain similarly with monoclonal antibodies Mc1 and Mc5; b) both the nipple and intraductal components stain with anti-FAS in a similar cytological pattern, but very different from that seen in keratinocytes; and c) ICL's are found in both nipple and intraductal components and not in keratinocytes. From all of the above, we are reassured that all Paget cells (both in the epidermis and in the intraductal carcinoma) share breast epithelial characteristics and not those of keratinocytes, or cells found in the dermis underlying the areola. A judicious use of immunohistochemical staining using monoclonal antibodies raised to components of breast epithelial cells prove an accurate means of identifying cell lineages as exemplified in this case.

REFERENCES

1. Ceriani, R.L., Thompson, K.E., Peterson, J.A. and Abraham, S.: Surface differentiation antigens of human mammary epithelial cells carried by the human milk fat globule. Proc. Nat. Acad. Sci. (U.S.) 74:582, 1977.
2. Peterson, J.A. Buehring, G., Taylor-Papadimitriou, J. and Ceriani, R. L.: Expression of human mammary epithelial (HME) antigens in primary cultures of normal and abnormal breast tissue. Int. J. Cancer 22:655, 1978.
3. Ceriani, R.L., Sasaki, M., Peterson, J.A. and Blank, E.W.: Mammary epithelial cell identification my means of cell surface antigens. In: Cell Biology of Breast Cancer (Charles McGrath, Michael J. Brennan, and Marvin A. Rich, eds.) Academic Press, N.Y., 1981. pp. 33-56.
4. Ceriani, R.L., Peterson, J.A., Blank, E. and Miller, S.: Use of mammary epithelial antigens as markers in mammary neoplasia. In: Tumour Markers: Impact and Prospects, (Boelsma, E. and Rumke, Ph., eds.), Elsevier/North-Holland Biomedical Press, 1979, p. [1].
5. Sebesteny, A., Taylor-Papadimitriou, J., Ceriani, R.L., Millis, R./, Schmitt, C. and Trevan, D.: Primary human breast carcinomas transplantable in the nude mouse. J. Nat. Cancer Inst. 63:1331, 1979.
6. Ceriani, R.L. Taylor-Papadimitriou, J. and Peterson, J.A.: Characterization of cell cultured from early lactation milk. In Vitro. 15:356, 1979.
7. Sasaki, M., Peterson, J.A. and Ceriani, R.L.: Quantitation of human mammary epithbelial antigens in cells cultured from normal and cancerous breast tissues. In Vitro 17:150, 1981.
8. Ceriani, R.L., Sasaki, M., Sussman, H., Wara, W.E. and Blank, E.W.: Circulating human mammary epithelial antigens (HME-Ags) in breast cancer. Proc. Nat. Acad. Sci., u./s. 79:5421, 1982.
9. Ceriani, R.L., Orthendhal, D., Sasaki, M., Kaufman, L., Miller, S., Wara, W. and Peterson, J.A.: "Use of mammazry epithelial antigens (HME-Ags) in breast cancer diagnosis". In: "Cancer Detection and Prevention: 1981". H.E. Nieburgs ed. Marcel Dekker, Inc., N.Y., 4:613, 1981.

10. Taylor-Papadimitriou, J., Peterson, J.A. Arklie, J., Burchell, J., Ceriani, R.L. Bodmer, W.F.: Moinoclonal antibodies to epithelium-specific components of the human milk fat globule membrane: production and reaction with cells in culture. Int. J. Cancer 28:17, 1981.
11. Ceriani, R.L. Peterson, J.A., Lee, J.Y., Moncada, F.R. and Blank, E.W. Preparation and characterization of monoclonal antibodies to normal human breast epithelial cells. Som. Cell Genet. 9:415, 1983.
12. Peterson, J.A. Bartholomew, J.C., Stampfer, M. and Ceriani, R.L.: Analysis of expression of human mammary epithelial antigens in normal and malignant breast cells at the single cell level by flow cytofluorimetry. Exp. Cell Biol. 49:1, 1981.
13. Lan, S., Smith, H.S., Ceriani, r.l. and Stampfer, M.R.: Clonal proliferation of cultured nonmalignant human breast epithelia. Cancer Res. 41:4637, 1981.
14. Peterson, J.A., Ceriani, R.L., Blank, E.W. and Osvaldo, L.: Human breast carcinoma cells have an increased rate of phenotypic variability in expression of surface antigens as compared to normal breast epithelial cells. Cancer Res. 43:4291, 1983.
15. Ceriani, R.L. Peterson, J.A. Blank, E.W. Variability in surface antigen expression of human breast epithelial cells cultured from normal breast, normal tissue peripheral to breast carcinomas, and breast carcinomas. Submitted for publication.
16. Azzopardi, J.G. Intracytoplasmic lumina in breast cancer cells. In: Problems in breast pathology. W.B. Saunders, London-Philadelphia, 1979, pp. 146-148.
17. Ozzello, L. Benign and malignant proliferations of the mammary epithelium: Ultrastructural observations. 1984. Monograph. Pathol. (25) : 106-38. 1984.
18. Battifora, H. Intracytoplasmic lumina in breast carcinona: A helpful histopathologic feature. Arch. Path. 99: 614-617, 1975.
19. Eusebi, V., A. Pich, E. Macchiorlatti and G. Bussolati. Morphofunctional differentation in lobular cacinoma of the breast. Histopath. 1:301-314. 1977.
20. Eusebi, V., C. Betts, d.e. Haagensen, P. Gugliotta, G. Bussolati and J.G. Azzopardi. Apocrine differentiation in lobular carcinoma of the breast: A morphologic,c, immunologic and ultrastructural study. Human Path. 15(2): 134-140. 1984.
21. Schlom, J., D. Colcher, P. Hand, D. Wunderlich, M. Nuti and Y.A. Teramoto. Antigenic heterogeneity, modulation and evolution in breast cancer lesions as defined by monoclonal antibodies. In: Understanding breast cancer. M.A. Rich, ed, Marcel Dekker, Inc., N.Y., 1983.
22. Ahmed, A. Atlas of the ultrastructure of human diseases. Churchill Livingstone, N.Y., 1978.
23. Ozzello, L. Ultrastracture of the human mammary gland. In: Pathology Annual, Sommers, S.C. ed. (6): 1-59, Butterworth, London, 1971.

Supported by Public Health Service grants CA-34630 and CA-33871 from the National Cancer Institute.

15

IMMUNOCYTOCHEMICAL LOCALIZATION OF ESTROGEN RECEPTORS WITH MONOCLONAL ANTIBODIES

GEOFFREY L. GREENE, WILLIAM J. KING AND MICHAEL F. PRESS

Monoclonal rat antibodies to MCF-7 human breast cancer estrogen receptor (estrophilin) have been used to study the structure and cellular location of receptor in reproductive tissues and cancers as well as to develop assays for receptor that do not depend on the binding of hormone to the receptor protein. Fusion of splenic lymphocytes from Lewis rats, immunized with affinity-purified estrogen receptor from MCF-7 cell cytosol, with two different mouse myeloma lines [1-3], provided 13 cloned hybridoma cell lines; each of these (with one possible exception) secretes a unique idiotype of antibody that recognizes a distinct region of the receptor molecule. These antibodies have high affinity ($K_d=10^{-9}-10^{-10}M$) for both steroid-occupied and unoccupied estrogen receptor and recognize nuclear as well as cytosol forms of the receptor molecule. Although they vary in their cross reactivity with estrogen receptors from various animal species, each antibody appears to be completely specific for the 65,000-dalton steroid-binding subunit of the estrogen receptor complex, as judged by extensive sucrose gradient and immunoblot analyses of cytosol and nuclear extracts from a variety of tissues and cell lines. Cross reactivity patterns indicate both sequence homology and heterogeneity among mammalian and nonmammalian estrophilins. Some determinants (eg. H222 and H226) are common to all tested estrogen receptors, including those from hen oviduct, whereas others (eg. D547 and D58) are present only in mammalian receptors and one (D75) appears to be restricted to primate estrophilin.

As part of our ongoing effort to elucidate the distribution and dynamics of the estrogen receptor protein (ER) in target tissues, as well as to establish new criteria for the assessment of prognosis and hormonal response in breast cancer, we have developed an immunocytochemical assay (ER-ICA) for visualizing receptor directly in tissues and cells. Five monoclonal antibodies (D547, D58, D75, H222, H226) have been used individually to localize estrophilin by an indirect immunoperoxidase technique in frozen, fixed sections of human breast tumors, human uterus, rabbit uterus, and in other mammalian reproductive tissues, as well as in fixed MCF-7 cell cultures [4-6]. Specific immunoperoxidase staining for receptor in estrogen-sensitive tissues is confined to the nucleus of all stained cells, regardless of hormone status. Staining is absent in nontarget tissues, such as colon epithelium, and in receptor-negative breast cancers; in addition, it can be abolished by the addition of highly purified receptor to primary antibody. Heterogeneous staining has been observed in MCF-7 cells as well as in receptor-poor and receptor-rich breast cancers, possibly reflecting either variations in cell cycle or the presence of estrogen-sensitive and insensitive cells. Little or no cytoplasmic staining for estrophilin has been observed in any of the tissues or tumor cells examined thus far, including those deprived of exogenous estrogens. In a study of 117 human breast cancers by the ER-ICA method, the presence or absence of nuclear staining was significantly associated with the concentration of cytosolic estrogen receptor determined by steroid-binding assay. Staining intensity, epithelial cellularity and the proportion of tumor cells stained also correlated significantly with receptor concentration.

The heterogeneous pattern of nuclear staining observed in many of the breast tumors analyzed by the ER-ICA method may reflect the polyclonal origins of such tumors, and it is possible that the failure of some ER-rich tumors to respond to endocrine therapy results from the survival of a subpopulation of ER-poor cells. Although it is not possible to rule out experimental artifact as a factor in staining patterns, the correlation between the degree of heterogeneity and the levels of receptor determined biochemically suggest that the staining patterns reflect the true distribution of receptor-containing cells. Clinical response data will help resolve this issue. In a recent study of approximately 100 patients with stage 2 breast cancer, the most significant prognostic indicator was the percentage of tumor cells that displayed nuclear staining for estrophilin by the ER-ICA method.

In view of the exclusively nuclear localization of specific immunoperoxidase staining for receptor in all estrogen-sensitive tissues and cells studied thus far, it appears that both cytosol and nuclear forms of the receptor may reside in the nuclear compartment in the presence and absence of steroid. We have seen little or no increase in nuclear staining intensity in MCF-7 cells and in uteri from immature rabbits or from postmenopausal women following short-term exposure of cells or tissue to estradiol. These observations are consistent with the hypothesis that unoccupied estrophilin recovered in the low salt cytosol fraction of a tissue homogenate represents receptor that is loosely associated with nuclear components and that binding of estradiol to receptor leads to a tighter association, a phenomenon previously interpreted as indicating translocation of the receptor from the cytoplasm to the nucleus.

In conclusion, preliminary data indicate a strong correlation between ER-ICA results and those of steroid-binding assays for estrogen receptors in breast cancers. In addition, our data suggest a significant relationship between several immunocytochemical staining parameters and time to recurrence or death. These parameters include 1) the presence or absence of specific nuclear staining for ER, 2) the intensity of staining, and 3) the proportion of tumor cells that are stained. Ongoing clinical studies will reveal the general utility of the ER-ICA method as an indicator of prognosis and therapy selection in breast cancer and may enable us to identify ER-rich tumors that contain subpopulations of hormone-unresponsive cells.

ACKNOWLEDGEMENTS

These studies were supported by Abbott Laboratories, the American Cancer Society (BC-86), the NCI (CA-02897) and by the Women's Board of the University of Chicago Cancer Research Foundation.

REFERENCES

1. Greene, G.L., Nolan, C., Engler, J.P. and Jensen, E.V.; Monoclonal antibodies to human estrogen receptor. Proc. Natl. Acad. Sci. USA (77); 5115-5119: 1980.

2. Miller, L.S., Tribby, I.I.E., Miles, M.R., Tomita, J.T. and Nolan, C.: Hybridomas producing monoclonal antibodies to human estrogen receptor. Fedn. Proc. (41); 520: 1982.

3. Greene, G.L., Sobel, N.B., King, W.J. and Jensen, E.V.; Immunochemical studies of estrogen receptors. J. Steroid Biochem. (20); 51-56: 1984.

4. King, W.J. and Greene, G.L.; Monoclonal antibodies localize estrogen receptor in the nucleus of target cells. Nature (307); 745-747: 1984.

5. Press, M.F. and Greene, G.L.; An immunocytochemical method for demonstrating estrogen receptor in human uterus using monoclonal antibodies to human estrophilin. Lab. Invest. (50); 480-486: 1984.

6. King, W.J., Desombre, E.R., Jensen, E.V. and Greene, G.L.; A comparison of immunocytochemical and steroid-binding assays for estrogen receptor in human breast tumors. Cancer Research, 1984, in press.

16

IMMUNOCYTOCHEMISTRY OF AN ESTROGEN-REGULATED PROTEIN (28K) IN ESTROGEN TARGET CELLS AND TISSUES

DANIEL R. CIOCCA

1. INTRODUCTION

The interaction between estrogens and their intracellular receptor molecule is the first step in the mechanism of action of these hormones, while the biological response is the final consequence of such interaction. Between these initial and final steps are many biochemical events which include the synthesis of several proteins. Some of these proteins have well characterized functions while others have unknown functions (1-7). The study of these estrogen-regulated proteins has been of interest because they are an end product of estrogen action in target cells. They might be useful tools for understanding postreceptor events in estrogen-regulated cells and tissues. As a consequence, it is possible that such marker proteins could serve as predictors of the hormonal responsiveness of endocrine-dependent tumors, thus complementing or replacing conventional measurements of estrogen receptors.

Recently, one of these estrogen-regulated proteins, of unknown function, was identified in the MCF-7 human breast cancer cell line (8). This protein was demonstrated by the double isotope gel electrophoresis method and gave a molecular weight of 24,000 (24K) on sodium dodecyl sulfate-polycrylamide gels. More recently, the molecular weight of this protein was corrected to 28K after purification with anion exchange and monoclonal antibody affinity chromatographies (9). Obtaining of monoclonal antibodies against the 28K protein, was important because these antibodies are useful in detecting the protein with using immunochemical (10) and immunohistochemical (11) techniques. With these methodologies, the 28K protein was detected not only in MCF-7 cells but also in other breast tumor cell lines and in certain human breast tumor biopsy samples. In addition, a retrospective study with several human normal and pathological tissues could be performed using immunohistochemistry (12). Such studies point out the value of the 28K protein as a marker of estrogen action in human estrogen target organs, tumors, and cell lines.

In this review, the current knowledge on the immunohistochemical detection of the 28K protein in human normal and neoplastic cells and tissues will be presented and the present diagnostic value of the 28K estrogen-regulated protein in immunohistopathology will be discussed.

2. IMMUNOHISTOCHEMICAL SPECIFICITY

Using the hybridoma technique, three monoclonal antibodies against 28K protein were generated (10). One of the first steps using these antibodies in immunohistochemistry, was to perform a careful evaluation of the immunostaining pattern during the interpretation and validation of the results. Although monoclonal antibodies are chemically homogenous (13, 14), sensitivity, efficiency and specificity of a given monoclonal antibody should still be tested (15). For example, in the case of the monoclonal antibodies against 28K protein, antibody dilution was found to greatly influence on immunohistochemical specificity (16). In such a case, a "titration curve" for a monoclonal antibody should be constructed like for a polyclonal antiserum (17). In addition, storage condition also affect immunostaining: when highly diluted monoclonal antibody to 28K was stored at 4 C, the activity was lost within 2 weeks if carrier proteins were not added (16). For these specificity tests, solid MCF-7 tumors grown in athymic nude mice were a valuable source of tissue. In this case, when the monoclonal antibodies were used at appropriate dilutions, the MCF-7 cells appeared immunostained while surrounding mouse tissues remained unstained.

The three monoclonal antibodies against 28K protein currently available seem to be identical based on their biochemical characterization (18) and immunostaining pattern.

3. DISTRIBUTION OF 28K PROTEIN

3.1 Cell lines

Once the presence of 28K protein was well established by immunocytochemistry in MCF-7 breast cancer cells, it was of interest to know if MCF-7 cells of different passage number or from another laboratory were also able to express the 28K protein. At the same time, other cell lines were tested not only to detect the 28K protein but also to detect the presence of estrogen receptors (ER) and progesterone receptors (PgR). It was found that only ER and PgR positive cell lines showed the 28K estrogen-regulated protein (12) (Table 1).

Table 1. Distribution of 28K protein in cell lines

Cell line	Tissue of origin	ER	PgR	28K protein
MCF-7-243	Breast carcinoma	+	+	+
MCF-7-353	Breast carcinoma	+	+	+
CG-5	Breast carcinoma	+	+	+
MCF-7	Breast carcinoma	+	+	+
MDA-MB-231	Breast carcinoma	-	-	-
T47D	Breast carcinoma	+	+	+
ZR-75	Breast carcinoma	+	+	+
HBL-100	"Normal" breast	-	-	-
KB	Esophageal carcinoma	NT	NT	-
T-24	Bladder carcinoma	NT	NT	-

NT: not tested
Table reproduced, with some modifications, from Cancer Research 43:1204-1210, 1983.

These results encouraged the study of 28K in human breast cancer samples, but they also indicated that cell heterogeneity was a problem in immunostaining analysis. When MC-7 cells were stained, 90 to 100% of the cells showed 28K protein (Fig. 1a), while other ER and PgR positive cells (T47D and ZR75 breast cancer cells) displayed low 28K immunostaining intensity in only 1 to 3% of the cells. Since these cell lines have low levels of ER, they were stimulated to determine if immunostaining of 28K could be enhanced. This was done using the estrogen rescue protocol: after 6 days of antiestrogen treatment some of the cells were continued on antiestrogen while others were switched to a medium containing estradiol for 4 days (8). Estradiol treatment increased both the intensity of 28K immunostaining and the percentage of 28K positive T47D and ZR75 cells (Fig. 1b)(12). However, about 40 to 50% of these cells remained unstained. Thus, an important question remains: when should 28K immunostaining be considered positive? The results obtained by

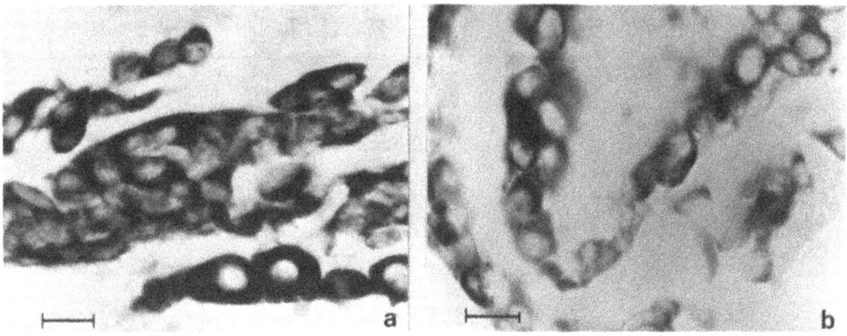

FIGURE 1. a) MCF-7 cells showing 28K protein. ABC staining. Bar=25 μm. b) ZR75 cells, note that 28K protein is not present in all of the cells even after estrogen stimulation. ABC staining. Bar=25 μm.

the estrogen rescue protocol suggested that even when a sample had a low percentage of immunostained cells it should be considered positive since under more favorable conditions, such as estrogen stimulation, the number of 28K immunostained cells increased. This point will be further elaborated when tumor biopsy samples are considered.

3.2 Normal Tissues

The fact that 28K protein could be detected in routine paraffin sections using an immunoperoxidase technique facilitated the study of numerous human normal and pathological tissues. Since 28K protein is regulated by estrogens, estrogen target organs were of particular interest for screening. The results obtained showed that the 28K protein was mainly restricted to normal estrogen target organs (12). However, neither all of the cells present in these tissues nor all of the estrogen target samples tested, displayed the 28K protein. Table 2 shows the cellular distribution of 28K protein in the normal tissues stained with the monoclonal antibodies.

The results of this study showed that 28K protein is not a tumor-specific marker, nor a milk-related protein (lactating breast samples were 28K negative) (12). In addition, the lack of reaction of the monoclonal antibodies with fetal tissues showed that this protein is not a fetal-associated antigen (12). This study also suggested that the presence of 28K protein in some of the estrogen target organs tested, may be due to variations in estrogen sensitivity during the ovarian cycle

Table 2. Cellular localization of 28K in non-malignant tissues.

Sample	Diagnosis	Cellular Localization
Breast	Normal	Cytoplasm of epithelial cells of some intralobular small ducts.
Breast	Fibrocystic	Cytoplasm of epithelial cells of some small ducts.
Uterus	Normal	Cytoplasm of epithelial cells lining the endometrium surface. Less intense in endometrial glands and myometrium. Predecidual cells.
Placenta	Normal	Cytoplasm of decidual cells.
Endometrium	Biopsy at caesarean operation	Cytoplasm of decidual cells.
Fallopian Tube	Normal	Cytoplasm of ciliated epithelial cells.
Vagina	Normal	Cytoplasm of epithelial cells.
Skin	Normal	Cytoplasm of epithelial cells and some ducts of sweat glands.

(12). This was confirmed when the presence of 28K protein was demonstrated in endometrial biopsies from regularly cycling women (19).

3.2.1. Modulation of 28K protein. Utilizing MCF-7 cells and a double-label electrophoresis technique, it was shown that 28K protein synthesis is specifically stimulated by estradiol (applying the estrogen rescue protocol) (20). This study showed that 28K protein is constitutively found in unstimulated MCF-7 cells, and that its synthesis is both time and estrogen-dose dependent. Knowing this, it was not surprising to find different 28K immunostaining intensity in endometrial cells of regularly cycling women (19). However, the immunostaining pattern revealed a striking cell distribution of 28K within the endometrium: three cell types appeared immunostained at specific times of the menstrual cycle. The cells in the superficial epithelium showed the highest 28K immunostaining intensity during the midsecretory phase (days 20-22 of the menstrual cycle). In these cells, 28K protein was clearly seen in the apical cytoplasm and the bulbous projections. On the other hand, glandular cells always appeared more weakly immunostained and they reached maximum 28K staining, in both intensity and cell number, around the late proliferative phase. Finally, predecidual cells located around spiral arterioles also showed 28K immunostaining.

These results indicate that 28K protein is a marker of hormonal events in human endometrium during the normal menstrual cycle. Since 28K protein appeared maximally expressed in the superficial epithelium during the midsecretory phase, and at this time progesterone levels are at their maximum (21), probably at least in the superficial epithelium, the protein is synthesized by the synergistic action of estrogen and progesterone. A similar situation might occur in human decidual cells, cells that show 28K immunostaining (12,19) and that are controlled mainly by progesterone (22).

It is interesting to note that the strongest 28K protein immunostaining, mainly in the superficial epithelium, was reached when the ER concentration had decreased (23). Lowest ER levels have been found in tissues showing decidual reaction (24), and these cells have 28K immunostaining (12,19). Therefore, it is possible that this negative quantitative correlation between ER and 28K protein might also be found in some endocrine-dependent tumors assessed for the presence of both ER and 28K protein.

3.3 Pathological Tissues

The distribution of 28K protein in pathological tissues was not restricted to classical estrogen-target organs. For instance, 28K immunostaining could be seen in some of the kidney, bladder and skin carcinomas tested (12). At present, there is not a clear explanation for the presence of 28K protein in some of these carcinomas. Therefore, the identification of 28K protein cannot be used as a tissue-specific marker for the determination of the histogenesis of a metastasis from an unknown primary carcinoma.

The problem now is to know if 28K identification may be useful to predict the hormonal responsiveness of endocrine-dependent tumors. Logically, breast carcinomas were among the first to be tested and approximately 25% of them showed 28K immunostaining (12). This percentage is lower than the 60% of ER positive breast carcinomas but is correlates well with the percentage of patients that respond objectively to endocrine therapy (25). However, by immunohistochemistry it is

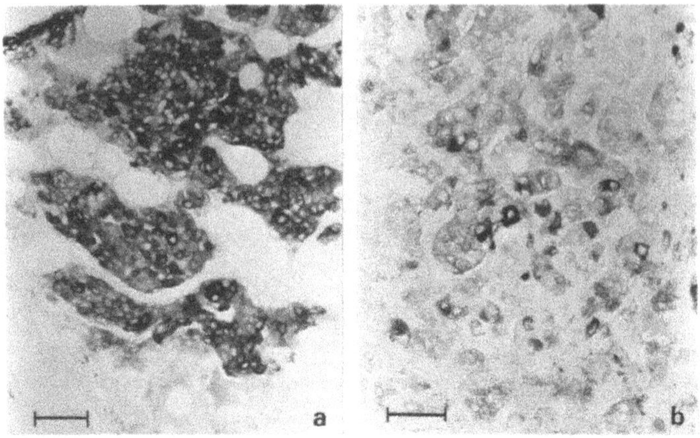

FIGURE 2. a) Human breast carcinoma biopsy sample showing 28K protein in several tumor cells. ABC staining. Bar=100 μm. b) This human breast carcinoma sample shows 28 K protein in only a few cells. ABC staining. Bar=75 μm.

difficult to evaluate the presence of 28K protein since several of the tumors showed a limited number of 28K positive cells (Fig. 2). Such tumor cell heterogeneity for 28K was seen in the cell lines with low levels of ER, but tumor samples cannot be treated with the estrogen rescue protocol to see if there is or not an evident increase in the number of 28K positive cells. This makes difficult an immunohistochemical study correlating the presence of 28K protein with ER and PgR determinations. In addition, ER and PgR heterogeneity has also been reported in human breast tumors analyzed by multiple intratumoral assays (26). At this point, immunohistochemistry may be too specific, showing only a very limited amount of tissue which sometimes was obtained from a different site to the tissue processed for ER and PgR assays. For a correlative study a quantitative immunoassay for 28K protein using the same cytosol sample assayed for ER and PgR might be better than the immunohistochemical examination. This has been recently achieved and the results obtained have shown that the presence of 28K protein correlates with that of steroid receptors, particularly ER (27). This quantitative immunoassay will also facilitate future correlative immunohistochemical studies using tumor samples obtained in close proximity to the tissue which is immunoassayed.

Additional evidence on the histopathological value of 28K protein as a marker of estrogen sensitive cells, came by the study of abnormal human endometrial samples (28). In this retrospective study, women with active forms of persistent proliferative endometrium and cystic hyperplasia showed the strongest 28K immunostaining, while 28K protein decreased in samples with adenomatous and atypical hyperplasia. Well-differentiated endometrial adenocarcinomas displayed more 28K reaction than moderately differentiated carcinomas, while poorly differentiated endometrial carcinomas were practically devoid of 28K protein (28). The study also showed that clear cells are highly estrogen sensitive and that they are precursors of ciliated cells. These results indicate that 28K protein is estrogen- and ciliated cell-related, and endometrial ciliogenesis and 28K protein are morphologic and biochemical markers, respectively of estrogenic endometrial response. In addition, the study supports the concept that early hyperplasia is highly sensitive to unopposed hyperestrogenism, reaching a maximum in active cystic hyperplasia. But with prolonged estrogenic stimulation there is an increase in architectural and cytologic atypia concomitantly with an increase in the cell populations that are independent of estrogenic influence. Therefore, 28K seems to be a protein marker expressed by those cells highly sensitive to estrogens and as an end product resulting from a differentiated cell function.

4. SUBCELLULAR LOCALIZATION OF 28K PROTEIN

In order to assess the subcellular localization of 28K protein, MCF-7 cells grown in tissue culture or in vivo in nude mice were examined light and electron microscopically using immunoperoxidase techniques. MCF-7 cells growing free in the ascites fluid of nude mice tended to form acinar structures like those reported when the cells grew in a tridimensional collagen-coated cellulose sponge (29). These cavitary structures were not true acini since the cells showed junctional complexes and microvilli at the outer surface but not in the lumen of the pseudoacini (29). When these pseudoacinar formations were examined under the light microscope using the antibody to 28K, the estrogen-regulated protein appeared localized in the apical cytoplasm (30). These cells displayed varying degrees of 28K immunoreactivity. On the other hand, cytocentrifuged MCF-7 cells taken from tissue culture showed 28K immunostaining in cytoplasmic granules (30). As opposed to paraffin sections, cytocentrifuged cells are not sectioned, they are lightly fixed, and they are not shriveled as occurs when the paraffin support is dissolved by xylene. This accounts for the different immunostaining pattern observed in MCF-7 cells processed for paraffin sections, where the reaction was not seen in cytoplasmic granules. Finally, the localization of 28K protein in cytoplasmic granules was confirmed by immunoelectronmicroscopy of MCF-7 cells grown both in culture and as solid tumors. The 28K reaction appeared in large cavities, some of them showing a few microvilli protruding into the lumina (30). In these granules, the 28K reaction also appeared with variable staining intensity. These findings of 28K protein in cytoplasmic granules, in the apical cytoplasm of the cells, with different immunostaining intensity from granule to granule and from cell to cell, strongly suggest that this protein undergoes phases of active synthesis, accumulation, and probably secretion. Recently, additional evidence for the secretory nature of 28K protein was presented (27) using an enzyme-linked immunosorbent assay (ELISA). With this methodology it was possible to show that estrogen stimulates the release of 28K by MCF-7 cells in culture.

5. IDENTITY WITH OTHER ESTROGEN-REGULATED PROTEINS

Based on the biochemical and immunohistochemical characteristics of 28K, the attempts to identify this protein with other estrogen-regulated proteins have led to the conclusion that 28K is not a milk-related protein, or one of the proteins found in breast cystic fluid (9,12,20). Moreover, 28K is different to the 52K (previously 46K) secreted glycoprotein (4) which is also found in estrogen receptor positive breast tumor and cancer cell lines. This 52K protein is not present in normal breast or normal uterus collected at different times of the menstrual cycle (31). In addition, 28K protein localization and cyclic fluctuations are different to those described for some endometrial enzyme systems (32,33) and to alpha-uterine protein (34).

On the other hand, it has been reported that cultured rat Leydig cells treated with hCG or estradiol show a 27K protein (35). The synthesis of this protein, investigated by the double-labeling technique, was inhibited by tamoxifen and the hCG effect occurred through increased estradiol production. It was therefore of interest to explore the cross-immunological identity of this 27K Leydig cell protein with the 28K protein. The study was done using the monoclonal antibody against 28K

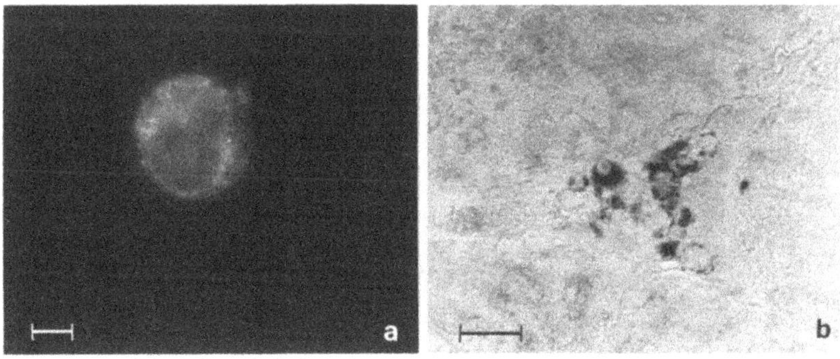

FIGURE 3. a) Positive 28K immunofluorescence is seen in this isolated human Leydig cell. Bar=5 μm. b) Rat testis showing 28K reactive Leydig cells. ABC staining. Bar=50 μm.

protein and immunocytochemical techniques (36). The Leydig cells from rat and human tissue showed specific immunofluorescence and immunoperoxidase staining upon incubation with the antibody to the 28K protein from MC-7 cells (Fig. 3). The immunostaining intensity increased when the cells were treated with estradiol or hCG and the intensity was reduced after tamoxifen treatment. The reaction was restricted to the cytoplasm of the Leydig cells. During the screening of human tissues reacting with the 28K antibodies (12), three testes were also tested and they did not show 28K staining; however, those testes were atrophic and probably lacking in healthy Leydig cells. The finding of 28K immunoreactivity in rat and human Leydig cells also shows that the monoclonal antibody against 28K has cross-species specificity which will facilitate studies using animal models.

ACKNOWLEDGEMENTS

I am very grateful to Dr. William L. McGuire, in whose laboratory I was introduced to the study of 28K protein using the hybridoma technology.

REFERENCES

1. Lyttle CR, DeSombre ER: Generality of estrogen stimulation of peroxidase activity in growth responsive tissues. Nature (268):337-339, 1977.

2. Horwitz KB, McGuire WL: Estrogen control of progesterone receptor in human breast cancer. Correlation with nuclear processing of estrogen receptor. J Biol Chem (253):2223-2228, 1978.

3. O'Malley BW, Tsai MJ, Tsai SY, Towle HC: Regulation of gene expression in chick oviduct. Cold Spring Harbor Symp Quant Biol (42):605-617,1978.

4. Westley B, Rochefort H: A secreted glycoprotein induced by estrogen in human breast cancer cell lines. Cell (20):353-362, 1980.

5. Mairesse N, Galand P: Estrogen-induced proteins in luminal epithelium, endometrial stroma and myometrium of the rat uterus. Mol Cell Endocrinol (28):671-679, 1982.

6. Chalbos D, Vignon F, Keydar I, Rochefort H: Estrogens stimulate cell proliferation and induce secretory proteins in a human breast cancer cell line (T47D). J Clin Endocrinol Metab (55):276-283,1982.

7. Adams DJ, Edwards DP, McGuire WL: Estrogen regulation of specific proteins as a mode of hormone action in human breast cancer. In: Nowotny A (ed) Pathological Membranes. Plenum Press, New York, 1983, pp. 389-414.

8. Edwards DP, Adams DJ, Savage N, McGuire WL: Estrogen induced synthesis of specific proteins in human breast cancer cells. Biochem Biophys Res Commun (93):804-812, 1980.

9. Adams DJ, Hajj H, Bitar KG, Edwards DP, McGuire WL: Purification of an estrogen-regulated breast cancer protein by monoclonal antibody affinity chromatography. Endocrinology (113):415-417, 1983.

10. Adams DJ, Hajj H, Edwards DP, Bjercke RJ, McGuire WL: Detection of a Mr 24,000 estrogen-regulated protein in human breast cancer by monoclonal antibodies. Cancer Res (43):4297-4301, 1983.

11. Ciocca DR, Adams DJ, Bjercke RJ, Edwards DP, McGuire WL: Immunohistochemical detection of an estrogen regulated protein by monoclonal antibodies. Cancer Res (42):4256-4258, 1982.

12. Ciocca DR, Adams DJ, Edwards DP, Bjercke RJ, McGuire WL: Distribution of an estrogen-induced protein with a molecular weight of 24,000 in normal and malignant human tissues and cells. Cancer Res (43):1204-1210, 1983.

13. Goding JW: Antibody production by hybridomas. J Immunol Meth (39): 285-308, 1980.

14. Edwards PAW: Some properties and applications of monoclonal antibodies. Biochem J (200):1-10, 1981.

15. Ciocca DR, Bjercke RJ: Immunohistochemical techniques using monoclonal antibodies. In: Di Sabato G, Langone JL, Van Vunakis H (eds) Immunochemical Techniques. Methods in Enzymology. Academic Press, New York (in preparation).

16. Ciocca DR, Adams DJ, Bjercke RJ, Sledge GW, Edwards DP, Chamness GC, McGuire WL: Monoclonal antibody storage conditions, and concentration effects on immunohistochemical specicity. J Histochem Cytochem (31):691-696,1983.

17. Petruz P: Essential requirements for the valididity of immunocytochemical staining procedures. J Histochem Cytochem (31):177-179, 1983.

18. McGuire WL, Adams DJ, Edwards DP: Estrogen-regulated protein in human breast cancer. J Steroid Biochem (20):73-75, 1984.

19. Ciocca DR, Asch RH, Adams DJ, McGuire WL: Evidence for modulation of a 24K protein in human endometrium during the menstrual cycle. J Clin Endocrinol Metab (57):496-499, 1983.

20. Edwards DP, Adams DJ, McGuire WL: Estradiol stimulates synthesis of a major intracellular protein in a human breast cancer cell line (MCF-7). Breast Cancer Res Treat (1):209-223, 1981.

21. Frolich M, Brand EC, van Hall EV: Serum levels of unconjugated aetiocholanolone, androstenedione, testosterone, dehydroepiandrosterone, aldosterone, progesterone and oestrogens during the normal menstrual cycle. Acta endocrinol(81):548-562, 1976.

22. Finn CA, Porter DG: Handbooks in Reproductive Biology. Elek Science, London, Vol 1, p. 27, 1975.

23. Sanborn BM, Kuo HS, Held B: Estrogen and progesterone binding site concentrations in human endometrium and cervix throughout the menstrual cycle and in tissue from women taking oral contraceptives. J Steroid Biochem (9):951-955, 1978.

24. Evans LH, Martin JD, Hahnel R: Estrogen receptor concentration in normal and pathological human uterine tissues. J Clin Endocrinol Metab (38):23-32, 1974.

25. Osborne CK, Yochmowitz MG, Knight WA, McGuire WL: The value of estrogen and progesterone receptors in the treatment of breast cancer. Cancer(46):2884-2888, 1980.

26. Davis BW, Zava DT, Locher GW, Goldhirsch A, Hartmann WH: Receptor heterogeneity in human breast cancer as measured by multiple intratumoral assays of estrogen and progesterone receptor. Europ J Cancer Clin Oncol (20):375-382, 1984.

27. Adams D, Chamness G, Edwards D, McGuire W: Quantitative immunoassay for 24K, a major estrogen-regulated protein in human breast cancer. 7th International Congress of Endocrinology, Quebec, Canada. 48A, 1984.

28. Ciocca DR, Puy LA, Edwards DP, Adams DJ, McGuire WL: The presence of an estrogen-regulated protein detected by monoclonal antibody in abnormal human endometrium. J Clin Endocrinol Metab (In press).

29. Russo J, Bradley RH, McGrath C, Russo IH: Scanning and transmission electron microscopy study of a human breast carcinoma cell line (MCF-7) cultured in collagen-coated cellulose sponge. Cancer Res (37):2004-2014, 1977.

30. Ciocca DR, Adams DJ, Edwards DP, Bjercke RJ, McGuire WL: Estrogen-induced 24K protein in MCF-7 breast cancer cells in localized in granules. Breast Cancer Res Treat (in press).

31. Garcia M, Salazar-Retana G, Richer G, Capony F, Domergue J, Laffargue F, Pujol H, Pau B, Rochefort H: Immunohistochemical detection of an estrogen-regulated 52,000 protein in human primary breast cancer but not in normal breast and uterus. J Clin Endocrinol Metab 1984 (in press).

32. Hall JE: Alkaline phosphatase in human endometrium. Am J Obstet Gynecol (60):212-223, 1950.

33. Elias EA, Elias RA, Kooistra AM, Roukema AC, Blacquiere JF, Barrowclough H, Meijer AEFH: Fluctuations in the enzymatic activity of the human endometrium. Histochemistry (77):159-170, 1983.

34. Horne CHW, Paterson WF, Sutcliffe RG: Localization of alpha-uterine protein in human endometrium. J Reprod Fert (65):447-450, 1982.

35. Nozu K, Dehejia A, Zawistowich L, Catt KJ, Dufau ML: Gonadotropin-induced receptor regulation and steroidogenic lesions in cultured Leydig cells. Induction of specific protein synthesis by chorionic gonadotropin and estradiol. J Biol Chem (258):12875-12882, 1981.

36. Ciocca DR, Dufau ML: Estrogen-dependent Leydig cell protein recognized by monoclonal antibody to MCF-7 cell line. Science (in press).

17

MONOCLONAL ANTIBODIES IN THE DIAGNOSIS OF SOLID TUMORS: STUDIES ON RENAL CARCINOMAS, TRANSITIONAL CELL CARCINOMAS AND MELANOMA

CARLOS CORDON-CARDO, M.D.,PH.D.

I. INTRODUCTION

Immunodiagnosis of cancer may provide an early and objective diagnosis, and aid in staging, monitoring treatment and clinical follow-up of cancer patients. It also may lead to a new classification of human neoplasia based on immunohistogenesis.

Two different approaches have been used to detect tumor-associated antigens of relevance in immunodiagnosis: 1) Immunohistochemistry (using tissue sections) (1,2); and 2) Immunochemistry of body fluids (especially blood plasma or serum and urine) (3,4). Unfortunately, serum and urine are not stored frequently at the initial diagnosis, whereas fixed and/or frozen tissues are usually available for most cancers.

Conventional histochemistry was used in an attempt to produce specific tissue and/or tumor markers, and it has been of some value in the classification of certain tumors. Unfortunately, these markers lack specificity and they have not been found to discriminate between normal and tumor cells.

In contrast, the introduction of immunohistochemical methods has permitted many applications where high resolution and sensitivity are required, using antibodies (Ab) as powerful probes for localization of tissue antigens (Ag).

Heterologous and autologous antisera raised against carcinoma and sarcoma lesions were used to distinguish tumor-associated Ags from other nonrelated Ags (5,6). With the advent of the hybridization technique and the production of monoclonal antibodies (mAb), described by Kohler and Milstein (7), immunohistochemical methods have become very powerful. Highly specific markers have been produced that offer promise in fundamental as well as applied aspects of human tumor biology and immunopathology (8-10).

It is becoming increasingly evident that differentiation Ags and tumor-associated Ags, as well as protein products encoded by oncogenes, play some role in the development of human cancer (11). Because they reflect the origin and function of the tumor, mAbs to these Ags are potentially of value to the pathologist to characterize and subclassify undifferentiated and like-appearing tumors of different origins or different clinical behavior. While it is possible that a single highly specific Ab will recognize a particular tumor, most cancer probably will require a battery or panel of several antibodies for their identification and subclassification.

Ultimately, we anticipate a new subclassification of human tumors based on their immunohistogenesis. The value of this subclassification will be determined by correlation with clinical and conventional pathologic features, rate of tumor progression and metastases, response to therapy and prognosis. If highly restricted Ags detected by these mAbs are identified it is conceivable that they may also be of value for clinical imaging (12) and/or immunotherapy (13,14).

2. GENERATION AND ANALYSIS OF MONOCLONAL ANTIBODIES

The strategy followed at Memorial Sloan-Kettering Cancer Center to analyze Abs which will be used in future research and clinical projects is as follows:

a) Antibody specificity is determined by serology on panels of over 100 established human cell lines. They include short term cultures of normal cells, as well as panels of carcinomas, sarcomas, melanomas and lymphomas.

b) Antigen characterization is studied by immunoprecipitation and/or immunoblotting tests.

c) Antigen distribution is analyzed using frozen and paraffin-embedded tissue sections on panels of normal human fetal and adult tissues.

d) Antigen expression and/or modulation is studied using frozen and paraffin-embedded tissue sections on panels of human tumors, including carcinomas and sarcomas.

The diversity of Ags and other molecules difficulty (if not impossible) to be identified using conventional histology and subjective interpretation, has been the main reason for the approach presented above. Detailed description of the methods used has been previously reported (15-17).

3. IMMUNOANATOMIC DISSECTION OF THE HUMAN NEPHRON

The analysis of mouse mAbs to human renal and bladder cancers has led to the definition of a large number of differentiation Ags of the urinary system (18,19). The microanatomy of the human urinary tract has been studied by the use of a panel of these Abs, and shown to define specific domains and structures of the human nephron (20). The antibodies recognize a series of glycoproteins different from other antigens previously described. None of the mAbs reacted with blood group antigens, as demonstrated by hemaglutination tests and solid phase enzyme-linked immunosorbent assay (ELISA) using purified blood group glycoproteins expressing A, B, H, Lewis a, Lewis b, X and Y determinants. These antibodies detect antigens characteristic of different cell types within the urinary system.

Table I summarizes the derivation of the mAbs comprising this panel and the characterization of the Ags detected. The immunoreactivity of these mAbs was assessed by the use of frozen sections of normal fetal and adult tissues (20). Figure 1 illustrates the immunostaining patterns of these mAbs in frozen sections of normal adult kidney and urinary bladder.

TABLE I. Description of mouse monoclonal antibodies detecting differentiation antigens of the urinary system

ANTIGEN DESIGNATION	ANTIBODY (Ig SUBCLASS)	IMMUNOGEN	ANTIGEN CHARACTERIZATION
URO 1	J143 (y_1)	253J BC	140/120/30
URO 2	S4 (y_{2a})	SK-RC-7 RC	160
URO 3	F23(y_{2a})	Normal Kidney	140
URO 4	S27 (y_1)	SK-RC-7 RC	120
URO 5	T16 (y_{2b})	T24 BC	48/42

BC Bladder Cancer
RC Renal Cancer
Antigen Characterization in Kilodaltons

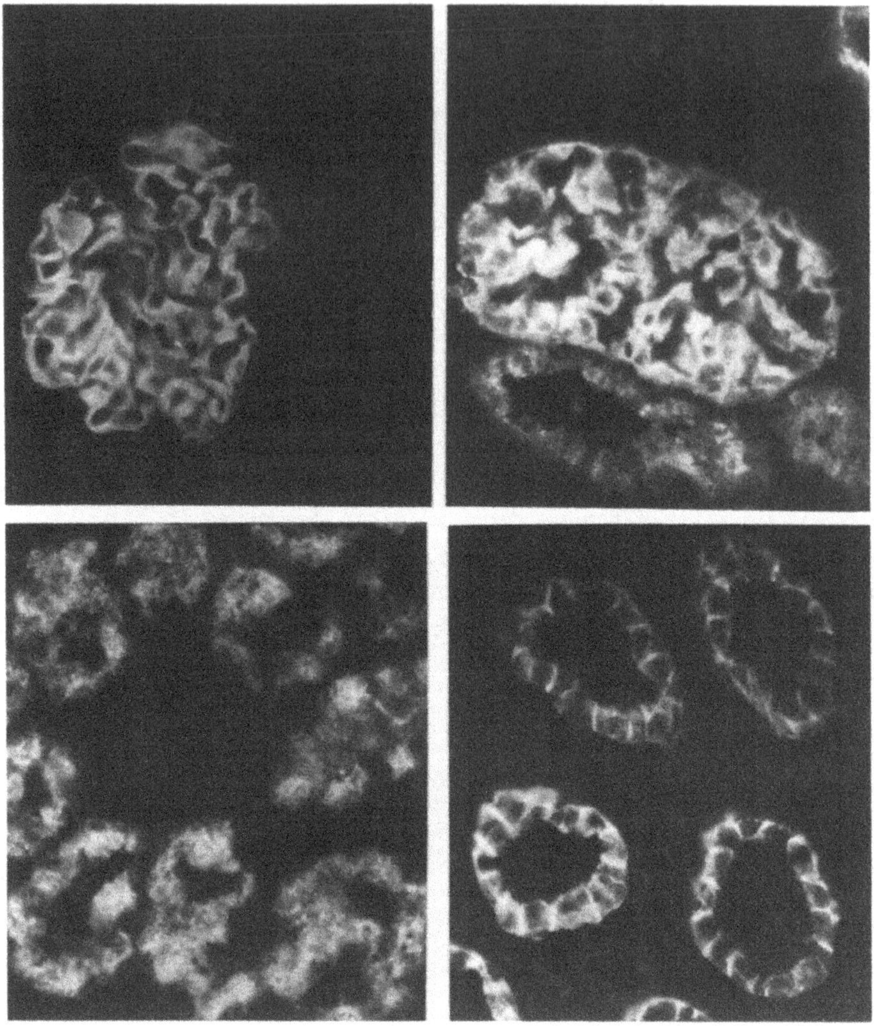

Figure 1. Immunostaining patterns of reactivity of URO monoclonal antibodies in frozen sections of normal adult kidney. The method applied was indirect immunofluorescence, using undiluted tissue culture supernatant as primary antibody, and goat anti-mouse flouresceinated antibodies (1:14 dilution) as secondary reagent. 1a: URO 1 staining with an evenly linear pattern the glomerulus, suggesting expression of the antigen in the basement membrane (x400). 1b: URO 2 staining the glomerulus and epithelial cells of the proximal tubules (x400). 1c: URO 3 staining epithelial cells of the proximal tubules. Note the non-stained glomerulus (x400). 1d: URO 5 staining epithelial cells of the collecting ducts (x400).

Uro 1 (J143) detects a glycoprotien with Mr 140,000/120,000/30,000 which has an evenly linear pattern of reactivity in the glomerulus, suggesting the expression of this Ag in the basement membrane (Figure 1a). Recently, the chromosomal assignment of Uro 1 has been reported as being concordant with chromosome 17 (21). Uro 2 (S4) recognizes a glycoprotein with Mr 160,000 found in epithelial cells of the glomerulus and proximal tubules (Figure 1b); biochemical, serological and immunopathologic data suggest that this Ag is not related with hematopoietic Ags reported (i.e: Common Acute Lymphoma Leukemia Antigen or CALLA), which also react with this urologic domain. Uro 3 (F23) identifies a glycoprotein Mr 140,000 expressed on epithelial cells of the proximal tubules (Figure 1c); it also reacts with fibroblasts. The chromosomal assignment of Uro 3 has been shown to be in chromosome 15 (21). Uro 4 (S27) detects a glycoprotein Mr 120,000 which has been reported to be the adenosine deaminase binding protein (ADAbp) (22). Uro 4 reacts with epithelial cells of the proximal tubules, Bowman's capsule epithelium, portion of the loop of Henle, prostatic epithelium and placental trophoblasts. Finally, Uro 5 (T16) detects a glycoprotein with Mr 48,000/42,000 found in the epithelial cells of the distal tubules of the cortex and medulla, collecting ducts (Figure 1d), weakly in loops of Henle, and in the transitional epithelium; it is also reacting with other epithelial cells, as previously reported (20).

Figure 2 illustrates the schematic representation of the domains of antigen expression through the human nephron.

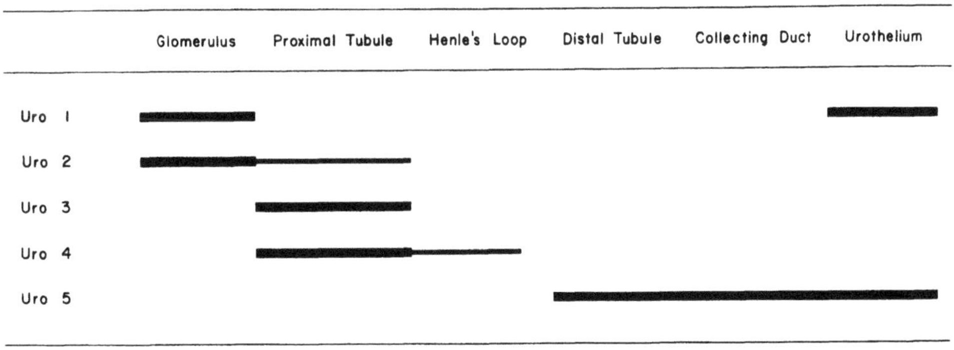

Figure 2. Immunoanatomic dissection of the human nephron by the panel of URO monoclonal antibodies.

4. IMMUNOPATHOLOGIC ANALYSIS OF RENAL CELL AND TRANSITIONAL CELL CARCINOMAS

The specificity analysis of the antibodies generated against renal cell and transitional cell carcinomas has been extended on human tumors. A number of antigens defined in the previous studies were not detected on normal tissues, or not found to be expressed in the human nephron; but were expressed by renal or transitional carcinomas "in vitro" and "in vivo" (18, 19). They were not discussed in the previous section because their restricted pattern of reactivity.

Table II summarizes the derivation of the mAbs comprising this second panel and the characterization of the Ags detected. Table III summarizes the immunopathologic analysis of human tumors tested with a combination of antibodies from the URO panel.

4.1 Renal Cell Carcinoma:

URO 7 (S22) is one of the mAbs generated during the study of cell surface antigens of renal cell carcinomas (18). URO 7 detects a glycoprotein of Mr 115,000 which has not been found in any normal fetal or adult tissue. Nevertheless, URO 7 has been found on a subset of renal cancers (see Table III). URO 2, URO 3 and URO 4 defined distinct domains of the human nephron, but they are all expressed by proximal tubular epithelial cell. Recently, a panel of 20 renal cell carcinomas was typed for expression of these antigens (Finstad CL, Cordon-Cardo, C et al, Proc. Natl. Acad. Sci., in press). Different phenotypes were distinguished with the URO2+/URO3+/URO4+/URO7+ or - phenotype being the most common (15 out of 20 cases). This finding suggests

TABLE II. Derivation and Characterization of mouse monoclonal antibodies detecting restricted differentiation antigens of the urinary system.

ANTIGEN DESIGNATION	ANTIBODY (Ig SUBCLASS)	IMMUNOGEN	ANTIGEN CHARACTERIZATION
URO 7	S22(γ1)	SK-RC-7 RC	115
URO 9	OM5(γ1)	Non-Cultured Bladder Papilloma	ND
URO 10	T43(γ1)	T24 BC	85

RC - Renal Cancer; BC - Bladder Cancer; ND - Not Determined; Antigen Characterization in Kilodaltons.

TABLE III. Reactivity of a selected panel of monoclonal antibodies detecting differentiation antigens of the urinary stystem of human cancers.[a]

	URO 2	URO 3	URO 4	URO 7	URO 9	URO 10
RENAL CARCINOMA	16/20[b]	18/20	19/20	10/20	0/8	3/8
BLADDER CARCINOMA	0/8	0/8	0/8	1/8	22/40	23/40
COLON CARCINOMA	0/5	0/5	0/5	0/5	0/5	2/5
LUNG CARCINOMA	0/5	1/5	0/5	0/5	0/5	4/5
BREAST CARCINOMA	0/5	1/5	0/5	0/5	0/5	3/5
MELANOMA	0/4	3/4	0/4	0/4	0/4	0/4
ASTROCYTOMA	0/3	1/3	0/3	0/3	0/3	1/3
LYMPHOMA	0/3	0/3	0/3	0/3	0/3	3/3
TERATOCARCINOMA	0/3	0/3	0/3	0/3	0/3	3/3

a) In direct Immunofluorescence and Immunoperoxidase (Avidin-Biotin Method) on frozen sections of human tumors. b) Results are shown as number of antigen-positive tumors specimens over total number of specimens tested.

that most renal cell carcinoma arise in epithelial cells of the proximal tubules. The significance of renal cancer subsets that lack expression of one or more URO differentiation antigens needs to be assessed. Antigen loss could account for these phenotypes or they may be derived from early progenitors, not detected by the present panel of mAbs. Much effort is actually devoted to expand the analysis of renal cell carcinomas, as well as correlate antigenic phenotype with clinical course and response to therapy (Bander N.H., Cordon-Cardo, C., Finstad, C.L. et al, manuscript in preparation). In addition to tissue studies, analysis are underway evaluating the detection of shed or secreted URO antigens in blood and urine. This would enhance our ability to detect and monitor renal disease, as recently reported for renal transplant rejection and drug-induced nephrotoxicity (23).

4.2 Transitional Cell Carcinoma:

The generation of characterization of the first panel of mouse mAbs against cell surface antigens of human bladder tumors has been recently reported (19). The antibodies were obtained by immunization with cultured human transitional cell carcinomas or lysates of human bladder papilloma. This new strategy allowed us to obtain Abs against tumor lesions that usually do not grow in culture as low grade transitional cell carcinomas. Initial screening for papilloma-specific antigens was carried out by indirect immunofluorescence on frozen sections. These sections were obtained from stored frozen tissue of the papilloma lesion used for immunization. A number of antigens defined in this study were found in bladder cancers "in vitro" and "in vivo" but were not detected on normal bladder urothelium. Three categories of antigens were identified in this analysis according to their reactivity with normal urothelium and other normal tissues: The first type is represented by a highly restricted urothelial antigen (URO 9); the second type is composed of a series of Ags not found in normal fetal and adult urothelium but expressed in subsets of aggressive transitional cell acarcinomas and other tumors (URO 10); the final type includes a set of Ags expressed in normal and transformed urothelium (URO 5) (Fradet Y., Cordon-Cardo C et al, manuscript in preparation).

URO 9 (OM5) shows a very restricted pattern of expression limited to bladder tumors and some normal urothelium. It has not been detected on any other normal cells or tissues even in individuals with URO 9+ urothelium, nor on any 60 non-bladder human tumor specimens studied. The fact that some normal urothelial tissues have been found positive and others negative for URO 9 is being evaluated with clinicopathological correlation. URO 9 has been found in 17 of 20 non-invasive papillary bladder tumors, 6 of 8 non-papillary carcinoma-in-situ (CIS), 3 of 15 invasive transitional carcinomas, and 0 of 6 bladder cancer metastases. URO 10 (T43) is not found in normal fetal and adult urothelium but is detected on proximal tubular epithelial cells of the kidney. URO 10 is expressed in tumors presenting signs of aggressiveness. It has been found in 4 of 20 non-invasive papillary bladder tumors, 3 of 8 CIS, 14 of 15 invasive transitional carcinomas, and 6 of 6 metastases. This study suggest that transitional cell carcinomas can be defined on the basis of their selective reactivity with the panel of mAbs generated. Preliminary data on the correlation with histologic criteria and clinical course suggests that cells with different potential may be identified by their phenotype.

5. IMMUNOPATHOLOGIC ANALYSIS OF MELANOMA

Melanomas are malignant neoplasms arising from melanocytes. These are the pigment-producing cells, synthesizing melanin; and are embryologically derived from the neural crest. Melanoma constitutes 3% of human cancers and the rising incidence of melanoma exceeds that of all other neoplasms, with the exception of bronchogenic carcinoma.

Melanoma has been the subject of much immunological study, serological analysis being the most prominent approach. The relevance of such immunologic analysis is due to several facts: a) Growth properties "In vitro" of normal melanocytes and melanoma cells, which facilitate serological and immunohistochemical studies; b) Spontaneous regression of a small percent of clinical cases of melanoma, suggesting immunogenic properties of this tumor; and c) Definition of "unique" or "tumor-specific" Ags expressed by melanomas. Heterologous and autologous antisera, and more recently mAbs against melanomas have been used to distinguish melanoma-specific and associated Ags from other non-related Ags (24, 25). Melanoma-associated Ags have been found in melanoma patients' sera (26), melanoma patients' urine (27, 28), the serum of cystic melanoma lesions (29), tissue culture supernatants of murine and human melanomas (30, 31), and in tissue sections of melanoma lesions (32, 34).

Despite these efforts and studies, no individual antibody has been found to possess the required specificity and sensitivity to assist realistically for the detection and management of patients with malignant melanoma. Nevertheless, there are some Abs showing a very restricted pattern of reactivity, being useful in the diagnosis and study of melanoma, and possibly in therapy.

Permanent melanoma cell lines can be established in 20-30% of metastatic lesions, and autologous typing has been applicable (35). Using this approach three classes of surface antigens have been defined in melanoma cells. Class 1 Ags are restricted to the autologous tumor cell; they are not found on any other normal or malignant cell type. Class 2 Ags are shared on autologous as well as in other tumor cells; some Class 2 Ags are found on a restricted set of normal cell types, while others have not been found in any normal cell type as yet. Class 3 antigens are widely distributed on malignant as well as normal cells.

The hybridoma technology has been applied extensively, and a large number of mouse and human mAbs reactive with melanoma have been produced. The definition of a differentiation pathway for normal and malignant melanocytes has been proposed, based on their antigenic expression and phenotypes (36). Several categories of antigens of particular interest for further analysis have been defined by mouse monoclonal antibodies. The first category represents Ags characteristic of differentiation stages in the neural crest and melanocyte lineage. Some of them are expressed only by melanocytes and melanoma cells at a late stage of differentiation. Because the restricted reactivity presented by Abs directed against these specific Ags, their use in diagnosis, imaging and treatment of melanoma is now being explored. Other antigens in this group are expressed on melanoma cells at early stages of differentiation as the major histocompatibility class II Ags. A second category of Ags has been related to malignant transformation of melanocytes or changes in properties of melanoma cells indicative of tumor progression; some of these Ags, including Ia Ag and tissue plasminogen activator, have been found on melanoma cells but not on melanocytes.

The antibodies of this series are not present in all melanoma lesions, dividing melanomas into distinguishable subsets. The diversity of melanoma phenotypes seems to reflects a corresponding diversity in the surface phenotype of normal cells undergoing melanocyte differentiation. It may be postulated that melanomas arise at different stages in the melanocyte pathway. Support for this hypothesis has been provided by the comparison of malignant melanomas vs. normal melanocytes (newborn and adult). A correlation was evident between cell surface antigenic phenotype, morphologic characteristics, pigmentation, and tyrosinase activity (36). The implication of these subsets of melanoma lesions expressing early, intermediate or late differentiation markers suggests a new classification of melanomas with potential clinical applications and clinico-pathologic correlations.

Two particular phenomena have been defined as characteristic features of melanomas. They include: a) Heterogeneity of antigen (37) and molecular-probe (38) expression; and b) Induction and modulation of antigenic systems (39). These two events may give rise to crucial problems in dealing with antibodies as immunodiagnostic reagents, and in clinical trials for immunolocalization and/or immunotherapy; especially the great variability in the phenotype of cells derived from patients with metastatic disease. Possible mechanisms for this heterogeneity may be the polyclonal origin of melanoma, genetic instability, and changes in the differentiation stages of tumor cells during transformation and progression of the disease.

The advances in hybridoma technology, especially the production of human mAbs, will provide new reagents that may lead to a precise serological dissection of highly restricted Ags. They are clearly important for future progress, and much effort is going into generating them. Extensive specificity analysis with some of these reagents has begun, and they will undoubtedly have considerable value for a range of clinical applications.

ACKNOWLEDGEMENTS

The author wishes to thank Drs. Old and Melamed for their guidance and fruitful discussions; Drs. Oettgen, Houghton, Bander, Fradet and Ms. Finstad for their invaluable help. In addition, Ms. Katheleen Weinstein and Ms. Mary Ellen McGroarti for their skillful technical assistance and Ms. Jannette Rios for expert secretarial help.

REFERENCES

1. Neville AM, Foster CS, Moshakis V, Gore M: Hum Pathol 13: 1067, 1982.
2. Osborn M, Weber K: Lab Invest 48:372, 1983.
3. Herberman RB: Cancer 37:549, 1976.
4. Bast RC, Klung TL, John E, Jenison E, Niloff JM, Lazarus H, Berkowitz RS, Leavitt T, Griffiths CT, Parker L, Zurawski VR, Knapp RC: N Engl J Med 309:883, 1983.
5. Metzgar RS, Bergoc PM, Moreno MA, Seigler HF: J Natl Cancer Inst 50:1065, 1973.
6. Shiku H, Takahashi T, Resnik LA, Oettgen HF, Old LJ: J Exp Med 145:784, 1977.
7. Kohler G, Milstein C: Nature 256:459, 1975.
8. Old LJ: Cancer Res 41:361, 1981
9. Lloyd KO: In Basic & Clinical Tumor Immunology, Martinus Nijhoff, Netherlands, 1983.
10. Wright GL: Monoclonal antibodies in cancer. Marcel Dekker, New York, 1984.
11. Salmon DJ, de Kernion JB, Verma IM, Cline MJ. Science 224:256, 1984.
12. Smedley HM, Finan P, Lennox ES, Ritson A, Takei F, Wraight P, Sikora K: Br J Cancer 47: 253, 1983.
13. Cobbold SP, Waldmann H: Nature 308: 460, 1984.
14. Houghton AN, Mintzer D, Cordon-Cardo C, Welt S, Fliegel B, Vadhan S, Carswell E, Melamed MR, Oettgen HF, Old LJ: Proc Natl Acad Sci (USA) (in press).
15. Ueda R, Shiku H, Pfreundschuh M, Takahashi T, Li LTC, Whitmore WF, Oettgen HF, Old LJ: J Exp Med 150:564, 1979.
16. Sternberger LA: Immunocytochemistry. John Wiley & Sons, New York, 1979.
17. Erlandson RA, Cordon-Cardo C, Higgins P: Am J Surg Pathol 11:803, 1984.
18. Ueda R, Ogata SI, Morrissey DM, Finstad CL, Szkudlarek J, Whitmore WF, Oettgen HF, Lloyd KO, Old LJ: Proc Natl Acad Sci (USA) 78:5122, 1981.
19. Fradet Y, Cordon-Cardo C, Thomason T, Daly ME, Whitmore WF, Lloyd KO, Melamed MR, Old LJ: Proc Natl Acad Sci (USA) 81:224, 1984.
20. Cardon-Cardo C, Bander NH, Fradet Y, Finstad CL, Whitmore WF, Lloyd KO, Oettgen HF, Melamed MR, Old LJ: J Histochem Cytochem 32:1035, 194.
21. Rettig W, Dracopoli NC, Goetzer TA, Spengler BA, Biedler JL, Oettgen, HF, Old LJ: Proc Natl Acad Sci (USA) (in press).
22. Any RJ,Finstad CL, Old LJ, Lloyd KO, Kornfeld R: J Biol Chem (in press).

23. Rubin RH, Thompson R, Piper D, Bander NH, Old LJ, Hansen WP, Tolkoff-Rubin NE: NSN Abstract, 1985.
24. Metzgar RS, Bergoc PM, Moreno MA, Seigler HF: J Natl Cancer Inst 50:1065, 1973.
25. Shiku H, Takahashi T, Resnik LA, Oettgen HF,Old LJ: J Exp Med 145: 784, 1977.
26. Ishii Y, Mavligit GM: Oncology 39:23, 1982.
27. Carrel S, Thailkaes L: Nature 242:609, 1973.
28. Huth RK, Morton DL: Cancer 47:2856, 1981.
29. Jehn UM, Nathanson L, Schwartz RS, Skinner M: N Engl J Med 283:329,1970.
30. Bystryn JC: J Immunol 116: 1302, 1976.
31. Grimm EA, Silver HKB, Roth JA, Chee DO, Gupta RK, Morton DL: Int J Cancer 17:559, 1976.
32. Reisfeld RA, Ferrone S (eds): Melanoma Antigens and Antibodies. Plenum Press, New York, 1982.
33. Garrigues HJ, Tilgen W, Franke W, Hellstrom KE. Int J Cancer 29:511, 1982.
34. Ruiter DJ, Bergman W, Welvaart K, Scheffer E, Vloten WA, Russo C, Ferrone S: Cancer Res 44:3930, 1984.
35. Old LJ, Cancer Res 41: 361, 1981.
36. Houghton AN, Eisinger M, Albino AP, Caincross JG, Old LJ: J Exp Med 156:1735, 1982.
37. Albino AP, Lloyd KO, Houghton AN, Oattgen HF, Old LJ: J Exp Med 154:1764, 1981.
38. Albino AP, Le Strange R, Oliff AI, Furth MG, Old LJ: Nature 308:69, 1984.
39. Houghton AN, Thomson TM, Groos D, Oattgen HF, Old LJ: J Exp Med 160:255, 1984.

18

IMMUNOHISTOCHEMISTRY OF OVARIAN TUMORS

ROBERT E. SCULLY, M.D.

1. INTRODUCTION

Almost all ovarian tumors can be diagnosed on routine examination of adequate numbers of sections stained with hematoxylin and eosin, with the occasional addition of mucin, glycogen, argyrophil or reticulum stains (1). Although electron microscopic studies have expanded our knowledge of the morphologic features of ovarian tumors, they have rarely yielded information of diagnostic significance. Immunohistochemistry has already contributed to our understanding of the biology of ovarian tumors, but up to the present time has likewise been of little diagnostic aid. It is probable, however, that, with the continuing identification of new and more specific antibodies and experience with larger numbers of cases, this approach will have on increasingly important role in the diagnosis of unusual ovarian tumors.

Several problems exist currently with regard to the use of immunohistochemistry for the diagnosis of ovarian neoplasms. Some of these problems apply to the field of immunohistochemistry in general, and have been well summarized in a recent editorial (2). They include variations in fixation and technique from one study to another, differences in the specificity of the antibodies being used, and experience with too few cases, leading to preliminary unwarranted claims of specificity for many antibodies. An additional problem with regard to ovarian tumors is that most of the diagnostic difficulties involve the interpretation of rare neoplasms, which often exhibit considerable variation from one specimen to another. For example, Sertoli-Leydig cell tumors have many patterns and cell types, so that experience with large numbers of cases will be necessary before generally applicable conclusions can be drawn about their immunohistochemical properties.

This chapter will review some of the many contributions in the field of immunohistochemistry of ovarian tumors, with an attempt to evaluate their biologic and diagnostic significance. Instead of discussing successively each antibody and its application to the entire range of ovarian neoplasms, the chapter will consider the published experience with various antibodies in relation to each of the major categories of ovarian tumor and most of the subtypes that are included in the classification of the World Health Organization (3). Several valuable reviews of the role of immunohistochemistry in ovarian (4) and gynecologic pathology (5-7) have appeared recently in the literature.

2. COMMON EPITHELIAL TUMORS

Carcinoembryonic Antigen. Carcinoembryonic antigen (CEA), which was initially identified in the serum of patients with adenocarcinoma of the colon, was found subsequently to be elevated in the serum in association with benign disorders and cancers of a variety of organs, including those of the female genital tract (8). Immunohistochemical investigations of CEA in ovarian tumors (9-14) have produced a wide range of findings, with the differences attributable largely to methodology and antibody specificity. For example, one team of investigators (14) found that 50 percent of common epithelial carcinomas, including almost all types, stained positively for CEA, while others (13) reported its absence in serous and undifferentiated carcinomas in contrast to the other forms of common epithelial tumor, whether benign, borderline or invasive (Fig. 1). In addition to its presence in neoplastic glandular epithelium in these neoplasms, CEA has been demonstrated in the transitional type epithelium

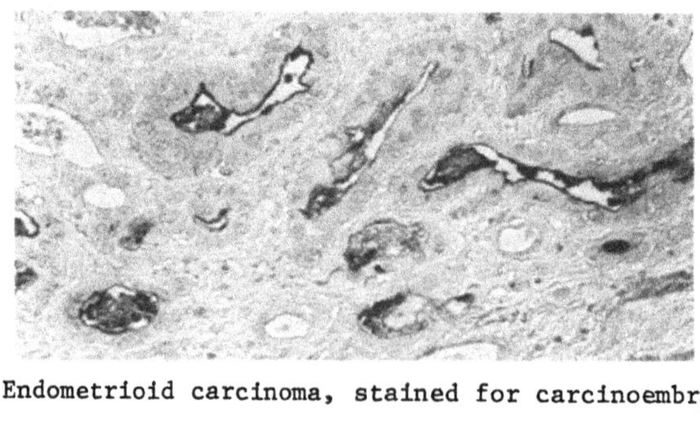

Figure 1. Endometrioid carcinoma, stained for carcinoembryonic antigen.

of Brenner tumors. A negative reaction for this antigen with the use of the more specific antibodies may be helpful, therefore, in differentiating serous from other common epithelial tumors. Also, since sex-cord stromal tumors have been uniformly negative for CEA except for mucinous elements in heterologous Sertoli-Leydig cell tumors (13), its absence may be of value in distinguishing this group of tumors from those of common epithelial type. Identification of CEA is not useful, however, in differentiating primary carcinomas from the most common forms of metastatic carcinoma in the ovary, which arise in the gastrointestinal tract and breast, since these tumors may also stain positively for this antigen (12,13).

Intestine-Associated Antigens. Intestinal mucous antigens have been demonstrated immunohistochemically in mucinous ovarian tumors (15,16), and a carbohydrate determinant (CA 19-9) recognized by a monoclonal antibody that was prepared against a colonic carcinoma cell line, has been identified significantly more often than CEA in common epithelial tumors, including those of serous type (13). Lysozyme, an enzyme that is widely distributed in the body and is encountered in Paneth cells of the small intestine as well as glandular cells of the pylorus, duodenum and endocervix, has also been demonstrated immunohistochemically in mucinous tumors of the ovary (17). Staining for these various antigens, therefore, is of no specific diagnostic help in establishing the ovarian origin of a mucin-secreting tumor.

Chorionic Gonadotropin and Other Placental Antigens. Because of cross reactivity of intact hCG with pituitary luteinizing hormone, identification of the specific beta subunit of hCG is the basis of most assays and immunohistochemical demonstrations of this hormone at the present time. The beta subunit is elevated in the serum not only during pregnancy and in association with trophoblastic neoplasia, but also in patients with benign disorders and malignant tumors of a variety of organs. Chorionic gonadotropin is a valuable marker for several types of gonadal primitive germ cell tumor, but has been demonstrated additionally in the serum of almost 40 percent of patients with ovarian carcinomas of common epithelial type (8). Immunohistochemical staining of common epithelial tumors for the beta subunit of hCG has yielded widely varying results (14,18,19). One team of workers (19) found an approximately 40 percent frequency of staining, with no significant differences among benign, borderline and invasive tumors, while another group (18) reported only a 10 percent frequency of staining of carcinomas and no staining of benign forms of these tumors. Because of its presence in a variety of ovarian tumors, including a single example of a granulosa cell tumor (18), the immunohistochemical identification of hCG is of relatively little help in differential diagnosis. Demonstration of its presence or absence may be of interest, however, in the evaluation of ovarian tumors with functioning stroma. These tumors, which can be benign or malignant, and primary or metastatic, are associated with endocrine effects that may be estrogenic, androgenic, progestagenic or of mixed types (1). One possible explanation for the secretion of steroid hormones by these tumors is stimulation of their stroma by hCG secreted by the neoplastic cells. This hormone has been demonstrated immunohistochemically in sporadic cases of tumors of this type (Fig. 2),

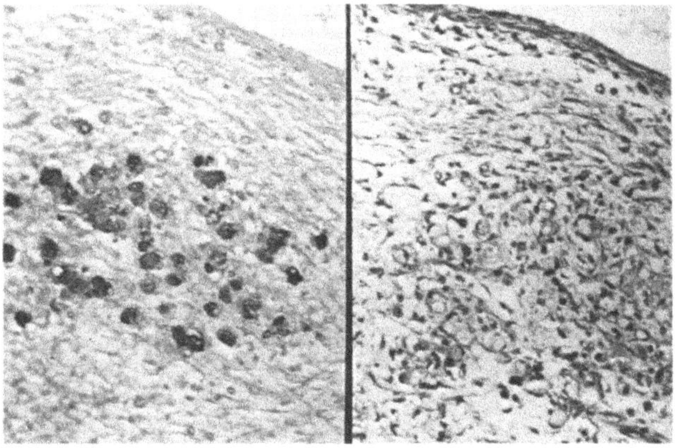

Figure 2. Krukenberg tumor of gastric origin, stained for chorionic gonadotropin (left) and with hematosylin and eosin (right). Courtesy of Dr. Robert J. Kurman, Washington, D.C.

but a systematic investigation of them from the viewpoint of their content of hCG has not been reported. If such a study is undertaken, however, it must be emphasized that the immunohistochemical demonstration of hCG or its beta subunit in a neoplastic cell does not indicate whether the hormone was being secreted or bound or whether, if secreted, it was biologically active (18).

Placental lactogen (hPL), a product of intermediate trophoblast and syncytiotrophoblast of the normal placenta, has been reported to be elevated in the serum in association with a variety of malignant tumors (20). In one study it was demonstrated immunohistochemically in 15 percent of common epithelial carcinomas of the ovary (14).

Placental-like alkaline phosphatase, (PLAP), which is normally present in the cytoplasm of syncytiotrophoblast cells, is elevated in the serum in association with a variety of cancers, including ovarian carcinomas, with which high levels have been found in approximately one-third of the cases (8,21,22). PLAP has also been demonstrated immunohistochemically in a number of malignant tumors (23), including a serous carcinoma (24) and the epithelial component of a malignant mesodermal mixed tumor of the ovary (25). It is almost certain that this enzyme will be identified immunohistochemically in other forms of common epithelial tumor as well.

Alpha-fetoprotein. Although this oncofetal protein, which is a product of the yolk sac and its derivatives, has been commonly regarded as a specific marker for several types of germ cell tumor, hepatocellular carcinomas and occasional carcinomas of the stomach and pancreas, it may be elevated additionally in the serum in patients with benign hepatic disease and rarely in those with other types of malignant tumors (26,27), including serous carcinomas of the ovary (28). All forms of common epithelial carcinoma except for the clear cell carcinoma have been reported to be positive for alpha-fetoprotein on immunohistochemical staining (14), and we have recently seen staining of this form of tumor.

Alpha-1-Antitrypsin. Among the common epithelial tumors, alpha-1-antitrypsin has been demonstrated in both the epithelial and mesenchymal components of malignant mesodermal mixed tumors (29); staining was present throughout the cytoplasm of the neoplastic cells as well as within intracellular hyaline bodies. Demonstration of this enzyme has little diagnostic signficance, however, since it has been identified in a variety of tumors as well as normal tissue (30).

Serous Ovarian Neoplastic Amylase. Amylase (SONA) may be elevated in the plasma, urine, ascitic fluid and cyst fluid of patients with serous tumors of the ovary, as well as with neoplasms of other organs, but it has been reported to be absent from the fluid of non-serous types of ovarian cyst (31,32). With the use of an antibody prepared against pancreatic amylase, SONA has been demonstrated immunohistochemically in benign, borderline and invasive serous tumors, as well as fallopian tube epithelium, but not in a mucinous cystadenoma (32,33). The specificity of amylase positivity for serous neoplasms of the ovary requires confirmation by examination of a larger series that includes other types of ovarian tumor.

Serotonin and Peptide Hormones. Serotonin and a variety of peptide hormones, including gastrin, somatostatin, neurotensin, glucagon, pancreatic polypeptide, secretin, enkephalin and adrenocorticotrophic hormone (ACTH), have been demonstrated immunohistochemically in benign, borderline and malignant mucinous tumors (Fig. 3) (17,34-37). The frequency with which one or more of these hormones have been stained has varied from 3 to 35 percent (17,34-37). Some of these hormones have also been identified immunohistochemically in Brenner tumors and endometrioid carcinomas (37,38). The relative frequency of demonstration of serotonin and peptide hormones in Brenner tumors resembles that

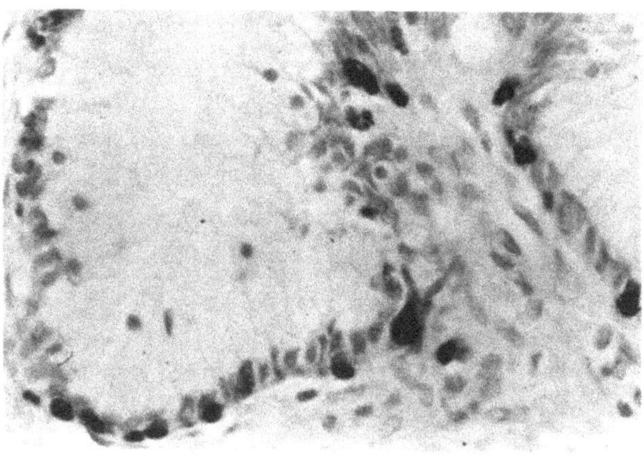

Figure 3. Mucinous cystadenoma of borderline malignancy, stained for somatostatin.

encountered in urinary transitional cell epithelium rather than in intestinal epithelium, i.e., a common finding of serotonin (32 percent) and an infrequent identification of peptide hormones (4 percent). The presence of peptide hormones in ovarian common epithelial tumors has clinical significance on rare occasions. For example, two examples of the Zollinger-Ellison syndrome have been described in association with mucinous cystic tumors of the ovary (39,40); one of these tumors was demonstrated to contain cells that stained immunohistochemically for gastrin (40).

Intermediate Filaments (Keratin, Vimentin and Desmin). The recent widespread use of antibodies prepared against intermediate filaments to differentiate epithelial from nonepithelial tumors, distinguish fibroblastic, myomatous and neural tumors from one another and identify various components of mixed tumors has involved investigation of ovarian neoplasms to a limited extent (41-49). The findings have varied depending on the methodology and the specificity of the antibody used. In most studies all types of common epithelial tumor have been positive for keratin (Fig. 4), whereas in one investigation (48) only the epithelial

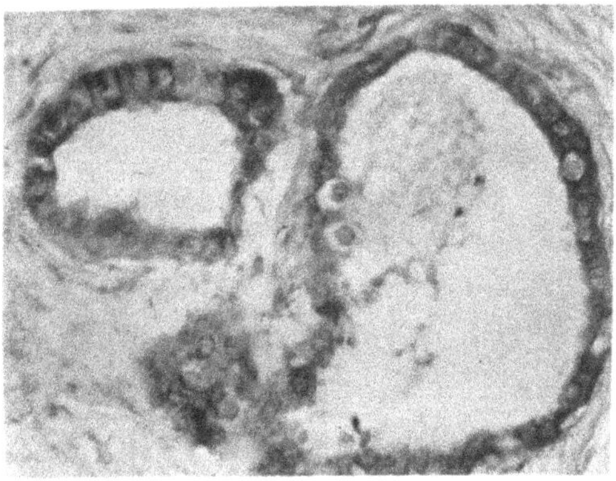

Figure 4. Endometrioid carcinoma simulating Sertoli cell tumor, stained for keratin.

component of Brenner tumors and the squamous component of endometrioid tumors were strongly positive. Vimentin, although typically a nonepithelial mesenchymal filament, has been reported to be present in the surface epithelium of the ovary (46) and in two serous carcinomas (41). The immunohistochemical demonstration of vimentin and desmin has also been useful in determining the nature of the mesenchymal components of carcinosarcomas and malignant mesodermal mixed tumors (49).

Involucrin. Involucrin, a precursor of the envelope protein in human stratum corneum (50), is thought to be a specific marker for squamous differentiation in tumors and non-neoplastic disorders. Although it has not been used, to the best of our knowledge, in the immunohistochemistry of ovarian tumors, it should be helpful in identifying squamous differentiation in adenocarcinomas and undifferentiated carcinomas, as it has proven to be in investigations of pulmonary and endometrial carcinomas (51,52).

Actin, Myosin and Myoglobin. Antibodies prepared against actin, myosin (53-55) and myoglobin (55-57) may be useful to varying extents in identifying smooth muscle and skeletal muscle elements in malignant mesodermal mixed tumors, and in pure sarcomas of the ovary, some of which may belong in the common "epithelial" category.

Monoclonal Antibodies Against Ovarian and Other Carcinomas. Several monoclonal antibodies that have been raised against ovarian carcinomas (58-62) as well as other types of carcinoma (62,63) have been shown to react immunohistochemically with the former. The antibody that has been studied most extensively from an immunohistochemical viewpoint is OC-125, a murine monoclonal antibody raised against a serous carcinoma of the ovary (59,60). It has reacted with serous, endometrioid and clear cell tumors and undifferentiated carcinomas of the ovary (Fig. 5), as well as

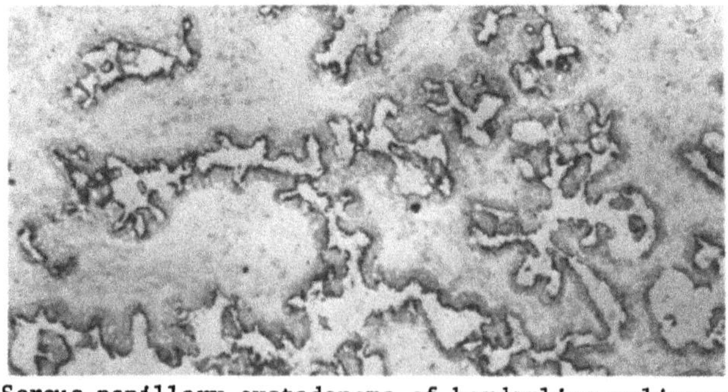

Figure 5. Serous papillary cystadenoma of borderline malignancy, stained with monoclonal antibody OC-125. Courtesy of Dr. Salim Kabawat.

with adenocarcinomas of the fallopian tube, endometrium and endocervix and mesotheliomas. Ovarian mucinous and Brenner tumors, however, have been unreactive. The antibody stains additionally the normal epithelium of the endocervix, endometrium and fallopian tubes and the mesothelial lining cells of the peritoneum, pleura and pericardium. Surprisingly, the surface epithelia of fetal and adult ovaries are unreactive, but surface papillary excrescences and epithelial inclusion cysts stain positively. Only 7 of 64 nongynecologic tumors, including some breast carcinomas and adenocarcinomas of the lung, have stained for OC-125. So far, the immunohistochemical demonstration of this antigen has required the use of fresh or frozen tissue.

Estrogen and Progesterone Receptors. An immunohistochemical method for demonstrating estrogen receptors, using a monoclonal antibody, has been been described recently (64). The antibody was prepared in the rat against human estrogen receptor protein derived from the cytosol of human breast cancer cells. It is anticipated that a similar staining method for progesterone receptors will be available in the near future. Since many common epithelial tumors of the ovary contain estrogen receptors, progesterone receptors or both (65-68), undoubtedly these tumors will be investigated immunohistochemically for their receptor content.

Basement Membrane Antibodies. Antibodies prepared against laminin (69,70) and type IV collagen (71), constituents of the basal lamina, have been used to investigate tumor invasion in various organs. Future studies of this type applied to borderline and invasive common epithelial tumors of the ovary may prove helpful in their differential diagnosis.

3. GERM CELL TUMORS, NONTERATOMATOUS

Chorionic Gonadotropin (hCG). Both hCG and its beta subunit have been demonstrated immunohistochemically in the syncytotrophoblastic elements of choriocarcinomas, polyembryomas, embryonal carcinomas, mixed primitive germ cell tumors and occasional dysgerminomas (72-78). Isolated mononucleate cells in embryonal carcinoma that are not recognizable as trophoblastic in routine sections may also stain positively (77). The finding of hCG in these tumors is significant since this hormone and its beta subunit are valuable markers in monitoring the clinical course of the patient and the secretion of this hormone explains a variety of associated endocrine manifestations including sexual precocity, postpubertal menstrual disturbances and virilization (79). These hormonal changes may result from gonadotropic stimulation of the stroma of the tumor, the ovarian stroma uninvolved by neoplasia, or residual ovarian follicles. Placental lactogen and various pregnancy specific proteins may also be identified in the syncytotrophoblast cells of germ cell tumors (80). None of these substances, however, is specific for either germ cell tumors, pregnancy or gestational trophoblastic tumors.

Alpha-Fetoprotein. This valuable tumor marker can be identified immunohistochemically in typical endodermal sinus tumors (81), foci of yolk sac differentiation within embryonal carcinomas (77) and yolk sac elements within polyembryomas (76). Demonstration of this antigen has also proved useful in confirming the existence of atypical forms of yolk sac tumor, including a hepatoid form (Fig. 6) (82) and a glandular form that resembles secretory endometrioid adenocarcinoma on routine staining (83).

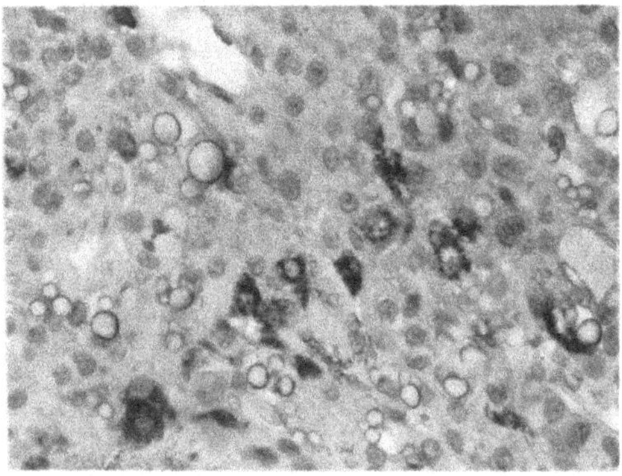

Figure 6. Hepatoid yolk sac tumor, stained for alpha-fetoprotein. The hyaline bodies do not stain.

Other Antigens in Nonteratomatous Germ Cell Tumors. Alpha-1-antitrypsin has been identified in various forms of yolk sac tumor both within the cytoplasm of the neoplastic cells and in the hyaline bodies that are commonly found in these tumors (84). This antigen, however, is also present in a wide variety of normal tissues and tumors, both benign and malignant (30). Ferritin, transferrin and placental-like alkaline phosphatase can be demonstrated in nonteratomatous germ cell tumors (72). PLAP has been found in dysgerminomas (23), yolk sac tumors, syncytiotrophoblast cells within germ cell tumors (Fig. 7) and the germ cell component of gonadoblastomas (85).

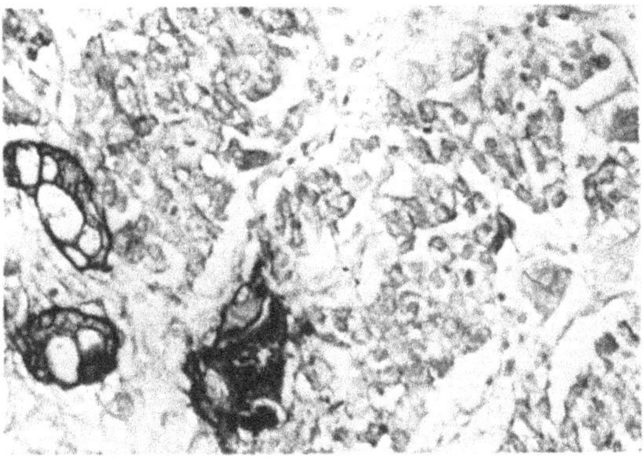

Figure 7. Dysgerminoma with syncytiotrophoblast cells, stained for placental-like alkaline phosphatase. Three large syncytiotrophoblast cells are stained diffusely; the surfaces of the dysgerminoma cells are also stained.

Very little investigation of intermediate filaments has been performed in cases of germ cell neoplasia of the ovary. A few dysgerminomas and yolk sac tumors have been reported to be negative for cytokeratin and desmin, but positive for vimentin (41). In the testis seminomas are said to be negative for keratin in contrast to teratomas, embryonal carcinomas, yolk sac tumors and choriocarcinomas, which are focally positive (86).

4. GERM CELL TUMORS, TERATOMATOUS

These tumors have been reported to contain almost all types of tissue in varying degrees of maturity, and to give rise to a variety of neoplasms that are typically encountered elsewhere in the body (1). Therefore, a positive immunohistochemical reaction with almost any type of antibody would not be surprising in a teratoma.

Alpha-fetoprotein has been demonstrated in endodermal elements, including liver cells, within teratomas. A wide variety of peptide hormones, including insulin, glucagon, gastrin, secretin, somatostatin and pancreatic polypeptide, have also been identified in these tumors (87,88). Primary carcinoid tumors of both insular (midgut) and trabecular type are encountered rarely in the ovary, accompanied by other teratomatous elements in most cases (89,90). In approximately one third of the cases, primary insular carcinoids are associated with the carcinoid syndrome. Both insular and trabecular carcinoids have been demonstrated to react positively immunohistochemically for a wide variety of peptide hormones (91). Strumal carcinoids are neoplasms composed of struma and carcinoid, which is usually of the trabecular type (92). Typically both elements are intimately admixed, with the carcinoid cells invading thyroid-type follicles and surrounding intraluminal colloid. Immunohistochemical staining has revealed evidence of thyroglobulin (Fig. 8) and thyroxin as

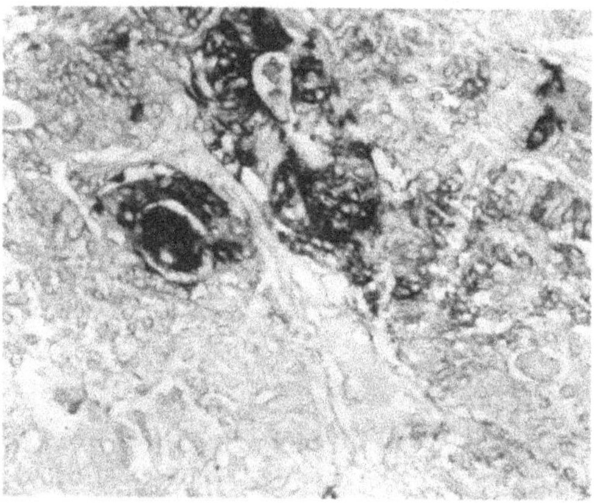

Figure 8. Strumal carcinoid, stained for thyroglobulin.

well as calcitonin in strumal carcinoids (93-98). One strumal carcinoid was associated with the carcinoid syndrome (97), and evidence suggestive of thyroid hyperfunction was reported in two cases (92). Carcinoid also reacts positively with antibodies against neuron-specific enolase (99-100) and human chromogranin A (101-102).

Anterior pituitary tissue has been identified rarely in the walls of dermoid cysts (103) and has been shown to react immunohistochemically with antibodies against a number of pituitary hormones (83,104). Pancreatic islet tissue, which stained for insulin, glucagon and somatostatin, has also been reported in an ovarian teratoma (105).

Thyroid tissue is encountered occasionally in the wall of a dermoid cyst, rarely forming a grossly recognizable mass (struma ovarii). Immunohistochemical staining has confirmed the thyroidal nature of struma by the demonstration of T3, T4, and thyroglobulin within it (106,107). Although thryoid tissue is usually evident on routine staining, a rare papillary tumor arising within a teratoma and containing little or no colloid may require immunohistochemical demonstration of thyroxin or thyroglobulin for its recognition (Fig. 9) (83).

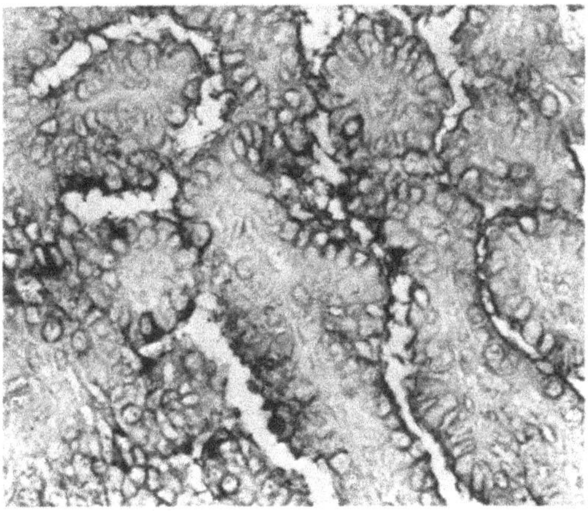

Figure 9. Papillary carcinoma arising in dermoid cyst, stained for thyroglobulin.

Neuroectodermal components of teratomas have been shown to react positively immunohistochemically for neural and glial filaments and myelin basic protein (108,109). Very rarely primitive neuroectodermal tumors and ependymomas have been reported to arise in the ovary or broad ligament (110-112). These neoplasms may be difficult to distinguish from other poorly differentiated small cell tumors, endometrioid carcinomas and serous carcinomas on routine staining, and in such cases a positive reaction for glial fibrillary acidic protein may confirm the diagnosis (Fig. 10).

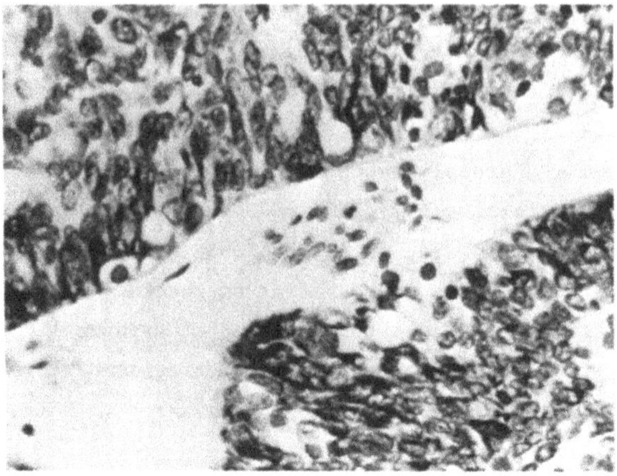

Figure 10. Ependymoma of broad ligament, stained for glial fibrillary acidic protein.

5. SEX CORD-STROMAL TUMORS

Estradiol, progesterone and testosterone have been localized immunohistochemically in the four major cell types of sex cord-stromal tumors (granulosa cells, theca cells, Sertoli cells and Leydig cells) as well as in nonspecific-appearing spindle-shaped cells found in some of these tumors (113-117). Kurman (7) has discussed problems in the interpretation of these reactions. It is impossible to be certain on the basis of immunohistochemical localization whether a positive reaction within the various types of neoplastic cells indicates synthesis, binding or storage of the hormone. Also, the same reactions that are demonstrable in these tumors may occur additionally in target organs of steroid hormones such as the breast and endometrium. Kurman concluded that at the present time the diagnosis of an ovarian neoplasm as a sex cord-stromal tumor is not warranted on the basis of immunohistochemical demonstration of steroid hormone content alone. Nevertheless, it is possible that steroid immunohistochemistry will be useful in the differentiation of tumors of endocrine type, such as thecomas, from non-endocrine neoplasms, such as fibromas; this approach may be helpful additionally in evaluating tumors with functioning stroma.

Immunohistochemical investigations of small numbers of sex cord-stromal tumors have indicated the presence of vimentin and the absence of keratin and desmin in all of them (41). In one report, however, granulosa cells of primordial and developing follicles were said to contain keratin (118). Additional study of larger numbers of cases with a wider variety of antibodies will be necessary to characterize the intermediate filament content of the various cell types in these tumors.

The mucinous and carcinoid components of heterologous Sertoli-Leydig cell tumors have reacted for serotonin and one or more polypeptide hormones on immunohistochemical examination (37). A few Sertoli-Leydig cell tumors have been associated with elevated levels of alpha-fetoprotein in the serum (119-121). In one case, immunohistochemical staining for this antigen was localized in liver cells within a retiform Sertoli-Leydig cell tumor with heterologous elements (Fig. 11) (120); in other cases there was staining of the mucinous epithelium or of the Sertoli and Leydig cell components of the neoplasm (121).

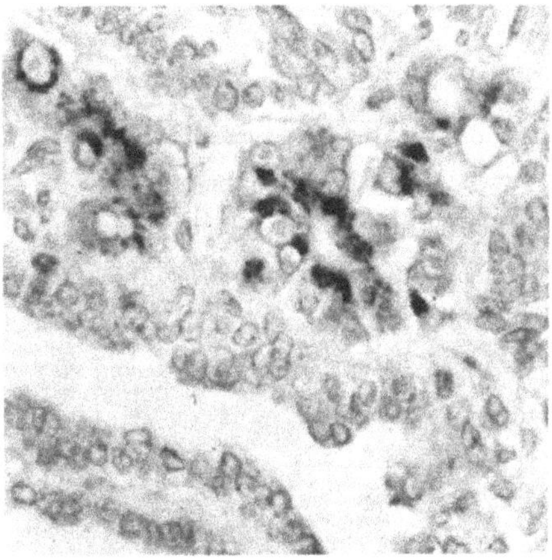

Figure 11. Clusters of hepatoid cells in retiform Sertoli-Leydig cell tumors, stained for alpha-fetoprotein. The cells lining the tubules are unstained.

6. UNUSUAL PRIMARY TUMORS AND SECONDARY TUMORS

The diagnosis of a wide variety of rare primary tumors of the ovary may be established or confirmed by immunohistochemical techniques. For example, we have recently encountered a pheochromocytoma of the ovary that created a diagnostic problem because of its resemblance to tumors in the steroid cell category. Positive staining for chromogranin confirmed the diagnosis (122); the use of antibodies against neuron-specific enolase and neurofilaments would also have been helpful in establishing the diagnosis.

Lymphomas growing in the ovary may have patterns resembling those of dysgerminoma and undifferentiated carcinoma. The various immunohistochemical reactions of lymphomas, discussed elsewhere, as well as those of dysgerminomas and undifferentiated carcinomas, mentioned earlier in this chapter, may be helpful in the differential diagnosis of difficult cases. The tumors that metastasize to the ovary most commonly and create problems in differential diagnosis are carcinomas originating in the gastrointestinal tract. We are not aware of any immunohistochemical method currently available that distinguishes these neoplasms from primary mucinous carcinomas in view of the cross-reactivity of ovarian mucinous and gastrointestinal carcinomas with various antibodies. The diagnosis of other rare metastatic tumors in the ovary, however, may be supported by immunohistochemical staining. For example, we have encountered recently an ovarian tumor in a patient with a remote history of cutaneous melanoma that caused a problem in diagnosis because of an unusual cystic pattern of growth. A positive reaction for S-100 (123) confirmed the suspected diagnosis of metastatic melanoma. Antibodies that are specific for breast carcinoma, which are discussed elsewhere, may be of value in distinguishing a primary ovarian carcinoma from a metastatic tumor of mammary origin.

7. CYTOLOGY OF OVARIAN TUMORS

Antibodies prepared against CEA (124), a monoclonal antibody to a component of milk-fat-globule membrane (MFG-2) (125,126) and monoclonal antibodies raised against ovarian (MOv2) and breast (MBr-1) carcinomas

(61,63) have been used with good to excellent results to differentiate reactive mesothelial cells, which are almost always negative on staining with these antibodies, and carcinoma cells, which are usually positive, in cytological smears of fluids from body cavities (Fig. 12). Since the cells of endometrioid and serous carcinomas of the ovary are derived

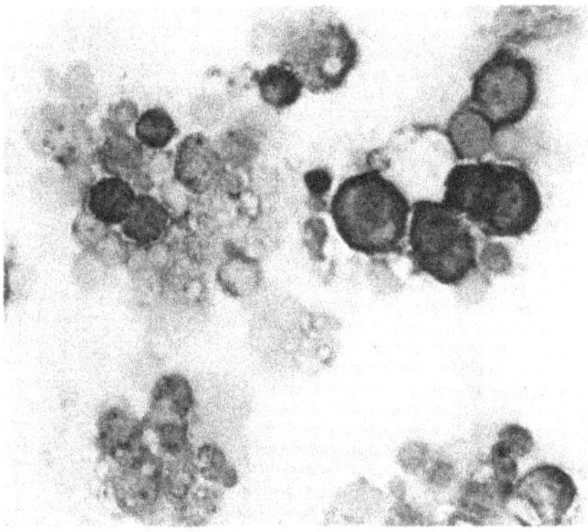

Figure 12. Carcinoma cells in abdominal fluid, stained for carcinoembryonic antigen.

ultimately from pelvic mesothelium and since the latter can undergo metaplasia into cells of endometrial and tubal type, one must exercise caution, however, in relying entirely on immunohistochemical findings in evaluating exfoliated cells in the female peritoneal cavity.

8. CONCLUSIONS

Immunohistochemistry is a rapidly evolving new approach to the refinement of diagnosis of human tumors. Although the results have not been spectacular to date in the area of ovarian neoplasms, undoubtedly the continuing availability of new and more specific antibodies and the application of batteries of antibodies to individual problem cases will enhance the usefulness of this technique in future years. In addition to its diagnostic contributions immunohistochemistry may be of great clinical value in identifying tumor markers for monitoring the course of the patient (127).

REFERENCES

1. Scully RE: Tumors of the ovary and maldeveloped gonads. Atlas of Tumor Pathology, Second series-Fascicle 6. Armed Forces Institute of Pathology, Washington, 1979, pp. 413.

2. Erlandson RA: Diagnostic immunohistochemistry of human tumors. Am J Surg Pathol (8):615-624, 1984.

3. Serov S, Scully RE, Sobin LH: Histological typing of ovarian tumours. International histological classification of tumours, no. 9. World Health Organization, Geneva, 1973. 56 pp.

4. Kurman RJ, Ganjei P, Nadji M: Contributions of immunocytochemistry to the diagnosis and study of ovarian neoplasms. Int J Gynecol Pathol (3):3-26, 1984.

5. Fenoglio CM: Antigens, enzymes and hormones. Their roles as tumor markers in gynecologic neoplasia. Diagn Gynecol Obstet (2):33-42, 1980.

6. Crum CP, Fenoglio CM: The immunoperoxidase technique. Review of its application to diseases of the female genital tract. Diagn Gynecol Obstet (2):103-115, 1980.

7. Kurman RJ: Contributions of immunocytochemistry to gynaecological pathology. Clin Obstet Gynaecol (11):5-23, 1984.

8. van Nagell JR, Donaldson ES, Hanson MB, Gay EC, Pavlik EJ: Biochemical markers in the plasma and tumors of patients with gynecologic malignancies. Cancer (48):495-503, 1981.

9. Marchand A, Fenoglio CM, Pascal R, Richart RM, Bennett S: Carcinoembryonic antigen in human ovarian neoplasms. Cancer Res (35):3807-3810, 1975.

10. Seppala M, Pihko H, Rouslahti E: Carcinoembryonic antigen and alpha fetoprotein in malignant tumors of the female genital tract. Cancer (35):1377-1381, 1975.

11. Heald J, Buckley CH, Fox H: An immunohistochemical study of the distribution of carcinoembryonic antigen in epithelial tumors of the ovary. J Clin Pathol (32):918-926, 1979.

12. Fenoglio CM, Crum CP, Pascal RR, Richart RM: Carcinoembryonic antigen in gynecologic patients. II. Immunohistological expression. Diagn Gynecol Obstet (3):291-299, 1981.

13. Charpin C, Bhan AK, Zurawski VR Jr, Scully RE: Carcinoembryonic antigen (CEA) and carbohydrate determinant 19-9 (CA19-9) localization in 121 primary and metastatic ovarian tumors: an immunohistochemical study with the use of monoclonal antibodies. Int J Gynecol Pathol (1):231-245, 1982.

14. Casper S, van Nagell JR, Powell DF, Dubilier LD, Donaldson ES, Hanson MB, Pavlik EJ: Immunohistochemical localization of tumor markers in epithelial ovarian cancer. Am J Obstet Gynecol (149):154-158, 1984.

15. DeBoer WGRM, Nayman J: Intestine-associated antigens in ovarian tumours: an immunohistological study. Pathol (13):547-555, 1981.

16. Ueda G, Tanaka Y, Hiramatsu K, Inoue Y, Yamasaki M, Inoue M, Kurachi K, Mori T: Immunohistochemical study of mucous antigens in gynecologic tumors with special reference to argyrophil cells. Int J Gynecol Pathol (1):41-45, 1982.

17. Aguirre P, Scully RE, Dayal Y, DeLellis RA: Mucinous tumors of the ovary with argyrophil cells. An immunohistochemical analysis. Am J Surg Pathol (8):345-356, 1984.

18. Fenoglio CM, Hayata T, Crum CP, Richart RM: The expression of human chorionic gonadotrophin in the female genital tract. Localization by the immunoperoxidase technique. Diagn Gynecol Obstet (4):94-97, 1982.

19. Mohabeer J, Buckley CH, Fox H: An immunohistochemical study of the incidence and significance of human chorionic gonadotrophin synthesis by epithelial ovarian neoplasms. Gynecol Oncol (16):78-84, 1983.

20. Muggia FM, Rosen SW, Weintraub BD, Hansen HH: Ectopic placental proteins in nontrophoblastic tumors. Cancer (36):1327-1337, 1975.

21. Nathanson L, Fishman WH: New observations on the Regan isoenzyme of alkaline phosphatase in cancer patients. Cancer (27):1388-1397, 1970.

22. Kellen JA, Bush RS, Malkin A: Placenta-like alkaline phosphatase in gynecological cancers. Cancer Res (36):269-271, 1976.

23. Uchida T, Shikata T, Iino S: Immunohistochemical localization of placental and intestinal alkaline phosphatases. In: DeLellis RA (ed) Advances in Immunohistochemistry, Masson Publishing, USA, New York, pp. 185-199.

24. Loose JH, Damjanov I, Harris H: Identity of the neoplastic alkaline phosphatase as revealed with monoclonal antibodies to the placental form of the enzyme. Am J Clin Pathol (82):173-177, 1984.

25. Takeda A, Matsuyama M, Kuzuya K, Chihara T, Tsubouchi S, Takeuchi S: Mixed mesodermal tumor of the ovary with carcinoembryonic antigen and alkaline phosphatase production. Cancer (53):103-112, 1974.

26. Tsung SH: Localization of α-fetoprotein synthesis in malignancies other than hepatoma. Arch Pathol Lab Med (101):572-574, 1977.

27. Yasunami R, Hashimoto Z, Ogura T, Hirao F, Yamamura Y: Primary lung cancer producing alpha-fetoprotein: A case report. Cancer (47):926-929, 1981.

28. Higuchi Y, Kouno T, Teshima H, Akizuki S, Kikuta M, Ohyumi M, Yamamoto S: Serous papillary cystadenocarcinoma associated with α-fetoprotein production. Arch Pathol Lab Med (108):710-712, 1984.

29. Dictor M: Ovarian malignant mixed mesodermal tumor: The occurrence of hyaline droplets containing α-1 antitrypsin. Hum Pathol (13):930-933, 1982.

30. Silva FG, Taylor WE, Burns DK: Demonstration of alpha-1-antitrypsin in yet another neoplasm. Hum Pathol (15):494, 1984.

31. van Kley H, Cramer S, Bruns DE: Serous ovarian neoplastic amylase (SONA): a potential useful marker for serous ovarian tumors. Cancer (48):1444-1449, 1981.

32. Hayakawa T, Kameya A, Mizuno R, Noda A, Kondo T, Hirabayashi N: Hyperamylasemia with papillary serous cystadenocarcinoma of the ovary. Cancer (54):1662-1665, 1984.

33. Bruns DE, Mills SE, Savory J: Amylase in fallopian tube and serous ovarian neoplasms. Immunohistochemical localization. Arch Pathol Lab Med (106):617-620, 1982.

34. Sporrong B, Alumets J, Clase L, Falkmer S, Hakanson R, Ljungberg O, Sundler F: Neurohormonal peptide immunoreactive cells in mucinous cystadenomas and cystadenocarcinomas of the ovary. Virchows Arch (Pathol Anat) (392):271-280, 1981.

35. Takeda A, Matsuyama M, Chihara T, Suchi T, Sato T, Tomoda Y: Ultrastructure and immunocytochemistry of gastroentero-pancreatic (GEP) endocrine cells in mucinous tumors of the ovary. Acta Pathol Jpn (32):1003-1015, 1982.

36. Louwerens JK, Schaberg A, Bosman FT: Neuroendocrine cells in cystic mucinous tumors of the ovary. Histopathology (7):389-398, 1983.

37. Scully RE, Aguirre P, DeLellis RA: Argyrophilia, serotonin, and peptide hormones in the female genital tract and its tumors. Int J Gynecol Pathol (3):51-70, 1984.

38. Ueda G, Yamasaki M, Inoue M, Tanaka Y, Hiramatsu K, Inoue Y, Saito J, Nishino T, Kurachi K: Argyrophil cells in the endometrioid carcinoma of the ovary. Cancer (54):1569-1573, 1984.

39. Cocco AE, Conway S: Zollinger-Ellison syndrome associated with ovarian mucinous cystadenocarcinoma. N Engl J Med (293):485-486, 1975.

40. Long TT, Barton TK, Draffin R, Reeves WJ, McCarty KS: Conservative management of the Zollinger-Ellison syndrome. Ectopic gastrin production by an ovarian cystadenoma. JAMA (243):1837-1839, 1980.

41. Miettinen M, Lehto VP, Virtanen I: Expression of intermediate filaments in normal ovaries and ovarian epithelial, sex cord-stromal, and germinal tumors. Int J Gynecol Pathol (2):64-71, 1983.

42. del Poggetto CB, Virtanen I, Lehto VP, Wahlstrom T, Saksela E: Expression of intermediate filaments in ovarian and uterine tumors. Int J Gynecol Pathol (1):359-366, 1983.

43. Ramaekers F, Huysmans A, Moesker O, Kant A, Jap P, Herman C, Vooijs P: Monoclonal antibody to keratin filaments, specific for glandular epithelia and their tumors. Lab Invest (49):353-361, 1983.

44. Nagle RB, Clark VA, McDaniel KM, Davis JR: Immunohistochemical demonstration of keratins in human ovarian neoplasms. A comparison of methods. J Histochem Cytochem (31):1010-1014, 1983.

45. Davis BW, Morassi LL, Locher GW, Wetherall N, Grigolato P: Cellular localization of keratin in proliferative epithelial processes and neoplasms of the human ovary. J Cancer Res Clin Oncol (106): 222-228, 1983.

46. Moll R, Levy R, Czernobilsky B, Hohlweg-Majert P, Dallenbach-Hellweg G, Franke WW: Cytokeratins of normal epithelia and some neoplasms of the female genital tract. Lab Invest (49):599-610, 1983.

47. Gown AM, Gabbiani G: Intermediate-sized (10-nm) filaments in human tumors. In: DeLellis RA, ed. Diagnostic immunochemistry. Masson Publishing, USA, New York, 1981, pp. 89-109. (Masson monographs in diagnostic pathology).

48. Ganjei P, Nadji M, Penneys NS, Averette HE, Morales AR: Immunoreactive prekeratin in Brenner tumors of the ovary. Int J Gynecol Pathol (1):353-358, 1983.

49. Ramaekers FCS, Verheijen RHM, Moesker O, Kant A, Vooijs GP, Herman CJ: Mesodermal mixed tumor. Diagnosis by analysis of intermediate filament proteins. Am J Surg Pathol (7):381-385, 1983.

50. Rice RH, Pinkus GS, Warhol MJ, Antonioli DA: Involucrin: Biochemistry and immunohistochemistry. In: DeLellis RA, ed. Diagnostic immunocytochemistry. Masson Publishing, USA, New York, 1981, pp. 111-125. (Masson monographs in diagnostic pathology).

51. Said JW, Nash G, Sassoon AF, Shintaku IP, Banks-Schlegal S: Involucrin in lung tumors. A specific marker for squamous differentiation. Lab Invest (49):563-568, 1983.

52. Warhol MJ, Rice RH, Pinkus GS, Robboy SJ: Evaluation of squamous epithelium in adenocanthoma and adenosquamous carcinoma of the endometrium: immunoperoxidase, analysis of involucrin and keratin localization. Int J Gynecol Pathol (3):82-91, 1984.

53. Mukai K, Rosai J: Application of immunoperoxidase techniques in surgical pathology. In Progress in surgical pathology, Vol 1, CM Fenoglio and M. Wolff, Eds. Masson, New York, 1980, pp. 15-49.

54. Bussolati G, Gugliotta P, Fulcheri E: Immunohistochemistry of actin in normal and neoplastic tissues. Diagnostic immunocytochemistry In: DeLellis RA, ed. Masson Publishing, USA, New York, 1981, pp. 325-342. (Masson monographs in diagnostic pathology).

55. deJong ASH, van Vark M, Albus-Lutter Ch E, van Raamsdonk W, Voute PA: Myosin and myoglobin as tumor markers in the diagnosis of rhabdomyosarcoma. Am J Surg Pathol (8):521-528, 1984.

56. Mukai K, Varela-Duran J, Nochomovitz LE: The rhabdomyoblast in mixed mullerian tumors of the uterus and ovary: an immunohistochemical study of myoglobin in 25 cases. Am J Clin Pathol (74):101-104, 1980.

57. Brooks JJ: Immunohistochemistry of myoglobin. In: DeLellis RA, ed. Diagnostic immunocytochemistry. Masson Publishing, USA, New York, 1981, pp. 343-358. (Masson monographs in diagnostic pathology).

58. Bhattacharya M, Chatterjee SK, Barlow JJ, Fuji H: Monoclonal antibodies recognizing tumor-associated antigen of human ovarian mucinous cystadenocarcinomas. Cancer Res (42):1650-1654, 1982.

59. Kabawat SE, Bast RC Jr. Bhan AK, Welch WR, Knapp RC, Colvin RB: Tissue distribution of a coelomic-epithelium-related antigen recognized by the monoclonal antibody OC125. Int J Gynecol Pathol (2):275-285, 1983.

60. Kabawat SE, Bast RC, Welch WR, Knapp RC, Colvin RB: Immunopathologic characterization of a monoclonal antibody that recognizes common surface antigens of human ovarian tumors of serous, endometrioid, and clear cell types. Am J Clin Pathol (79):98-104, 1983.

61. Rilke F: Carcinoma of the breast and ovary as a model for the application of monoclonal antibodies to diagnostic pathology. Presented at XV International Congress of Int Acad Pathol, Miami Beach, Fla, 1984.

62. Mattes MJ, Cordon-Cardo C, Lewis JL Jr, Old LJ, Lloyd KO: Cell surface antigens of human ovarian and endometrial carcinoma defined by mouse monoclonal antibodies. Proc Natl Acad Sci USA (81):568-572, 1984.

63. Mariani-Costantini R, Colnaghi MI, Leoni F, Menard S, Cerasoli S, Rilke F: Immunohistochemical reactivity of a monoclonal antibody prepared against human breast carcinoma. Virch Arch (Pathol Anat) (402):389-404, 1984.

64. Press MF, Greene GL: Methods in laboratory investigation. An immunocytochemical method of demonstrating estrogen receptor in human uterus using monoclonal antibodies to human estrophilin. Lab Invest (50):480-486, 1984.

65. Holt JA, Caputo TA, Kelly KM, Greenwald P, Chorost S: Estrogen and progestin binding in cytosols of ovarian adenocarcinomas. Obstet Gynecol (53):50-58, 1979.

66. Creasman WT, Sasso RA, Weed JC Jr., McCarthy KS Jr.: Ovarian carcinoma: histologic and clinical correlation of cytoplasmic estrogen and progesterone binding. Gynecol Oncol (12):319-327, 1981.

67. Hahnel R, Kelsall GRH, Martin JD, Masters AM, McCartney AJ, Twaddle E: Estrogen and progesterone receptors in tumors of the human ovary. Gynecol Oncol (13):145-151, 1982.

68. Kauppila A, Vierikko P, Kivinen S, Stenback F, Vihko R: Clinical significance of estrogen and progestin receptors in ovarian cancer. Obstet Gynecol (61):320-326, 1983.

69. Liotta L: Biochemical mechanisms of tumor invasion. Presented at XV International Congress of Int Acad Pathol, Miami Beach, Florida, 1984.

70. Haglund C, Roberts PJ, Nordling S, Ekblom P: Expression of laminin in pancreatic neoplasms and in chronic pancreatitis. Am J Surg Pathol (8):669-676, 1984.

71. Gusterson BA, Warburton MJ, Mitchell D, Kraft N, Hancock WW: Invading squamous cell carcinoma can retain a basal lamina. An immunohistochemical study using a monoclonal antibody to type IV collagen. Lab Invest (51):82-87, 1984.

72. Kurman RJ, Scardino PT, McIntire KR, Waldmann TA, Javadpour N, Norris HJ: Malignant germ cell tumors of the ovary and testis. An immunohistologic study of 69 cases. Ann Clin Lab Sci (9):462-466, 1979.

73. Kurman RJ, Scardino PT: Alpha-fetoprotein and human chorionic gonadotropin in ovarian and testicular germ cell tumors. In: DeLellis RA, ed. Diagnostic immunocytochemistry. Masson Publishing, USA, New York, 1981, pp 277-298. (Masson monographs in diagnostic pathology)

74. Kurman RJ, Norris HS: Malignant mixed germ cell tumors of the ovary. A clinical and pathologic analysis of 30 cases. Obstet Gynecol (48):579-589, 1976.

75. Beck JS, Fulmer HF, Lee ST: Solid malignant ovarian teratoma with "embryoid bodies" and trophoblastic differentiation. J Pathol (99):67-73, 1969.

76. Takeda A, Ishizuka T, Goto T, Goto S, Ohta M, Tomoda Y, Hosino M: Polyembryoma of ovary producing alpha-fetoprotein and HCG: immunoperoxidase and electron microscopic study. Cancer (49):1878-1889, 1982.

77. Kurman RJ, Norris HJ: Embryonal carcinoma of the ovary. A clinicopathological entity distinct from endodermal sinus tumor resembling embryonal carcinoma of the adult testis. Cancer (38):2420-2433, 1976.

78. Zaloudek CJ, Tavassoli FA, Norris HJ: Dysgerminoma with syncytiotrophoblastic giant cells. A histologically and clinically distinctive subtype of dysgerminoma. Am J Surg Pathol (5):361-367, 1981.

79. Case Records of the Massachusetts General Hospital. Case 11. N Engl J Med (286):594-600, 1972.

80. Horne CHW, Rankin R, Bremmer RD: Pregnancy-specific proteins as markers for gestational trophoblastic disease. Int J Gynecol Pathol (3):27-40, 1984.

81. Kurman RJ, Norris HJ: Endodermal sinus tumor of the ovary. A clinical and pathologic analysis of 71 cases. Cancer (38):2404-2419, 1976.

82. Prat J, Bhan AK, Dickersin GR, Robboy SJ, Scully RE: Hepatoid yolk sac tumor of the ovary (Endodermal sinus tumor with hepatoid differentiation). A light microscopic, ultrastructural and immunohistochemical study of seven cases. Cancer (50):2355-2368, 1982.

83. Scully RE: Personal observation.

84. Palmer PE, Safaii H, Wolfe HJ: Alpha$_1$-antitrypsin and alpha-fetoprotein. Protein markers in endodermal sinus (yolk sac) tumors. Am J Clin Pathol (65):575-582, 1976.

85. Aguirre P, Scully RE, DeLellis RA: Unpublished data.

86. Battifora H, Sheibani K, Tubbs RR, Kopinski MI, Sun T-T: Antikeratin antibodies in tumor diagnosis. Distinction between seminoma and embryonal carcinoma. Cancer (54):843-848, 1984.

87. Bosman FT, Louwerens JWK: APUD cells in teratomas. Am J Pathol (104):174-180, 1981.

88. Calame J, Bosman FT, Schaberg A, Louwerens JWK: Immunocytochemical localization of neuroendocrine hormones and oncofetal antigens in ovarian teratomas. Int J Gynecol Pathol (3):92-100, 1984.

89. Robboy SJ, Norris HJ, Scully RE: Insular carcinoid primary in the ovary. A clinicopathologic analysis of 48 cases. Cancer (36):404-418, 1975.

90. Robboy SJ, Scully RE, Norris HS: Primary trabecular carcinoid of the ovary. Obstet Gynecol (49):202-207, 1977.

91. Sporrong B, Falkmer S, Robboy SJ, Alumets J, Hakanson R, Ljungberg O, Sundler F: Neurohormonal peptides in ovarian carcinoids: an immunohistochemical study of 81 primary carcinoids and of intraovarian metastases from six mid-gut carcinoids. Cancer (49):68-74, 1982.

92. Robboy SJ, Scully RE: Strumal carcinoid of the ovary. An analysis of 50 cases of a distinctive tumor composed of thyroid tissue and carcinoid. Cancer (46):2019-2034, 1980.

93. Ueda G, Sato Y, Yamasaki M, Inoue M, Hiramatsu K, Kurachi K, Amino N, Miyai K: Strumal carcinoid of the ovary. Histological, ultrastructural, and immunohistological studies with anti-human thyroglobulin. Gynecol Oncol (6):411-419, 1978.

94. Greco MA, LiVolsi VA, Pertschuk LP, Bigelow B: Strumal carcinoid of the ovary. An analysis of its components. Cancer (43):1380-1383, 1979.

95. Dayal Y, Tashjian AH Jr, Wolfe HJ: Immunocytochemical localization of calcitonin-producing cells in a strumal carcinoid with amyloid stroma. Cancer (43):1331-1338, 1979.

96. Blaustein A: Calcitonin-secreting struma-carcinoid tumor of the ovary. Hum Pathol (10):222-228, 1979.

97. Ulbright TM, Roth LM, Ehrlich CE: Ovarian strumal carcinoid. An immunocytochemical and ultrastructural study of two cases. Am J Clin Pathol (77):622-631, 1982.

98. Senterman MK, Cassidy PN, Fenaglio CM, Ferenczy A: Histology, ultrastructure and immunohistochemistry of strumal carcinoid: a case report. Int J Gynecol Pathol (3):232-240, 1984.

99. Dranoff G, Bigner DD: A word of caution in the use of neuron-specific enolase expression in tumor diagnosis. Arch Pathol Lab Med (108):535, 1984.

100. Vinores SA, Bonnin JM, Rubinstein LS, Marangos PJ: Immunohistochemical demonstration of neuron-specific enolase in neoplasms of the CNS and other tissues. Arch Pathol Lab Med (108):536-540, 1984.

101. O'Connor DT, Burton D, Deftos LH: Immunoreactive human chromogranin A in diverse polypeptide producing human tumors and normal endocrine tissues. J Clin Endocrinol Metab (47):1084-1086, 1983.

102. Kumar NB, Cookingham CL, Lloyd RV, Appelman HD: Detection of human chromogranin with a monoclonal antibody in carcinoid secretory granules and its comparison with the generic silver stains and with serotonin. Lab. Invest. (50):33A, 1984.

103. Akhtar M, Young J, Brody H: Anterior pituitary component in benign cystic ovarian teratomas. Am J Clin Pathol (64):14-19, 1975.

104. McKeel DW, Askin FB: Ectopic hypophyseal hormonal cells in benign cystic teratoma of the ovary. Light microscopic histochemical dye staining and immunoperoxidase cytochemistry. Arch Pathol Lab Med (102):122-128, 1978.

105. Ueda G, Yamasaki M, Inoue M, Tanaka Y, Hiramatsu K, Saito J, Nishino T: A rare malignant ovarian mixed germ cell tumor containing pancreatic tissue with islet cells. Int J Gynecol Pathol (3):1220-1231, 1984.

106. Haselton TS, Kelehan P, Whittaker JS, Burslem RW, Turner L: Benign and maligant struma ovarii. Arch Pathol Lab Med (102):180-184, 1978.

107. Livolsi VA, Loferfo P, Feind C: Thyroglobulin in struma ovarii. J Surg Res (25):12-14, 1978.

108. Steeper TA, Mukai K: Solid ovarian teratomas: An immunocytochemical study of thirteen cases with clinicopathologic correlation. Pathol Ann (19):81-92, 1984.

109. Trojanowski JQ, Hickey WF: Human teratomas express differentiated neural antigens. An immunohistochemical study with anti-neurofilament, anti-glial filament, and anti-myelin basic protein monoclonal antibodies. Am J Pathol (115):383-389, 1984.

110. Aguirre P, Scully RE: Malignant neuroectodermal tumors of the ovary, primary and metastatic. A report of five cases. Am J Surg Pathol (6):283-292, 1982.

111. Kleinman GM, Young RH, Scully RE: Ependymoma of the ovary: report of three cases. Hum Pathol (15):632-638, 1984.

112. Bell DA, Woodruff JM, Scully RE: Ependymoma of the broad ligament. a report of two cases. Am J Surg Pathol (8):203-209, 1984.

113. Kurman RJ, Andrade D, Goebelsmann U, Taylor CR: An immunohistological study of steroid localization in Sertoli-Leydig tumors of the ovary and testis. Cancer (42):1772-1783, 1978.

114. Kurman RJ, Goebelsmann U, Taylor CR: Steroid localization in granulosa-theca tumors of the ovary. Cancer (43):2377-2384, 1979.

115. Gaffney EF, Majmudar B, Hertzler GL, Zane R, Furlong B, Breding E: Ovarian granulosa cell tumors--immunohistochemical localization of estradiol and ultrastructure, with functional correlations. Obstet Gynecol (61):311-319, 1983.

116. Gaffney EF, Majmudar B, Hewan-Lowe K: Ultrastructure and immunohistochemical localization of estradiol in three thecomas. Hum Pathol (15):153-160, 1984.

117. Kurman RJ, Goebelsmann U, Taylor CR: Localization of steroid hormones in functional ovarian tumors. In: DeLellis RA (ed). Diagnostic immunohistochemistry. Masson Publishing, USA, New York, 1981. pp. 137-148, (Masson monographs in diagnostic pathology).

118. Czernobilsky B: Immunohistochemistry of normal tissues of the female genital tract. Presented at XV International Congress of Int Acad Pathol, Miami Beach, Fla, 1984.

119. Benfield GFA, Tapper-Jones L, Stout TV: Androblastoma and raised serum α -fetoprotein with familial multinodular goitre. Case report. Br J Obstet Gynaecol (89):323-326, 1982.

120. Young RH, Perez-Atayde AR, Scully RE: Ovarian Sertoli-Leydig cell tumor with retiform and heterologous components. Report of a case with hepatocytic differentiation and elevated serum alpha-fetoprotein. Am J Surg Pathol (8):709-718, 1984.

121. Chumas JC, Rosenwaks Z, Mann NJ, Finkel G, Pastore J: Sertoli-Leydig cell tumor of the ovary producing α -fetoprotein. Int J Gynecol Pathol (3):213-219, 1984.

122. Lloyd RV, Shapiro B, Sisson JC, Kalff V, Thompson NW, Beierwaltes WA: An immunohistochemical study of pheochromocytomas. Arch Pathol Lab Med (108):541-544, 1984.

123. Nakajima T, Watanabe S, Sato Y, Kameya T, Hirota T, Shimosato Y: An immunoperoxidase study of S-100 protein distribution in normal and neoplastic tissues. Am J Surg Pathol (6):715-727, 1982.

124. Watts AE, Said JW, Banks-Schlegal S: Keratin and carcinoembryonic antigen in exfoliated mesothelial and malignant cells: an immunoperoxidase study. Am J Clin Pathol (80):671-676, 1983.

125. Epenetos AA, Canti G, Taylor-Papadimitrio UJ, Curling M, Bodmer WF: Use of two epithelium-specific monoclonal antibodies for diagnosis of malignancy in serous effusions. Lancet (2):1004-1006, 1982.

126. Battifora H, Kopinski MI: Distinction of mesothelium and reactive mesothelial cells from adenocarcinoma: an immunohistochemical study. Lab Invest (50):4A-5A, 1984.

127. Bast RC Jr, Klug TL, Schaetzl E, Lavin P, Niloff JM, Greber TF, Zurawski VR Jr, Knapp RC: Monitoring human ovarian carcinoma with a combination of CA125, CA 19-9, and carcinoembryonic antigen. Am J Obstet Gynecol (149):533-559, 1984.

19

IMMUNOPATHOLOGY OF TESTICULAR TUMORS

F.K. MOSTOFI, M.D., I.A. SESTERHENN, M.D. AND C.J. DAVIS, JR., M.D.

I. INTRODUCTION

The incidence of testicular tumors in general populations is 2 per 100,000, but in the age group of 18 to 34 deaths from testicular tumors are 7 per 100,000 the highest incidence of deaths from malignancy in this group.

Testicular tumors are generally classified as sex cord/stromal tumors, germ cell tumors, secondary tumors and adnexal tumors. The last two groups are quite rare and the presentation will be limited to the first two groups.

2. SEX CORD/STROMAL TUMORS

Sex cord/stromal or gonadal stromal tumors constitute about 6% of testicular tumors. They consists of Leydig cell, Sertoli cell, theca and granulosa cell tumors and admixtures. Leydig and Sertoli cells are present normally in the testes, granulosa, theca and lutein cells in the ovary. Leydig cells produce androgenic and estrogenic substances and corticosteroids. Sertoli cells are the main sources of estrogenic hormones in man but may produce androgens as well. In the female theca and granulosa cells are the main source of estrogens and lutein cells may produce androgenic hormones as well. The tumors of these cell types occur in either sex and recapitulate the hormone production in the normal.

In children, Leydig cell tumors have been invariably associated with macrogenitosomia; in adults about 40% of men manifest feminizing symptoms consisting of uni or bilateral gynecomastia and loss of libido. In older men with Leydig cell tumors or with Leydig cell tumor metastases, there may be a sensation of well being.

Serum and urine demonstration of markers in these tumors has been of limited value in the clinical management of these patients because unless the patient manifests some endocrine disturbances, he is apt to have an orchiectomy before these markers are investigated.

Tissue demonstration of the markers may be valuable in defferential diagnosis of these tumors especially in patients without endocrine disturbances. Testosterone, androstenedione, estradiol and progesterone can be demonstrated in Leydig cell tumors and estrogenic hormones in the others.

3. GERM CELL TUMORS

Germ cell tumors constitute 94% of testicular tumors. Pathological classification of these tumors, their histogenesis, the role of tumor markers in diagnosis and prognosis, the exact site of the markers, have all elicited much diagreement, discussion and confusion.

As far as the classification is concerned, throughout the years there have been several American and British classifications, a Scandinavian, a French and a Russian classification.

In the American Testicular Tumor Registry sponsored by the American Urological Association at the AFIP we have employed the WHO International Histological Classification of Testicular Tumors. This classification separates the tumors into those of a single histological type and those of more than one histological type. Seven basic histologic types are recognized: Seminoma (S), Spermatocytic Seminoma (SS), Embryonal Carcinoma (EC)), Yolk Sac Tumor (YST), Polyembryoma, Choriocarcinoma (CC) and Teratoma. Teratoma is subgrouped into mature (MT), immature (IT), and teratoma with malignant areas. These constitute 38% of tumors. Tumors of more than one histological type constitute 62% of neoplasms. We list all the components that are present and give a rough estimate of each. The classification recognizes syncytio-trophoblasts and intratubular malignant germ cells.

In England and some European countries the classification initially proposed by Collins & Pugh (2), and later modified by Pugh & Cameron (3) is used. This divides the tumors into seminoma, spermatocytic seminoma and teratoma. Teratoma is subclassified into teratoma differentiated; malignant teratoma intermediate; malignant teratoma undifferentiated; malignant teratoma trophoblastic and combined tumors. YST is recognized in infants and children but not in adults. Syncytiotrophoblasts and intratubular malignant germ cells are not recognized.

A number of tumor markers have been employed in the clinical and pathological management of germ cell tumors. These are alpha fetoprotein

(AFP), beta fraction of human chorionic gonadotropin (HCG), human placental lactogen (HPL), pregnancy specific beta globulin (SP1), placental alkaline phosphatase (PLAP), carcinembryonic antigen (CEA), lactic acid dehydrogenase (LDH), gamma glutamyl transpeptidase (GGT), ferritin and fibronectin. CEA, LDH, and GGT are elevated in some tumors and PLAP is demonstrated in a few seminoma cells but none of these have been useful in clinical and pathological diagnoses.

The two most frequently utilized markers are AFP and HCG. The markers have been used not only in clinical and pathological diagnoses but in monitoring the course of the disease. These have also been valuable in evaluating the applicability of the two pathological classifications.

This report is based on a study of over 800 successive tumors received in our laboratory within the last 4 years, in which we have used an indirect immunoperoxidase technic on paraffin embedded tissue.

4. ALPHAFETOPROTEIN (AFP)

A detailed discussion of physicochemical properties of AFP is beyond the scope of this presentation and the reader is referred to the excellent review of the subject by Rouslahti & Hirai (4) and Rouslahti & Engvall (5). For our purpose suffice it to say that human AFP is composed of a single polypeptide chain with a molecular weight of about 69,000, slightly larger than that of albumin. It contains about 4% carbohydrate. Heterogeneity based on variations in structure of carbohydrate moiety has been reported in human AFP. Its half life is 4-6 days. In the fetus AFP is produced by yolk sac, liver, and to some extent by mucous glands of gastrointestinal tract. The concentration of AFP in nonpregnant human sera may range from 24 to 25 ng/ml. Whether fetal AFP is identical to human adult AFP has not been resolved.

Rouslahti & Hirai (4) have listed conditions associated with abnormally elevated AFP: primary liver cancer, germ cell tumors, some tumors of upper gastrointestinal tract, hepatitis, hepatic cirrhosis, partial hepatectomy, liver damage due to hepatotoxins, hereditary tyrosinemia, ataxia-telangiectasia and others.

Elevation of serum AFP has been reported in a number of testicular germ cell tumors. The initial reports described the tumors as teratoblastoma, and more recently, teratocarcinoma, malignant undifferentiated teratoma and embryonal carcinoma. Teilum (6) and Talerman et al (7) must be credited with attempts to clarify the confusion. Our studies have contributed to this effort.

AFP elevation in serum and its presence in tumor cells is most frequently associated with testicular yolk sac tumor. This tumor constitutes about 60% of germ cell tumors encountered in infants and children. As of this writing 19 of our 20 yolk sac tumors in this age group were associated with elevated AFP and demonstration of the marker in tumor cells. The level of AFP was dependent on tumor load.

In adult patients, pure yolk sac tumor (i.e., where no other elements are present but YST) is infrequent, constituting about 2.7% of tumors. Its frequency in association with other tumors, although reported by Teilum (6) and Mostofi & Price (8) had escape attention until Talerman (9) found it in 42% of a prospective study of adult germ cell tumor. We found it in 41%. AFP was demonstrable in 93% of these tumors.

One of the factors responsible for the confusion about the source of AFP has been failure to recognize YST. Whether in infants and children, or in adults, YST presents a variegated histological appearance which is often missed. Most frequently it consists of anastomosing tubulo-glandular structures and spaces lined by flattened, cuboidal, or low columnar cells. The tumor may be papillary cystic covered by small or intermediate sized cells. An unusual papillary structure may be seen, referred to as Schiller-Duval bodies. The tumor may have a reticular or vesicular myxoid appearance. In other areas it may consist of solid sheets and in still others it may have a hepatocytic appearance. AFP is demonstrable in any one of these cells, (Fig.1A&B) however, not all the cells give a positive reaction.

As mentioned earlier, elevation of AFP has been reported in teratocarcinoma (TCA), malignant teratoma undifferentiated (MTU) and embryonal carcinoma (ECA) where it has been claimed that the carcinomatous elements are the source of AFP, that the presence of metastases of these tumors can be detected and the progression of metastases, could be monitored by the levels of AFP. Our studies indicate a different source for the AFP.

Embryonal carcinoma is present in pure form in about 3% of testicular germ cell tumors but it is found in 47% of the tumors constituting a frequent accompanier of other germinal tumors. In 356 embryonal carcinomas either pure or mixed with other histologic types, only 47 gave a positive reaction for

AFP, comprising about 13% of the tumors. AFP is demonstrable only in individual or small clones of cells and scattered cells (Fig. 2A&B).

The main source of AFP in those that had elevated levels of AFP was YST which was often overlooked in these neoplasm (Fig. 3A&B).

We have demonstrated that some mucous glands of teratomas (whether mature or immature) also produce AFP (Figs. 4A&B & 5A&B) and may contribute to the pool of elevated AFP. It should be emphasized that while teratomas constitute only 3% of germ cell tumors, teratomatous areas are found in 47% of testicular tumors and 19% of these gave positive reaction for AFP. This may contribute to the pool of AFP in serum and urine.

None of our 466 seminomas pure or mixed with other histologic types was positive for AFP. In all cases where S was associated with elevated AFP we were able to demonstrate YST elements (Fig. 6A&B). The same held true for ECA.

In summary in testicular germ cell tumors, AFP is predominantly produced by YST. ECA and teratoma also contribute to the AFP pool. None or our ECA either pure or mixed with other histologic types was associated with elevated AFP unless there was also YST or teratomatous elements. AFP is a reliable monitor for YST, it may be elevated before there is clinical evidence of metastasis; AFP may be normal even though histologically the metastatic tumor appears viable, and chemotherapy may lead to disappearance of AFP in tumor cells of the metastases. AFP is not a reliable monitor for tumors that consist entirely of ECA or of those without YST elements.

5. PLACENTAL GLYCOPROTEINS

Four placental glycoproteins have been utilized in monitoring testicular germ cell tumors. These are placental alkaline phosphatase (already referred to earlier); human chorionic gonadotropin (HCG); human placental lactogen (HPL) and pregnancy specific beta globulin (SP1). These may be synthesized by the placental, trophoblastic and non trophoblastic tumors. Eutopic or specific production of these glycoproteins is seen in the placenta, trophoblastic tumors and certain testicular germ cell tumors. Heterotrophic or non specific production is seen in non germinal tumors. The subject has been extensively discussed elsewhere (10,11,12,13).

The most important of these placental glycoproteins is HCG. This has a molecular weight of about 38,000. Its half life is 24-36 hours. Two subunits have been identified with dissimilar polypeptide chains (Alpha and Beta). The

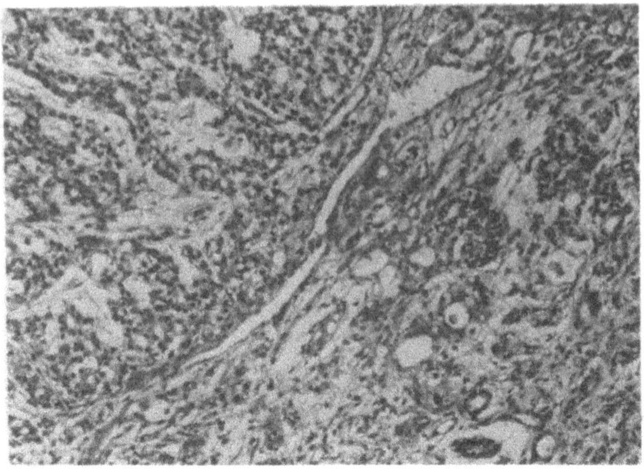

Figure 1A. Testicular yolk sac Tumor. AFIP Neg. 85-5156 H&E X 70.

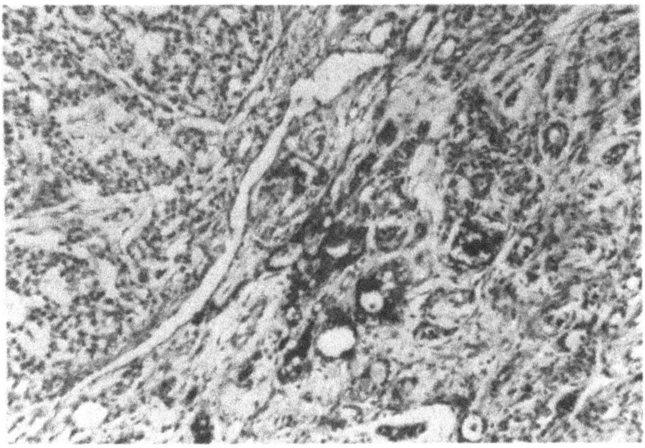

Figure 1B. From another field of the same tumor demonstrating positive reaction with AFP stain. AFIP Neg. 85-5157 AFP X 70.

Alpha subunit resembles pituitary luteinizing hormone.

The demonstration of Beta subunit in blood and serum is more specific since there is less concern about cross reactivity with L.H.

In testicular tumors there is universal agreement that choriocarcinoma, whether pure or in association with other germ cell tumors is manifested by elevated levels of Beta unit of HCG, and that syncytiotrophoblasts are the cells responsible for its synthesis (Fig.7A&B).

Disagreement exists, however, about elevation of HCG in several other germ cell tumors. Elevation of HCG, reported in teratomas, can be dismissed since the term has been applied to non seminomatous testicular tumors and no information is available as to the precise structure of these neoplasms.

More specifically, a number of reports have claimed elevated levels of HCG in "pure" seminoma and embryonal carcinoma (14,15). In all such tumors that we have studied the neoplasms were not pure (i.e. consisting only of one histological type). They all had clones of syncytiotrophoblasts (Fig. 8A&B).

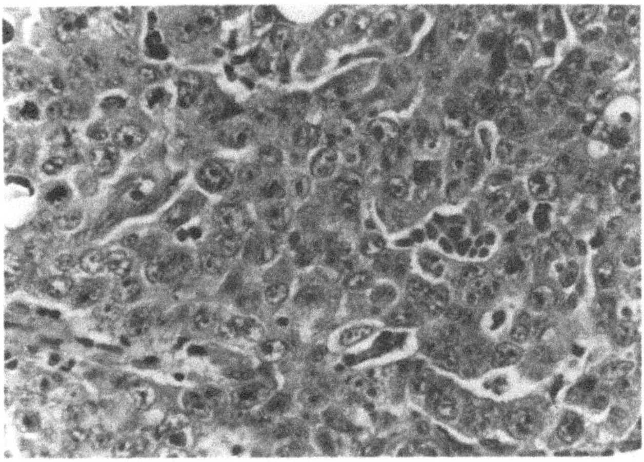

Figure 2A. Pure embryonal carcinoma. AFIP Neg. 85-5158 H&E X 100.

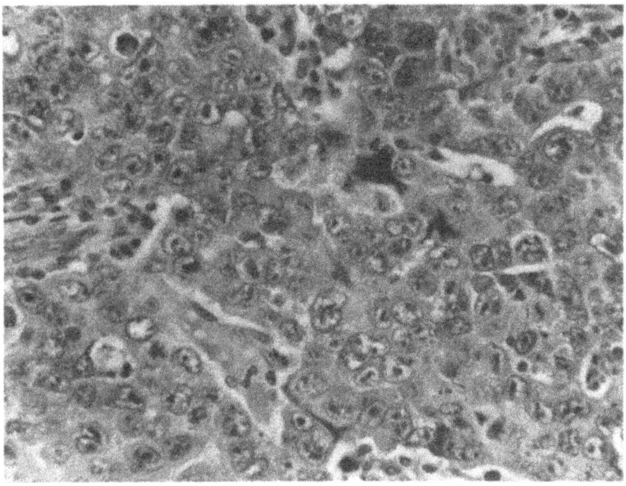

Figure 2B. From another field of same tumor showing only 2 cells that react positively with AFP. AFIP Neg. 85-5159 AFP X 100.

Failure to demonstrate these cells in such tumors may result from inadequate sampling. We have found clones of syncytiotrophoblasts in one of 12 sections with the first 11 being negative. Another reason for failure to recognize syncytiotrophoblasts is dependence on H&E stain alone. These cells can be identified almost four times as frequently with HCG stain as without such stain.

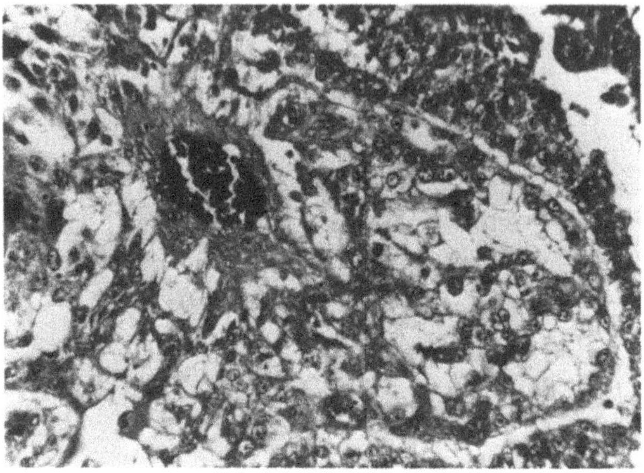

Figure 3A. Embryonal carcinoma at the periphery and yolk sac tumor in the center of the field. AFIP Neg. 85-5160 H&E X 100.

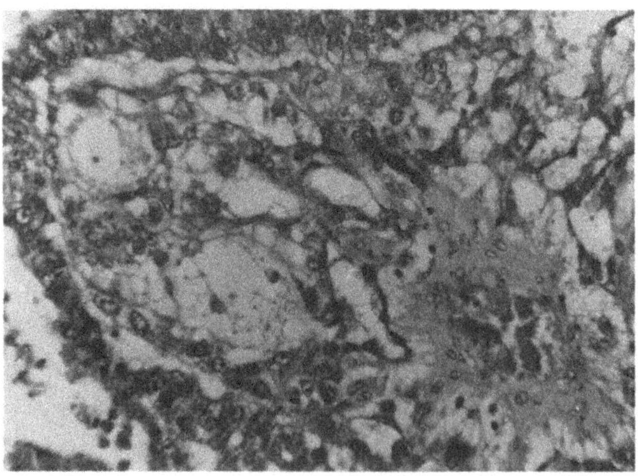

Figure 3B. From another field of the same tumor. YST reacts positively with AFP; ECA is negative. AFIP Neg. 85-5161 AFP X 100.

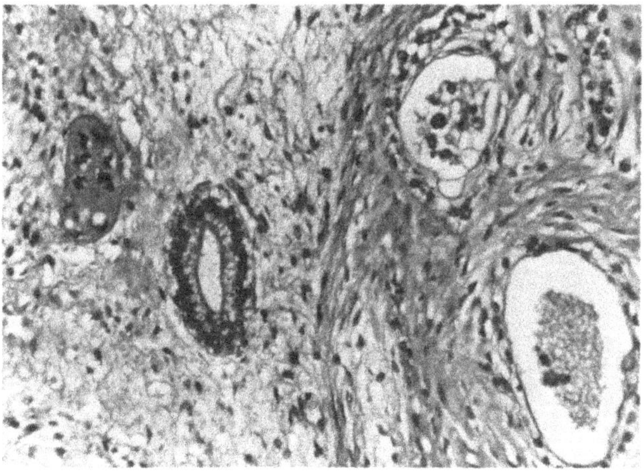

Figure 4A. Mature teratoma. Note the syncytiotrophoblast. AFIP Neg. 85-5162.

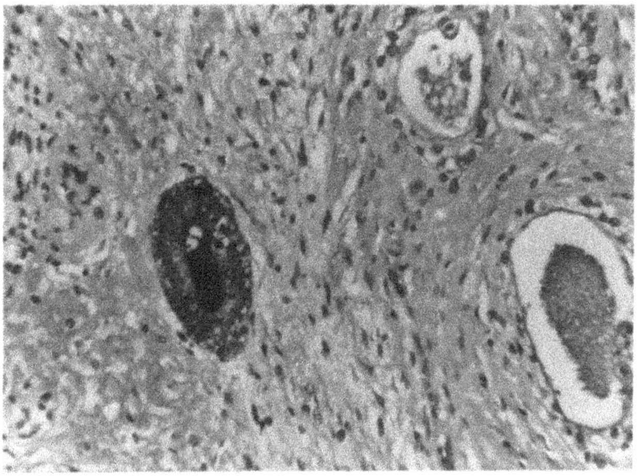

Figure 4B. From another field of the same tumor. The columnar epithelium of mucous glands reacts positively with AFP. AFIP Neg. 85-5163. AFP X 100.

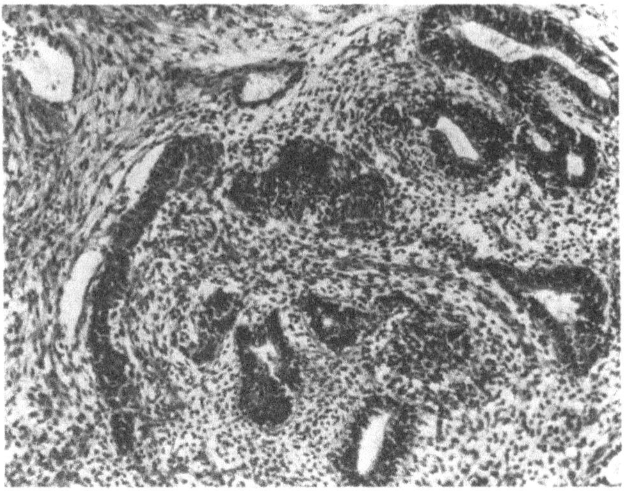

Figure 5A. Immature teratoma. AFIP Neg. 85-5164 H&E X 70.

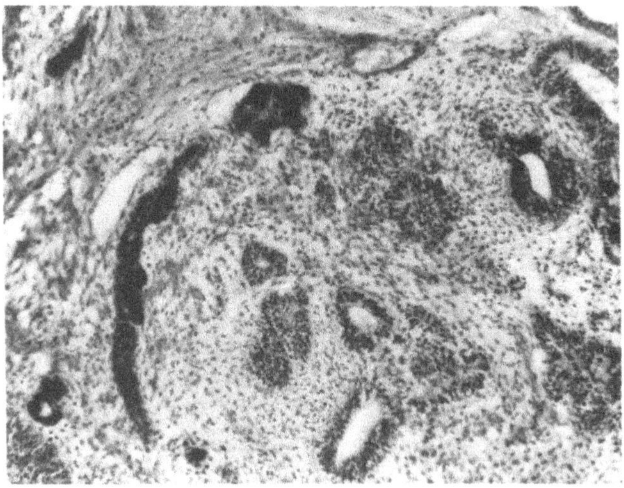

Figure 5B. From another area of the same tumor. The cells of several of the tubular structures react positively with AFP. AFIP Neg. 85-5165. AFP X 70.

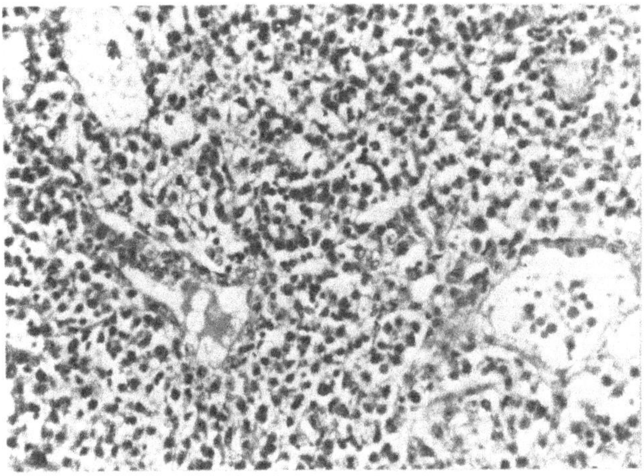

Figure 6A. Seminoma YST from patient with elevated AFP. Intermingled with seminoma cells are several spaces lined by small cuboidal or flattened cells. These are often overlooked or dismissed. AFIP Neg. 85-5166. H&E X 100.

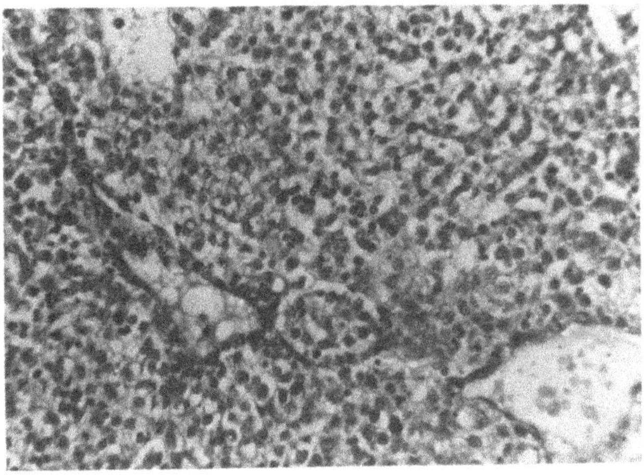

Figure 6B. From another area of the same tumor. The cells lining the spaces react positively with AFP. Note that the seminoma cells are all negative. AFIP Neg. 85-5167. AFP X 100.

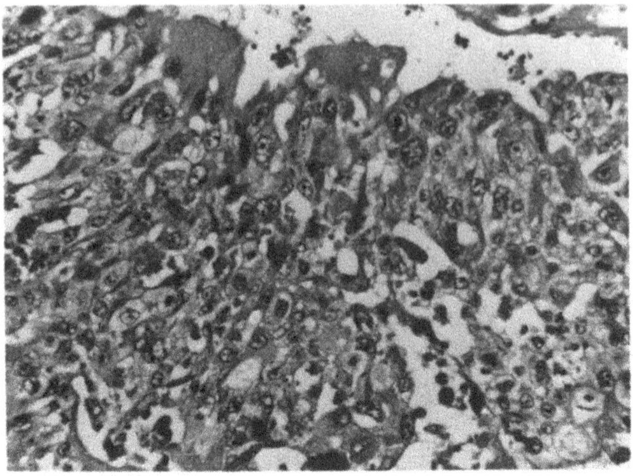

Figure 7A. Testicular choriocarcinoma. AFIP Neg 85-5168 H&E X 100.

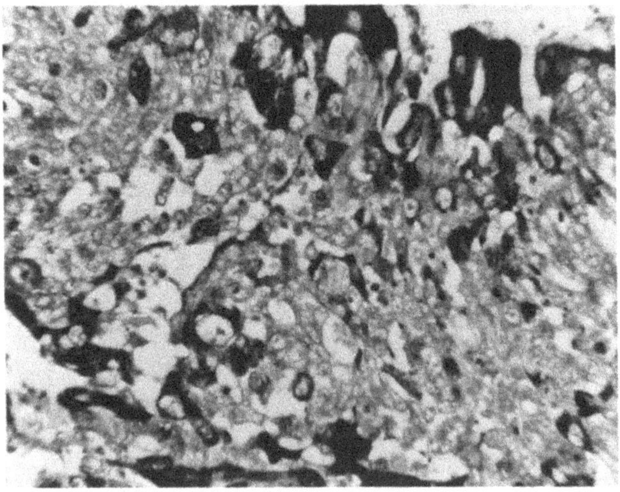

Figure 7B. Syncytiotrophoblasts react positvely with HCG stain. AFIP Neg. 85-5169 HCG X 100.

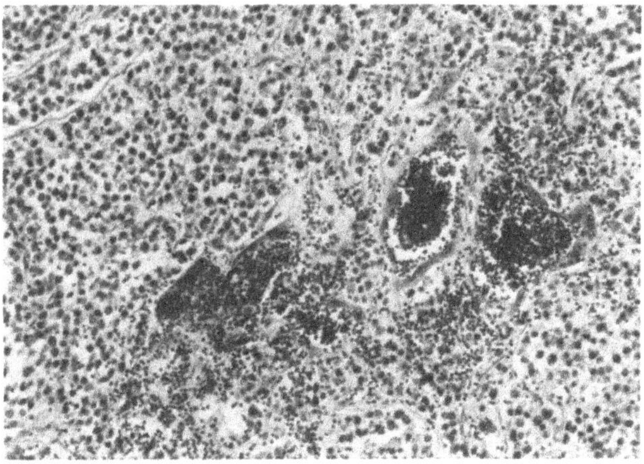

Figure 8A. Seminoma from patient with elevated HCG level showing several hemorrhagic areas. No other elements are identifiable. AFIP Neg. 85-5170 H&E X 70.

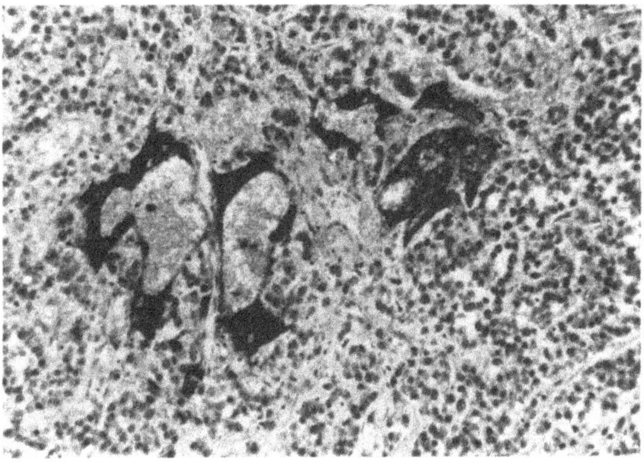

Figure 8B. From another areas of the same tumor. The cells lining the hemorrhagic areas react positively with HCG stain. The existence of these syncytiotrophoblasts could be detected only with HCG stains. Note that none of seminoma cells are positive. AFIP Neg. 85-5171 HCG X 70.

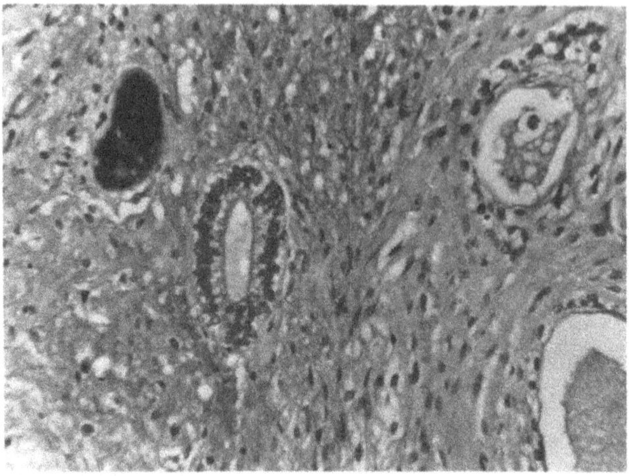

Figure 9. Syncytiotrophoblast in a teratoma. HCG stain of the section shown in Figures 4A and B that demonstrated AFP in teratoma, reveals the presence of HCG production in syncytiotrophoblast. Such observations clarify the presence of both markers in a tumor. AFIP Neg. 85-5155 X70.

Another reason is ignorance of the variable forms that syncytiotrophoblasts may manifest. In testicular tumors these cells manifest the same cytological variations that are seen in the placenta. The cells may be mononuclear or multinucleated with or without vacuolization, or they may be elongated endothelial-like.

Syncytiotrophoblasts may be seen in testicular tumors either as choriocarcinoma or individual cells. They may be intermingled with other tumor cells (embryonal carcinoma or seminoma or yolk sac tumor), they may be in the stroma of the tumor (Fig.9) or in the adjacent seminiferous tubules. Syncytiotrophoblasts were found in 42% of testicular tumors and 93% of these were positive for HCG. Not a single one of our syncytiotrophoblasts gave a positive reaction for AFP.

In 466 seminomas and 356 embryonal carcinoma occurring as pure or mixed with other histologic types, not a single cell was positive for HCG.

HPL is produced by placenta, its level in the serum is increased from the 8th week until termination of pregnancy. Cross reactivity is demonstrable with pituitary growth hormone. Its half life is 20 minutes. HPL is demonstrable in syncytiotrophoblasts producing HCG.

We have seen HPL in a number of embryonal carcinoma cells where it occurs in many of the cells.

SP1 has a molecular weight of 90,000. Its level shows a positive correlation with placental weight and HPL level. It has a half life of 34-60 hours. In testicular tumors SP1 is present only in syncytiotrophoblasts producing HCG.

Immunopathology of testicular tumors has contributed to evaluation of the two classifications. The demonstration of tumor markers can readily be correlated with the WHO categories. Elevated HCG is present in syncytiotrophoblasts either as choriocarcinoma or as individual cells. AFP is usually correlated with YST but embryonal carcinoma and teratoma may contribute to the pool. Elevated levels of AFP and HCG are correlated respectively with YST, and syncytiotrophoblasts, either alone or as choriocarcinoma.

Such correlation is impossible with the Pugh-Cameron (3) classification because it does not recognize syncytiotrophoblasts or yolk sac elements that may be present in a tumor. Thus a seminoma, differentiated teratoma, malignant teratoma undifferentiated, or a combined tumor may be positive or negative for AFP or HCG, depending on whether there were YST elements or syncytiotrophoblasts, respectively, in the tumor. Malignant teratoma trophoblastic will be positive for HCG but the levels may vary from low to very high, and the AFP may be negative or positive, depending on whether YST elements are present in the tumor.

5. SUMMARY

Immunopathology of testicular tumors has primarily been a study of AFP and HCG in tumor tissue. Our studies, based on over 800 germ cell tumors have shown that AFP is present principally in YST; HCG in syncytiotrophoblasts. Pure seminoma is negative for both but may give a positive reaction with PLAP. Embryonal carcinoma is negative for HCG but it is weakly positive for AFP in 19%. HPL may be positive in many ECA cells. AFP is demonstrable in 93% of YST. Pure YST is negative for HCG. Syncytiotrophoblasts occurring along or as choriocarcinoma react with HCG in 93% of cases. Mucous glands of teratoma react positively with AFP in 19% of cases, but pure teratoma is negative for HCG. Tumors of more than one histological type may react with one and/or the other marker, depending on the structure of the tumor.

REFERENCES

1. Mostofi FK and Sobin LH: International Histological Classification of Testis Tumors (16) WHO Geneva, 1977.
2. Collins DH and Pugh RCB: The pathology of testicular tumors. Br J Urol (Suppl. to 36) 1964.
3. Pug RCB and Cameron KM: Teratoma. Ch 6 pp 199-244. In Pathology of Testis (Ed) Pugh, RCB, Oxford, London. Blackwell Scientific Publications, 1976.
4. Rouslahti E. and Hirai H: Purification of the AFP and its physical and chemical properties. Scand J Immunol 8, Suppl 8:3-26, 1978.
5. Rouslahti E and Engvall E: Alphafetoprotein, Scand J Immunol. Supple 6, 1-17, 1978.
6. Teilum G: The concept of endodermal sinus (yolk sac tumor). Scand J Immunol 8, Suppl. 8:75-89, 1978.
7. Talerman A, Haije WG and Baggerman L: Histological patterns of germ cell tumors associated with raised serum alphafetoprotein (AFP). Scand J Immunol 8 Suppl. 8:97-102, 1978.
8. Mostofi FK and Price EB, Jr: Tumors of the Male Genital Syste (Fasc. 8) Atlast of Tumor Pathology, 2nd Series. Armed Forces Institute of Pathology, Washington, D.C., 1973.
9. Talerman A: Endodermal sinus (yolk sac) tumor elements in testicular germ cell tumors in adults. Comparison of prospective and retrospective studies. Cancer 46:1213-1217, 1980.
10. Braunstein GD, Vaitukaitis JL, Carbone PP and Ross GT: Ectopic production of human chorionic gonadotropin in neoplasms. Ann Int Med 78: 39-45, 1973.
11. Goldstein DP, Kosasa TS and Skarim AT: The clinical application of a specific radium-immunoassay for human chorionic gonadotropin in trophoblastic and non trophoblastic tumors. Surg Gynecol Obstet. 138: 747-754, 1974.
12. Rrsen SW, Weintraub BD, Vaitukaitis JL, Sussman HH and Muggia FM: Placental proteins and their subunits as tumor markers. Ann Intern Med 82:71-83, 1975.
13 Arends J: Limitation in the specificity of the assay of human chorionic gonadotropin using B subunit antiserum. Scan J Immunol (Suppl) 8:587-590, 1978.
14. Kurman RJ, Scardino PT, McIntire KR, Waldmann TA and Javadpour N: Cellular localization of alphafetoprotein and human chorionic gonadotropin in germ cell tumors of the testes using indirect immunoperoxidase technique. Cancer 40:2136-2151, 1977.
15. Javadpour N: Tumor markers in urologic cancer. In Principles and Management of Urologic Cancer. (2nd Edition) Williams and Wilkins, Baltimore, 1983.

20

IMMUNOPATHOLOGY OF PROSTATE AND BLADDER TUMORS

I SESTERHENN, M.D., FK MOSTOFI, M.D., CJ DAVIS, JR., M.D.

I. INTRODUCTION

The prostate consists of fibromuscular stroma with tubuloalveolar glands. Three basic cell types comprise the epithelial elements: a) basal cells, b) secretory prostatic acinar cell, c) transitional epithelium (and occasionally squamous epithelium).

The acini are lined by both the basal and secretory cells. Prostatic "ducts" contain all three cell types: basal, secretory, and transitional cells. The prostatic urethra is lined by transitional epithelium and intermingled prostatic secretory cells: the latter may occur either isolated or in groups of cells. Most new growths result in glandular and stromal hyperplasia.

Most carcinomas of the prostate are adenocarcinomas with cellular features of the mature secretory cell referred to as "prostatic carcinoma." Distressing for clinician as well as pathologist is the inability to predict the behavior in an individual patient. This is reflected in the fact that there are no universally accepted treatment modalities and over 30 histologic grading systems (1). Tumors which appear very similar with regard to cellular anaplasia and glandular differentiation, may metastasize and kill in one patient, whereas, in another, will remain localized. Much effort is being undertaken to more accurately assess a given tumor with respect to its metastatic potential and responsiveness to treatment.

2. PROSTATIC ACID PHOSPHATASE (PAP)

2.1 Historical:

Dmochowski and Assenhajm (2) discovered a high acid phosphatase content in

---

The opinions or assertions contained herein are the private views of authors and are not to be construed as official or as reflecting the views of the Department of the Army or the Department of Defense.

some patients. Kutscher and Wolbergs (3) and Kutscher and Worner (4) in 1935 and 1936 were able to identify the prostate of adult males as the source of a high acid phosphatase content with a maximum pH of 5.0. About the same time, Gutmann and his co-workers (5) reported about the significance of increased acid phosphatase activity at the site of bone metastases from prostatic carcinomas. These discoveries led to extensive work on the clinical significance of prostatic acid phosphatase (PAP) (6).

2.2 Biochemistry:

Biochemical characterization of PAP by Choe and his co-workers (7,8) and Lin (9) revealed that PAP is an enzyme with a molecular weight of 100,000 and several isomers. It is of interest to note that patients with highly elevated serum levels of PAP have predominately iso-enzymes with different pI values than those with low levels.

In contrast to other phosphatases, which are lysosomal in nature, PAP is a secretory enzyme, and is antigenically different from lysosomal acid phosphatases of other organs (7,8) as shown by the use of purified PAP and monoclonal antibodies. According to Choe and his co-workers, there is no cross-reactivity between the iso-enzymes of PAP and acid phosphatases of other organs, as determined by immunochemistry and immunohistochemistry (10). This is in contrast to the findings of Yam (11) and his associates and Li and his co-workers (12), who reported a weekly positive reaction with the unlabeled peroxidase-antiperoxidase method by Sternberger (13) in some granulocytes, islet cells of pancreas, parietal cells of stomach, liver cells, occasional tubular epithelial cells of the kidney and carcinoma of breast. The antigenic binding site differs from the enzymatically active site (9,14). Also, the chromosomal coding for PAP and lysosomal acid phosphatase appears to be at different gene loci (15).

2.3 Clinical:

A number of reliable assays have been developed to determine PAP activity in patients with prostatic carcinoma (16,17,18,19). Initially high levels of PAP herald a poor prognosis (20,21). PAP determinations in bone marrow aspirates are still controversial; it appears that detectable levels indicate the presence of microscopic metastatic disease (22,23).

3. PROSTATE SPECIFIC ANTIGEN (PSA)

3.1 Biochemical:

Wang and his associates (24,25), attempting to find new antigenic markers for prostatic acinar carcinoma, identified an antigen different from prostatic acid phosphatase. It can be isolated from prostatic tissue and seminal vesicle fluid. It is a glycoprotein with a molecualr weight of 33 - 34.000 Daltons. It does not have subunits. Although there are several isomers, the antigen identified has a pI of 6.9. Treatment with neuraminidase results in shifts of the pI indicating the presence of sialic acid. PSA has proteolytic activity capable of cleaving casein (Wang).

3.2 Clinical:

Serum levels of PSA are elevated in benign prostatic hyperplasia and prostatic carcinoma. The serum levels are independent from those of PAP. Recently, Guinan and co-workers (26) evaluated serum levels of PAP and PSA on 23 untreated patients with prostatic carcinoma and 23 control patients, and found PSA to be more sensitive than PAP.

4. IMMUNOHISTOCHEMISTRY

The advent of specific antibodies against PAP and PSA has led to histochemical demonstration of both enzymes in formalin-fixed and paraffin embedded material. Jöbsis (21) reported that 29 of 30 primary prostatic carcinomas and all 20 metastatic prostatic carcinomas showed a positive reaction for PAP. None of 55 tumors of non-prostatic origin were positive. Choe and co-workers were unable to detect positive staining in non-prostatic carcinoma, except for one case of a malignant islet cell tumor of the pancreas (10). Lam (28), Yam (11), and Li (12) reported some degree of cross reactivity expressed by a weakly positive reaction in other organs. The specificity of PSA for prostatic acinar calls has been shown by Nadji (29) and Wang (25). Papsidero (30) and his associates were unable to identify cross-reactivity with other organs.

Our experience is based on 1200 cases examined for PAP by the unlabeled peroxidase-antiperoxidase method (13) and 550 cases for PSA. We utilized an antibody against PAP developed by Mahan and Doctor (18) at the Walter Reed Army Institute of Research, and from Eureka Laboratories (California). We were fortunate enough to receive antibodies against PSA from Doctors Wang and Chu.

Recently, we have also utilized anti-PSA available from Dako Laboratories. Our results are similar to those in the literature.

4.1 Definition of positive reaction:

We interpret a reaction as positive if the cytoplasm shows a distinct granular color. All cases in which the cytoplasm has an indistinct hue and in which the staining intensity is similar to that of stromal cells are regarded as negative. Normal prostates show a strongly positive reaction for both PAP and PSA in secretory cells lining prostatic acini, prostatic ducts, and the prostatic urethra. The reaction is uniformly strong in all cells. Chromaffin cells not infrequently encountered in normal prostates are also positive for PAP and PSA. Basal cells of prostatic acini do not contain PAP or PSA, which substantiates the fact that PAP and PSA are markers for cell maturity. Transitional epithelium of prostatic ducts and prostatic urethra do not react with either one. Seminal vesicles and ejaculatory ducts are also negative.

4.2 Benign lesions:

In hyperplasia, the reaction is identical to that of the normal prostate (Figs. 1,2,3).

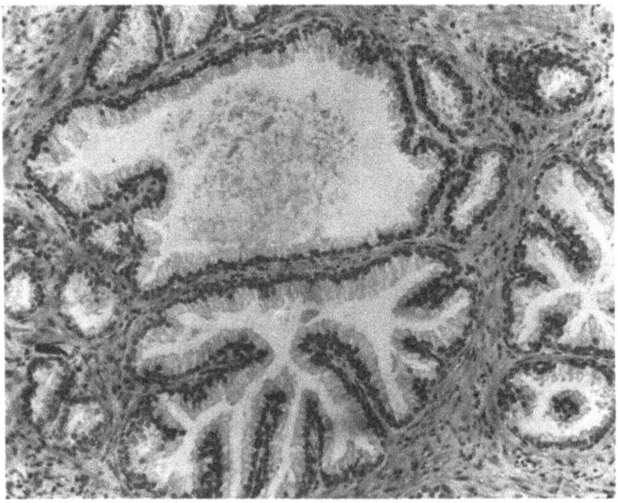

Figure 1. Hyperplasia H&E X 70 AFIP Neg. 85-5141.

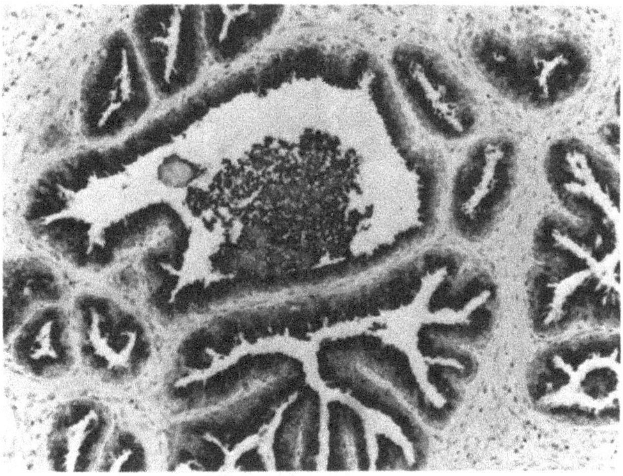

Figure 2. Same field PAP X 70. AFIP Neg. 85-5143.

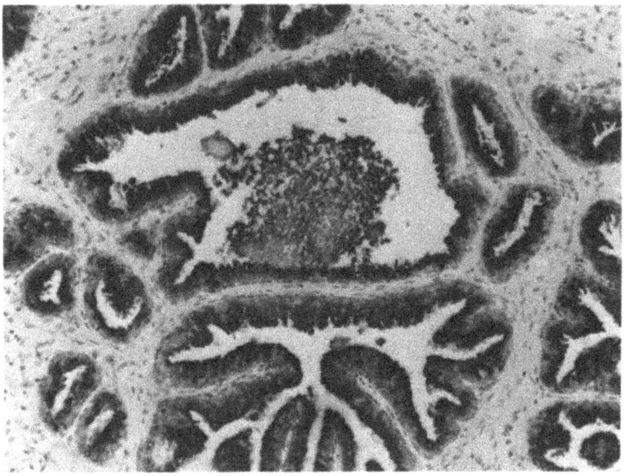

Figure 3. Same field PSA X 70 AFIP Neg. 85-5142.

In basal cell hyperplasia, only cells with secretory differentiation are positive for PAP and PSA. In atrophic acini, the reaction is variable depending on the degree of cellular atrophy.

4.3 Malignant tumors:

In our laboratory, prostatic carcinomas are graded according to the WHO nonenclature of prostatic tumors, which includes both the structural differentiation and degree of nuclear anaplasia (31). In contrast to normal and benigh lesions, in carcinoma, the positive reaction for PAP and PSA is variable.

Since PSA appears to be specific for prostatic acinar cells, it was suggested to utilize only PSA as marker for prostatic carcinoma. All tumors evaluated with anti-PSA were also studied with anti-PAP in consecutive sections; very soon, it became apparent that prostatic carcinomas which appeared to consist of a homogeneous cell population on H&E stained sections were markedly heterogeneous with respect to their functional differentiation. Some cells are positive for both PAP and PSA; others may be positive for one or the other, and some negative for both.

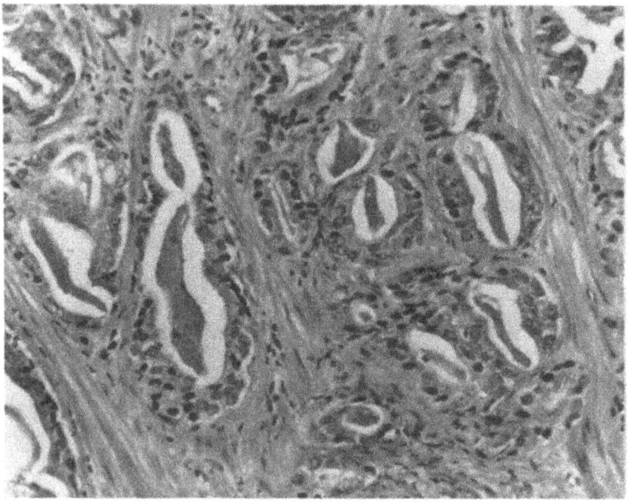

Figure 4. Well differentiated carcinoma H&E X 100 AFIP 85-5145.

In general, in well differentiated, simple gland-forming carcinomas, PAP and PSA are demonstrable in most cells, although the intensity of staining varies (Figs. 4,5,6). Moderately differentiated carcinomas (cribriform and fused-gland pattern) frequently reveal a strongly positive reaction in the apical cytoplasm of cells forming glandular structures in addition to cytoplasmic staining in many of the other tumor cells. Poorly differentiated carcinomas show the greatest degree of cell heterogeneity. Whereas some

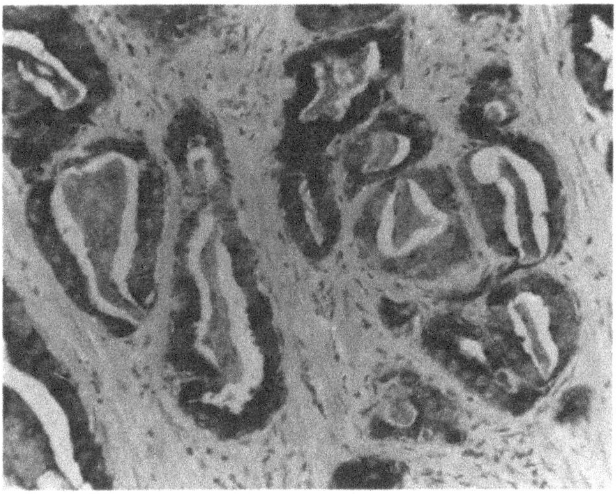

Figure 5. Same tumor PAP X 100 AFIP 85-5144

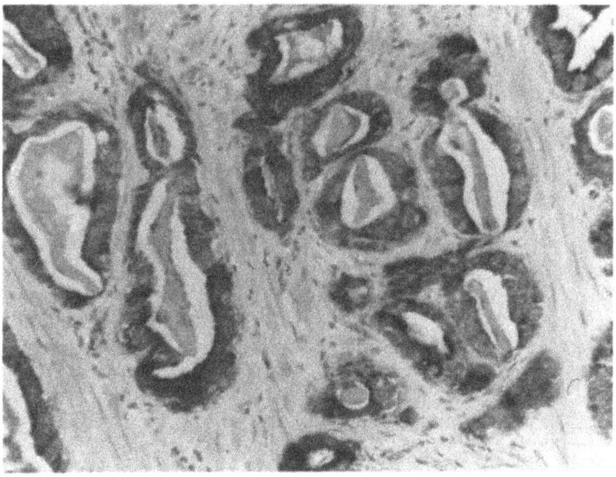

Figure 6. Same tumor PSA X 100 AFIP 85-5148.

tumors are strongly positive in most of the cells. Others show clones of cells, positive and negative for PAP and/or PSA (Figs. 7,8,9). A rare tumor is negative for both.

4.4 Nuclear Grade:

The degree of nuclear anaplasia correlates roughly with degree of glandular differentiation and enzyme production. Tumors consisting prodominantly of cells with a high degree of nuclear anaplasia contain fewer

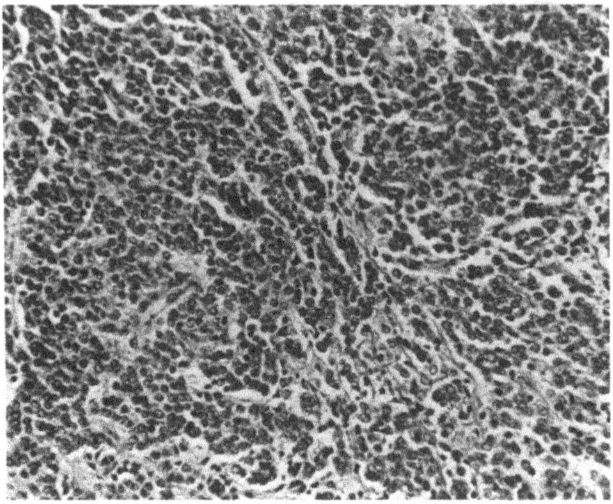

Figure 7. Undifferentiated carcinoma, H&E X 100 AFIP 85-5151.

cells positive for PAP and/or PSA than those with mild nuclear anaplasia. However, individual cells with marked nuclear anaplasia are not infrequently positive for PAP and/or PSA.

4.5 Special Types

Papillary carcinomas of prostatic acinar origin ("endometrioid" carcinomas) have a characteristic pattern of positive reaction for PAP and PSA at the apical portion of the cell, and in many cases also at the basal portion of the cell (Figs. 10,11,12). Papillary carcinomas frequently are associated with a simple gland and gland-in-gland pattern, and in the latter, intense diffuse cytoplasmic staining is also present.

Mucinous prostatic acinar carcinomas are positive for PAP and PSA in most tumor cells.

Cystadenocarcinomas are strongly positive in most cells.

Prostatic carcinomas with large numbers of chromaffin cells resembling carcinoids are positive for PAP and PSA, although the number of positive cells varies greatly.

Transitional cell carcinomas involving the prostate are negative for PAP and PSA.

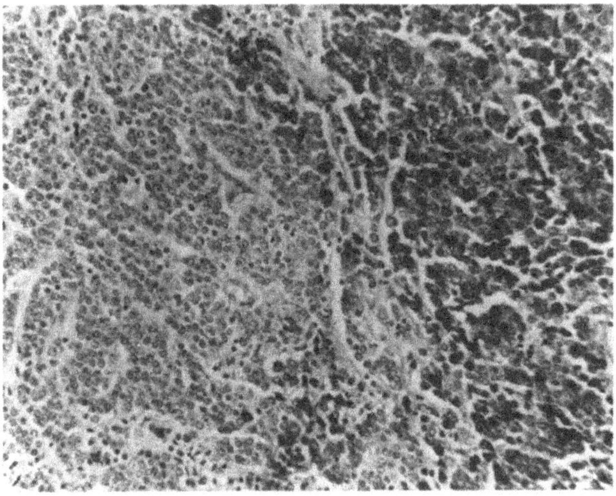

Figure 8. Same tumor PAP X 100 AFIP 85-5149

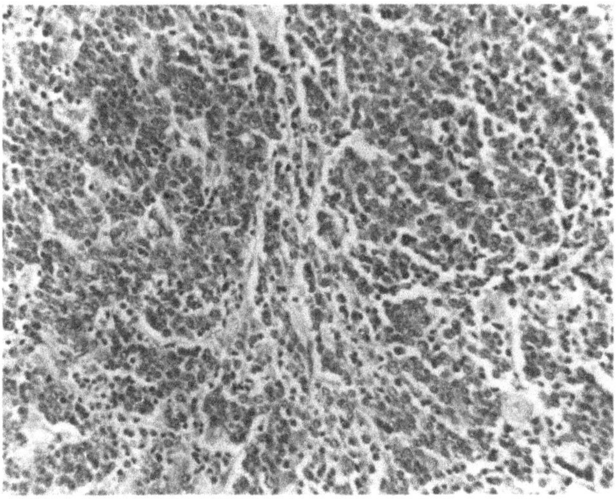

Figure 9. Same tumor PSA X 100 AFIP 85-5147.

As indicated before, prostatic ducts are lined by three cell types: secretory cell, transitional epithelium, and basal cell. Thus, the term "ductal carcinoma," without specifying the cell type, is of no clinical value, since treatment modalities vary.

Basal cell carcinoma of the prostate is negative for both PAP and PSA.

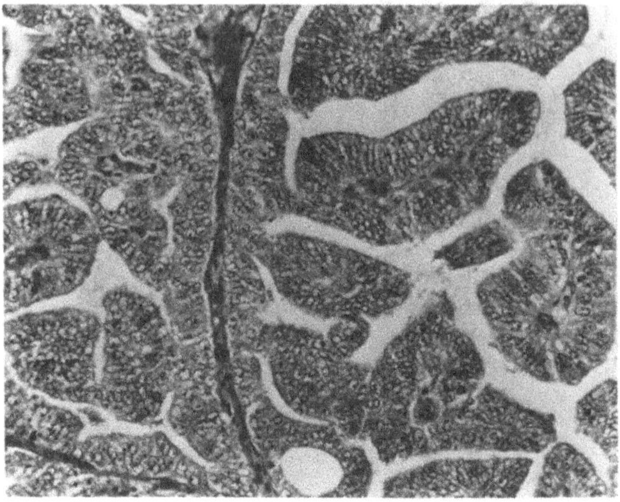

Figure 10. Carcinoma, papillary type, H&E X 100 AFIP 85-5152.

Pure squamous cell carcinoma is negative for PAP and PSA. However, prostatic acinar carcinomas may show variable degree of squamous differentiation, often after previous longterm estrogen treatment and occasionally spontaneously. In these instances, some cells with squamous features can be positive for PAP or PSA. We have encountered rare pleomorphic carcinomas of the prostate simulating sarcoma. The presence of PAP and/or PSA in a few of the pleomorphic cells supports the origin from secretory cells of the prostate. In these tumors, extensive sampling and use of PAP method on many blocks is often necessary.

4.6 Treatment Effect

In our experience, PAP and PSA are demonstrable in benign and carcinoma cells revealing radiation and estrogen effect. The use of immunohistochemistry in irradiated prostatic carcinomas is particularly helpful in identifying tumor cells. It is as yet undetermined if the presence of PAP or PSA in cells showing treatment effect denotes viability. The presence of a positive reaction for HCG in necrotic syncytiotrophoblasts in testicular germ cell tumors seems to indicate cell death before the hormone is released. The same may be true for prostatic carcinomas.

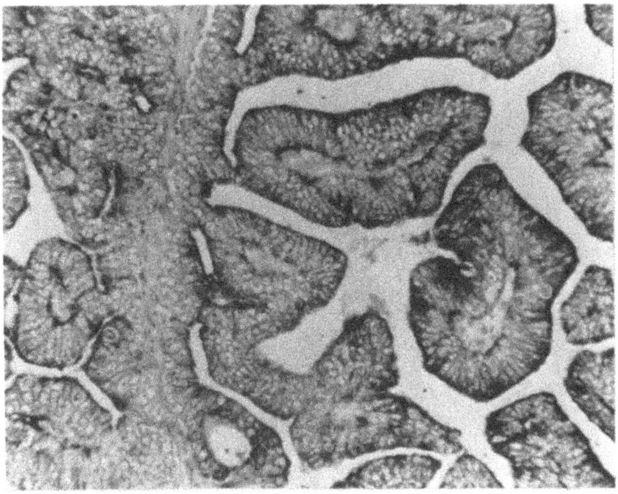

Figure 11. Same field PAP X 100 AFIP 85-5137.

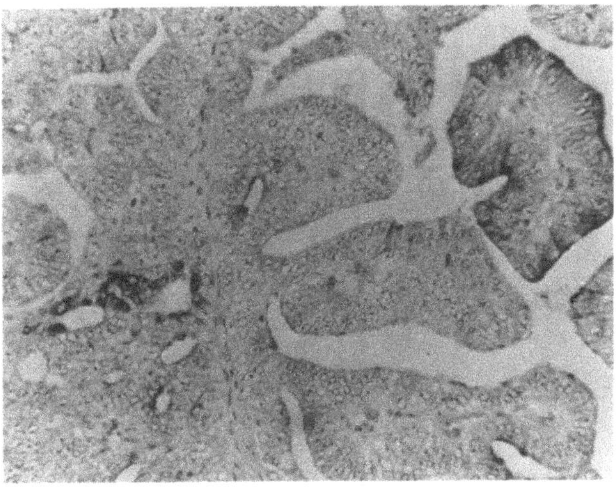

Figure 12. Same field PSA x 100 AFIP 85-5138.

4.7 Metastases

Most metastases of prostatic acinar carcinomas show a positive reaction for PAP and PSA.

If the primary tumor shows a markedly heterogeneous cell population with respect to PAP and PSA secretion, different metastatic sites can express one or several subpopulations of cells; that is, metastases in the lung may contain

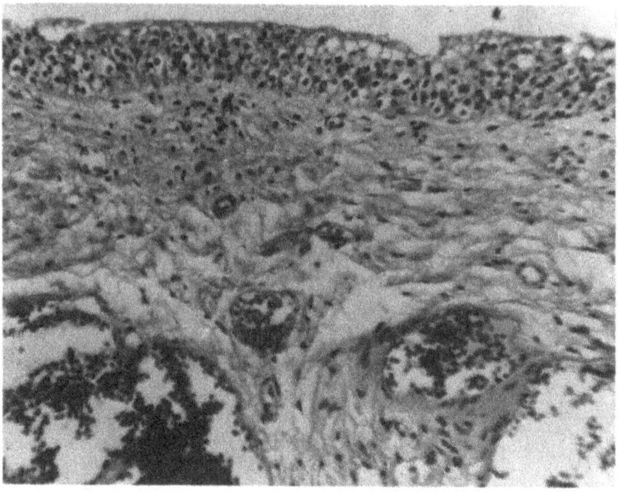

Figure 13. Normal bladder H&E X 100 AFIP 85-5140.

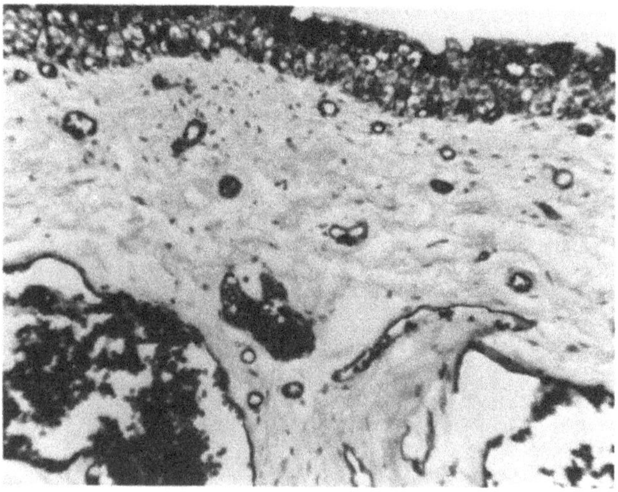

Figure 14. Same field Anti BG-A X 100 AFIP 85-5139.

cells positive for both PAP and PSA in contrast to lymph node or liver metastases, which may be positive for only one of the enzymes or even completely negative for both. Therefore, if a metastasis from prostatic acinar carcinoma is suspected, and the H&E stained sections are strongly suggestive of prostatic carcinoma, but both enzymes are not demonstrable, it is often helpful to examine the primary for a subset of cells explaining the negative metastases for both PAP and PSA. These findings are reminiscent of morphometric studies done by Lundberg (32) in autopsies of prostatic cancer patients. He found variations in morphometric values between different metastatic sites.

4.8 Differential Diagnosis

The two PAP antibodies (WRAIR and Eureka) show a positive reaction in carcinoids of the rectum. The reaction, using DAB as chromogen, is weaker than in prostatic acinar cells; more yellowish-brown and indistinct. Carcinoids from other sites are negative, with few exceptions, in which rare individual cells show a weakly positive reaction. PSA is negative in all carcinoids.

We did not encounter difficulties with unwanted staining in leukocytes, renal tubular epithelium, and pancreatic islet cells.

5. OTHER ANTIGENS AND LECTINS

Basal cells give a positive reaction for keratin, whereas secretory cells are negative, using a polyclonal antibody without predigestion. In our experience, atrophic acini also show a strongly positive reaction.

Recently, Brawer (33) and co-workers applied different monoclonal antibodies against keratin to prostatic acinar carcinomas, and were unable to demonstrate a positive reaction. Mammary epithelial membrane antigen (34) is demonstrable in basal cells and some transitional cells of the normal prostate. It is also present, especially in poorly differentiated prostatic acinar carcinomas.

Blood group iso-antigens can be demonstrated in secretory cells of the prostate as well as transitional epithelium. The distribution in secretory cells is irregular in normal prostates indicating a "heterogeneous" cell population in normal prostate.

The same applies to the distribution of peanut lectins. Peanut lectin receptors are demonstrable in most cells of the infant prostate (35). With maturation, the lectin receptors diminish greatly in number, and are predominately located in basal cells and some secretory cells. We can confirm these findings. This does not correlate with the presence or intensity of staining for PAP, PSA, or blood group iso-antigens. The staining is usually cytoplasmic.

Prostatic acinar carcinomas also reveal markedly heterogeneous staining for peanut lectin. The reaction can be seen at the cell surface, in a paranuclear "dot" or within the cytoplasm.

Studying three parameters: PAP, PSA, and peanut lectin contents, numerous subsets of cell types can be identified. An attempt to correlate the presence of peanut receptors to metastatic potential or metastatic site has been unsuccessful.

In our experience, CEA is rarely demonstrable in prostatic acinar carcinoma.

6. HORMONES

ACTH was demonstrated in undifferentiated prostatic carcinomas resembling "oat" cell carcinomas of the lung (Mendelsohn) (36). We have seen chorionic gonadotropin in a prostatic acinar carcinoma with marked nuclear anaplasia. HCG was demonstrable in the same cells which were positive for PAP.

7. HORMONES RECEPTORS

The prostate is a target organ for androgens. Carcinomas of the prostate respond to hormonal manipulations. Therefore, determinations of androgen receptors are of clinical significance. At the present, androgen receptors are being determined in cytosoles of fresh tissue (39, 40). Recently, the presence of estrogen and progesterone receptors, albeit in small numbers, have been identified in cytosoles of fresh tissue (37, 38). Estrogen receptors can be demonstrated by use of fluorescent ligands (41). Prolactin receptors have been found in normal prostate and carcinomas. Their value for treatment modalities and prognosis is currently being explored (42,43,44).

8. IMMUNOPATHOLOGY OF URINARY BLADDER

As far as immunopathology of urinary bladder is concerned, the work involves mainly two areas: distinction between cancerous and non-cancerous lesions, and detection of malignant potential of the tumor. Doctor Cardon-Cardo has discussed the former. I would like to limit my comments mostly to the latter - detection of malignant potential of tumors.

A large majority of tumors of bladder is epithelial, and most are transitional. About 80% are noninvasive, and 20% are invasive; however, most noninvasive tumors tend to show multiple recurrences, and some of these eventually become invasive. The behavior of these noninvasive tumors and of flat mucosal changes referred to as carcinoma-in-situ or dysplasia has been a problem. We are constantly asked about the invasive potential of these lesions. Bladder tumors kill primarily by their invasion and metastases.

To date, pathologists have utilized two methods of prognosticating the behavior of bladder tumors; grading and staging. We recognize three grades of malignancy - Grade I having good prognosis, Grade III having poor prognosis. Staging has also been used for prognostication. We recognize papillary tumors that have not broken through the basement membrane, those which are confined to lamina propria, those that have invaded superficial muscle, those with deep muscle invasion, those that have invaded adjacent organs and structures, and those that are fixed (45).

Both systems are valuable, but the are of limited value. While there is an 80% correlation between grade and depth of infiltration in the bladder wall it is not unusual to see a low-grade tumor invade and metastasize, and a high-grade tumor remain confined to the bladder.

In recent years, several methods have been introduced for detection of malignant potential: (a) blood group iso-antigens, (b) monoclonal antibodies, (c) tumor ploidy, either by flow cytometry or cytophotometry, (d) chromosomal analysis and (e) morphometry.

a) Blood group antigens are glycolipids or proteins, not only expressed in erythrocytes, but also in cell membranes of a wide variety of tissues (46). It has long been known that alterations in cell membranes occur during malignant transformation of the cell (47). Blood group iso-antigens A, B, and O have been extensively studied since Davidsohn's (48) classical work on gastrointestinal carcinoma.

The chemical properties of blood group iso-antigens A,B, and O (H-structure) have been described by Hakomiri (459). The H structure is the precursor for type A and B. The addition of N-acetylgalactoseamine by a specific glycosyltransferase results in BG-A and galactose in BG-B (50). Since glycolysation is incomplete, most persons with BG-A and/or B also express some H-antigen. The expression of ABH antigens on epithelial cells depends on the secretor status of an individual. The ABH antigens occur in tissues in two forms: the alcohol soluble form found in red blood cells, vascular endothelium, and epithelial cells, and the water soluble form in epithelial mucin (51).

In nonsecretors and tumors, the alcohol soluble forms of ABO antigens are more sensitive to lipid solvents used during the fixation and embedding process (52). Most studies of ABO antigens have been done by means of the specific red blood cell adherence test (SRCA) (53). Immunoperoxidase techniques appear to be more sensitive (54). We have utilized polyclonal, and, more recently, monoclonal antibodies against BG-A and B, developed by Lemieux and Baker in Edmonton, Canada. We use ulex-europaeus lectin to demonstrate BG-O. Endothelial cells and red blood cells are built-in controls (Figs. 13,14). If there are no transitional cells showing a positive reaction, we always alert the clinician that the "loss" of BG antigens may be false, due to fixation and embedding artifacts. A number of authors have correlated the deletion of BG iso-antigens with the clinical behavior, the largest series by Davidsohn (55) and his co-authors, and Limas and Lange (56). Most have shown similar results.

The prognostic value appears to be best for low-stage carcinomas. About 95% of BG antigen-positive tumors fail to infiltrate muscle within five years, in contrast to 66% of patients with BG antigen negative tumors, which will infiltrate muscle during the same time interval. The degree of cellular anaplasia does not necessarily correlate with the deletion of BG iso-antigens. Most carcinoma-in-situ cases are A,B,O negative (57). Sadoughy and his co-authors (58), and Srinivas and his co-workers (59) used the SRCA test to evaluate bladder washings with success. In our experience, most tumors show a heterogeneous cell population consisting of BG antigen-positive and negative cells. We record the estimated per cent of each group, rather than to designate a tumor as BG-antigen positive if at least 30-35% of tumor cells are positive.

The T-antigen (Thomsen-Friedenreich) is a precursor of the MN blood group system. In normal tissues, including transitional epithelium, the antigen is masked by sialic acid residues, and can be demonstrated only after predigestion with neuraminidase. The masked T-antigen is referred to as "cryptic" T-antigen, and the unmasked form as "T-antigen." The T-antigen can be demonstrated by use of peanut-lectin (Arachis hypogaea) (60,61). Aberrations from the normal, either emergence of the T-antigen or loss of cryptic T-antigen in low-stage and low-grade tumors correlate with aggressive behavior. Coon and his co-workers found that 39% of 23 Grade I and II carcinomas, which were either T AG positive or cryptic T-antigen positive carcinomas. They also found that evaluation of both ABO substance and T-antigen had an additive effect in prognosticating aggressive behavior (62). As with the ABO system, most tumors show a heterogeneous cell population with regard to the T-antigen (Figs. 15,16,17). An excellent review of modifications of various blood group antigens in cancer is the recent article by Hakomori (63).

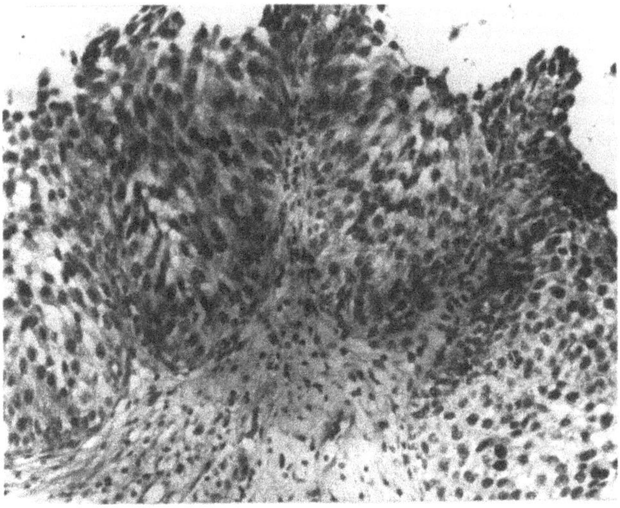

Figure 15. Transitional cell carcinoma in-situ H&E X 100 AFIP 85-5135.

b) The usefulness of monoclonal antibodies derived from transitional epithelium and transitional cell carcinomas has been discussed in detail by Dr. Cordon-Cardo in one of the chapters of this book.

c) Determination of DNA and RNA content by flow-through cytometry is of great prognostic importance. Over 90% of the patients with carcinoma and carcinoma-in-situ of the bladder have aneuploid cell population, and about 50% of Grade I papillary carcinomas and papillomas (64,65). Cytophotometry yields similar results, and is applicable to paraffin sections (66).

d) Chromosomal analysis has revealed the presence of marker chromosomes. Their presence is associated with poorer prognosis (67,68).

CEA can be demonstrated in the developing bladder from the 10th week of gestation, and disappears after the 22nd week, according to Hofstadter and his co-workers (69). Wahren and her co-workers (70) demonstrated CEA in

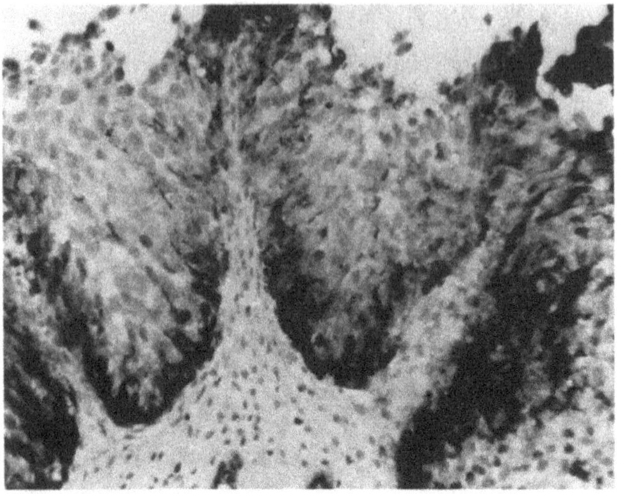

Figure 16. Deeper section Anti BG-A X 100 AFIP 85-5136.

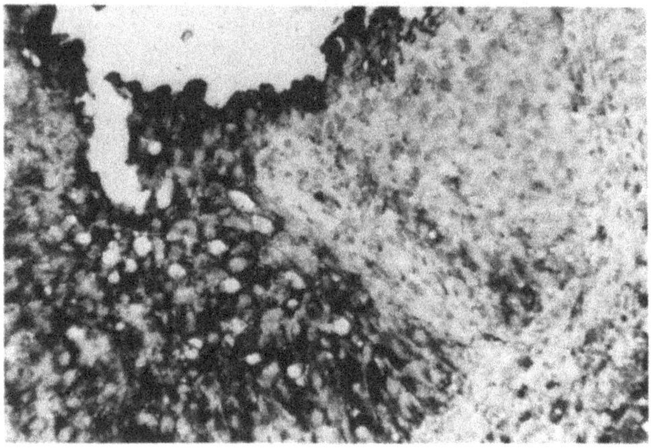

Figure 17. Deeper section Peanut and lectin after predigestion. Cryptic T antigen X100 AFIP 85-5134.

transitional cell carcinomas of the bladder. It was more prevalent in better differentiated tumors than in poorly differentiated carcinomas. Zimmerman and his co-authors (71) reported a correlation between rising CEA levels and tumor recurrence.

Urachal adenocarcinomas are associated with elevated serum levels of CEA (72). Those we have studied show a positive reaction for CEA in tissue sections (Figs. 18,19). In our experience, CEA is frequently present in bladder carcinomas with glandular differentiation, and in cells, whether normal or neoplastic, which show mucin production. Keratin can be demonstrated in transitional epithelium, though inconsistently, unless the sections have been predigested with trypsin (Figs. 20,21). Epithelial membrane antigen (34) is not infrequently demonstrable in transitional cell carcinomas (Figs. 22,23),

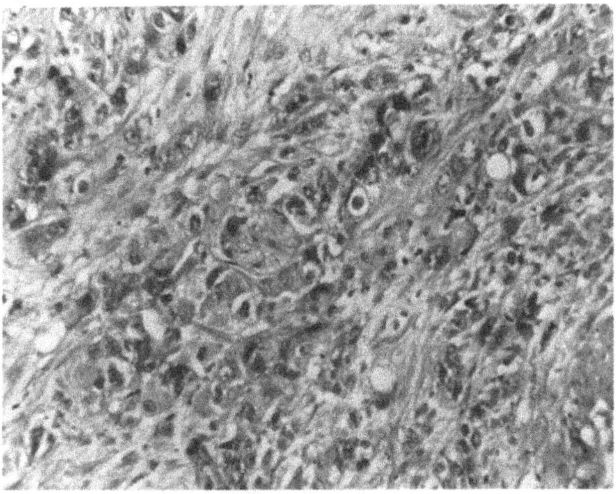

Figure 18. Urachal carcinoma H&E X100 AFIP 85-5132.

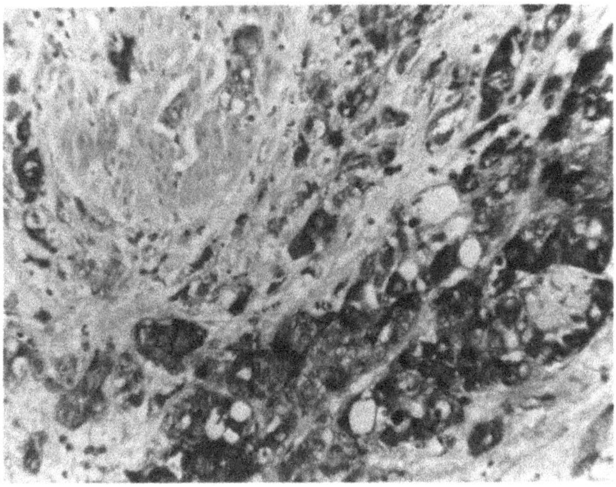

Figure 19. Same tumor CEA X 100 AFIP 85-5133.

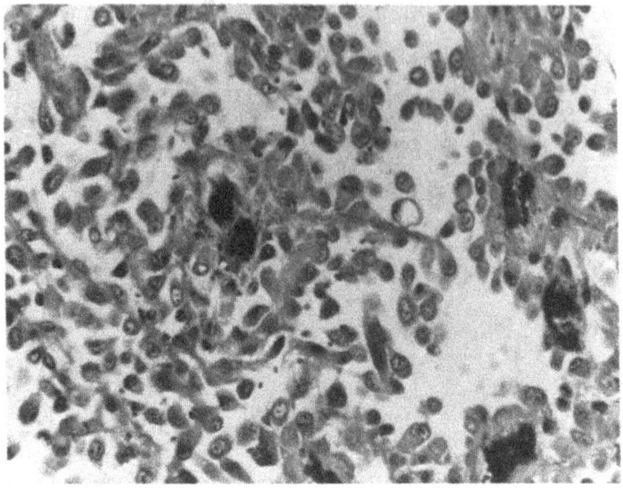

Figure 20. Poorly differentiated squamous cell carcinoma. H&E X 100 AFIP.

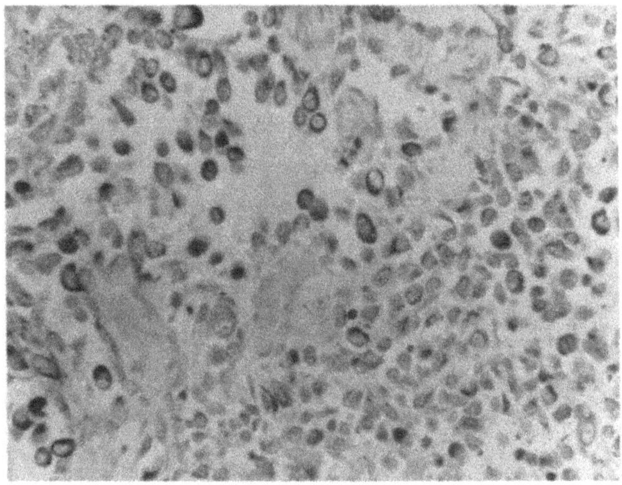

Figure 21. Same tumor Anti-keratin X 100 AFIP 85-5131.

and in normal epithelium. Ectopic hormone production, such as HCG (73) or HPL or SP1 can he found in pleomorphic carcinomas. In undifferentiated small cell carcinomas, ACTH or other hormones can be demonstrated. Soft tissue tumors of the bladder show the same immunohistochemical reactions as soft tissue tumors elsewhere.

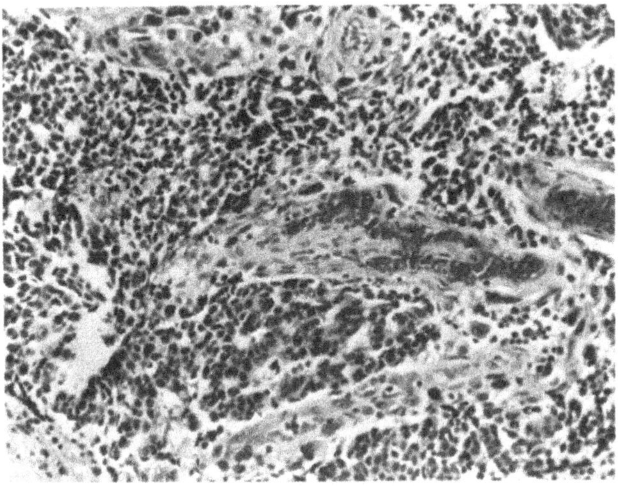

Figure 22. Undifferentiated carcinoma, H&E X 100 AFIP 85-5154.

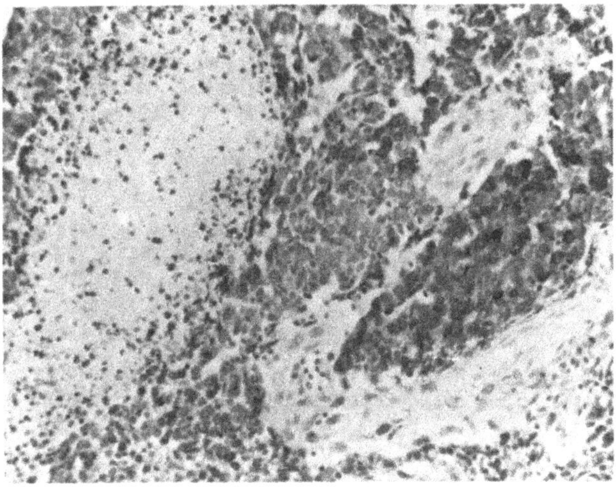

Figure 23. Same tumor Anti-EMA X 100 AFIP 85-5153.

REFERENCES

1. Mostofi FK: Problems of grading carcinoma of prostate. Seminars in Oncology (3) No. 2:161-169, 1976.
2. Dmochowski A, Assenhamj D: Uber Harn und Blutphosphatase, Naturwissenschaften 23:501, 1935.
3. Kutscher W, Wolbergs H: Prostataphosphatase. Z. Physiol Chem 236:237-240, 1935.

4. Kutscher W, Worner A: Prostataphosphatase. Z. Physiol Chem 239: 109-126, 1936.
5. Gutman EB, Sproul EE, Gutman AB: Significance of increased phosphatase activity of bone at the site of osteoplastic metastases secondary to carcinoma of the prostate gland. Am J Cancer 28:485-495, 1936.
6. Sullivan TJ, Gutman EB, Gutman AB: Theory and application of the serum "acid" phosphatase determination in metastasizing prostatic carcinoma: early effects of castration. J Urol 48:426-458, 1942.
7. Choe BK, Pontes JE, McDonald J, Rose Nr: Purification and characterization of human prostatic acid phosphatase. Preparative Biochemistry 8:73-89, 1978.
8. Choe BK, Pontes JE, Lillehej HS, Rose NR: Immunological approaches to human prostatic epithelial cells. The Prostate 1:383-398, 1980.
9. Lin MF, Lee CL, Wojcieszyn FW, Wang MC, Valenzuela LA, Murphy GP, Chu TM: Fundamental biochemical and immunological aspects of prostatic acid phosphatase. The Prostate 1:415-425, 1980.
10. Choe BK, Pontes EJ, Rose NR, Henderson MD: Expression of human prostatic acid phosphatase in a pancreatic islet cell carcinoma. Invest Urol 15:312-318, 1978.
11. Yam LT, Janckila AJ, Lam WKW, Li CY: Immunohistochemistry of prostatic acid phosphatase. The Prostate 2:97-107, 1981.
12. Li CY, Lam WKW, Yam LT: Immunohistochemical diagnosis of prostatic cancer with metastasis. Cancer 46:706-712, 1980.
13. Sterberger LA, Hardy PH, Cuculis JJ, Meyer HG: The unlabeled antibody enzyme method of immunohistochemistry. Preparation and properties of soluble antigen-antibody complex (horseradish peroxidase-antihorseradish peroxidase) and its use in identification of spirochetes. J Histochem Cytochem 18:315-333, 1970.
14. Lee CL, Wang MC, Killian CS, Slack NH, Murphy GP, Chu TM: Solid-phase immunofluorescent and immunoadsorbent assays of serum prostatic acid phosphatase. The Prostate 1:427-439, 1980.
15. Ferguson-Smith MA, Newman FB, Ellis PM, Thomson DMG, Riley ID: Assignment by deletion of human red cell acid phosphatase gene locus to the short arm of chromosome 2. Nature (New Biol) 24:271-274, 1973.
16. Shulman S, Mamrod L, Gonder MS, Soanes WA: The detection of prostatic acid phosphatase by antibody reactions in gel diffusion. J Immunol 93:473-480, 1964.
17. Foti AG, Cooper JF, Herschman H, Malvaez R: Detection of prostatic cancer by radioimmunoassay of prostatic acid phosphatase. N Engl J Med 297: 1351-1361, 1977.
18. Mahan DE, Doctor BP: A radioimmune assay for human prostatic acid phosphatase levels in prostatic disease. Clin Biochem 12:10-17, 1979.
19. Romas NA, Hsu KC, Tomashefsky P, Tannenbaum M: Counterimmunoelectrophoresis for detection of human prostatic acid phosphatase. Urology 12:79-83, 1978.
20. Ganem EJ: The prognostic significance of an elevated serum acid phosphatase level in advanced prostatic carcinoma. J Urol 76: 179-181, 1956.
21. Johnson DE, Scott WW, Gibbons RP: Clinical significance of serum acid phosphatase levels in advanced prostatic carcinoma. Urology 8:123-126, 1976.
22. Bruce AD, Mahan DE, Bellville WD: Radioimmunoassay of bone marrow prostatic acid phosphatase. The Prostate 1:457-463, 1980.

23. Pontes JE: Clinical significance of serum and bone marrow acid phosphatase. The Prostate 1:465-470, 1980.
24. Wang MC, Valenzuela LA, Murphy GP, Chu TM: Purification of a human prostatic specific antigen. Invest Urol 17:159-163, 1979.
25. Wang MC, Papsidero LD, Kuriyama M, Valenzuela LA, Murphy GP, Chu TM: Prostate antigen: An new potential marker for prostatic cancer. The Prostate 2:89-96, 1981.
26. Guinan P, Rubenstein M, Rashid B, Abramowitz J, Shaw M, Ojeda L: An assessment of prostatic specific antigen in prostate cancer patients. J Urol 131 (Abstr 87), 1984.
27. Jobsis AC, DeVries GP, Anholt RR, Sanders GTB: Demonstration of the prostatic origin of metastases. An immunohistochemical method for formalin-fixed embedded tissue. Cancer 41: 1788-1793, 1978.
28. Lam WKW, Yam LT, Wilbur HJ, Taft E, Li CY: Comparison of acid phosphatase iso-enzymes of human seminal fluid, prostate and leukocytes. Clin Chem 25:1285-1289, 1979.
29. Najdi M, Tabei SZ, Castro A, Chu TM, Wang MC, Murphy GP, Morales AR: Prostatic specific antigen, an immunohistologic marker for prostatic neoplasma. Cancer 48:1229-1232, 1981.
30. Papsidero LD, Kuriyama M, Wang LC, Horoszewicz J, Leong SS, Valenzuela LA, Murphy GP, Chu TM: Prostate antigen: A marker for human prostate epithelial cells, J Natl Cancer Inst 66:37-42, 1981.
31. Mostofi FK, Sesterhenn I, Sobin LH: International classification of tumors of prostate. WHO, Geneva, 1981.
32. Lundberg Sven: Personal communication, 1980.
33. Brawer MK, Bostwick DG, Peehl DM, Stamey TA: Keratin protein in normal, hyperplastic and neoplastic prostatic tissues. J Urol 131 (Abstr 830), 1984.
34. Sloane JP, Ormerod MG: Distribution of epithelial membrane antigen in normal and neoplastic tissues and its value in diagnostic tumor pathology. Cancer 47:1786-1795, 1981.
35. Bischof W, Aumuller G: Age dependent changes in the carbohydrate pattern of human prostatic epithelium as determined by peroxidase labeled lectins. The Prostate 3:507-513, 1982.
36. Vuitch MF, Mendelsohn G: Relationship of ectopic ACTH production to tumor differentiation. A morphologic and immunohistochemical study of prostatic carcinoma with Cushing's syndrome. Cancer 47:296-299, 1981.
37. Pousette A, Borgstom E, Hogberg B, Gustafsson JA: Analysis of the androgen receptor in needle biopsies from human prostatic tissue. In: Murphy GP, Sandberg AA, Karr JP (eds) The prostatic cell: Structure and function, Part B. Alan R. Liss, NY. 1981, pp 299-311.
38. Ekman P, Barrack ER, Walsh PC: Simultaneous measurement of progesterone and androgen receptors in human prostate. A microassay. J Clin Endocrinol 55:1089-1099, 1982.
39. Ekman P, Barrack ER, Burjnovsky P, Walsh PC: Steroid receptor profiles on subcellular fractions of different human prostatic tissues. J Urol 131 (Abstr 71), 1984.
40. Wolf RM, Schneider SL, Englander LS, Ruben RP, Sandberg AA, Murphy GP, Pontes JE: Progesteron and estrogeron receptor analysis of prostatic cancer and benign prostatic hyperplasia using sucrose density gradient centrifugation techniques. J. Urol 131 (Abstr 70), 1984.

41. Martin PM, Magdelenat HP, Benyahia B, Rigoud O, Katzenellenbogen JA: New approaches for visualizing inherently fluorescent ligands and image intensification. Cancer Res 43:4956-4965, 1983.
42. Keenan EJ, Ramsey Ee, Kemp ED: The role of prolactin in the growth of the prostate gland. In: Murphy GP, Sandberg AA, Karr JP (eds). The prostate cell. Structure and function, Part B. Alan R. Liss, NY. 1981, pp 9-18.
43. Webber MM: Polypeptide hormones and the prostate. ibid. pp. 63-88.
44. Witorsch RJ: Visualization of prolactin binding sites in prostate tissue. ibid pp. 89-113.
45. Mostofi FK: Pathology and spread of carcinoma of the urinary bladder. In: Johnson DE, Samuels ML (eds) Cancer of the genitourinary tract. Raven Press, New York 1979. pp. 303-308.
46. Glynn LE, Holborow EJ: Distribution of blood group substances in human tissues. Brit Med Bull 15:150-153, 1959.
47. Hakomori SI: Glycolipids of tumor cell membrane. Advanc Cancer Res 18:265-315, 1973.
48. Davidsohn I, Kovarik S, Lee Ch L: A, B,and O Substances in gastrointestinal carcinoma. Arch Path 81:381-390, 1966.
49. Hakomori SI: Blood Group ABH and I: Antigens of human erythrocytes: Chemistry, polymorphism and their developmental change. Sem Hematol 18:39-62, 1981.
50. Stellner K. Kakomori SI, Warner GA: Enzymatic conversion of h-glycolipid to A or B-glycolipid and deficiency of these enzyme activities in adenocarcinoma. Biochem Biophys Res Commun 55:439-445, 1973.
51. Kent SP: The demonstration and distribution of water soluble blood group O (H) antigen in tissue sections using a fluorescein labeled extract of ulex europaeus seed. Histochem Cytochem 12:591-599, 1964.
52. Limas C, Lange PH: A,B, H antigen detectability in normal and neoplastic urothelium. Influence of methodological factors. Cancer 49:2476-2484, 1982.
53. Kovarik S, Davidsohn I, Stejskal R: ABO antigens in cancer. Detection with the mixed cell agglutination reaction. Arch Path 86:12-21, 1968.
54. Coon JS, Weinstein RS: Detection of ABH tissue iso-antigens by immunoperoxidase methods in normal and neoplastic urothelium. Am J Clin 76:163-171, 1981.
55. Davidsohn I, Stejskal R, Lill P: The loss of iso-antigens A,B,and H in carcinoma of the urinary bladder. Lab Invest 28:382, 1973.
56. Limas C. Lange PH, Fraley EE, Vessella RL: A,B,H antigens in transitional cell tumors of the urinary bladder. Correlation with the clinical course. Cancer 44:2099-2107, 1979.
57. Lange PH, Limas C: Molecular markers in the diagnosis and prognosis of bladder cancer. Urology 23:46-54, 1983.
58. Sadoughi N, Rubenstone A, Milsna J, Davidsohn I: The cell surface antigens in bladder washing specimens in patients with bladder tumors. A new approach. J Urol 123: 19-21, 1980.
59. Srinivas V, Orihuela EO, Llyod K, Old LJ, Whitmore WF Jr: Quantitative estimation of ABO (H) Iso-antigens in bladder tumors. J Urol 131 (Abstr 649), 1984.
60. Lotan R, Skutelsky E. Danon D, Sharon N: The purification, composition, and specificity of the anti-T lectin from peanut (Arachis-Hypogaea). J. Biol Chem 250:8518-8523, 1975.

61. Klein PJ, Newman RA, Muller P. Uhlenbruck G, Schaefer HE, Lennartz KJ, Fischer R: Histochemical methods for the demonstration of Thomsen-Friedenreich antigen in cell suspensions and tissue sections. Klin Wschr 56:761-765, 1978.
62. Coon JS, Weinstein RS, Summers JL: Blood group precursor T-antigen expression in human urinary bladder carcinoma. Am J Clin Path 77:692-699, 1982.
63. Hakomori SI: Philip Levine Award Lecture: Blood group glycolipid antigens and their modification as human cancer antigens. Am J Clin Pathol 82:635-648, 1984.
64. Klein FA, Herr HW, Sogani PC, Whitmore WF, Melamed MR: Detection and followup of carcinoma of the urinary bladder by flow cytometry. Cancer 50:389-395, 1982.
65. Klein FA, Melamed MR, Whitmore WF Jr, Herr HW, Sogani PC, Darzynkiewicz Z: Characterization of bladder papilloma by two parameter DNA-RNA flow cytometry. Cancer Res 42:1094-1097, 1982.
66. Tavares AS, Costa J, DeCarvalho A, Reis M: Tumor ploidy and prognosis in carcinomas of the bladder and prostate. Brit J Cancer 20:438-441, 1966.
67. Sandberg AA: Chromosomes in bladder cancer. In: Bonney WW, Prout GR Jr (eds) Williams and Wilkins, Baltimore, 1982, pp 81-84.
68. Gibas Z, Pontes JE, Sandberg AA: Non random chromosomal rearrangements in transitional cell carcinoma of the bladder. J Urol 131 (Abstr 29), 1984.
69. Hofstadter F, Feichtinger H, Jackse G: CEA and blood group iso-antigens of the human bladder urothelium during embryonal development. J Urol 131 (Abstr 660), 1984.
70. Wahren B, Esposti P, Zimmerman R: Characterization of urothelial carcinoma with respect to the content of carcinoembryonic antigen in exfoliated cells. Cancer 40:1511-1518, 1977.
71. Zimmerman R. Wahren B, Edsmyr F: Assessment of serial CEA determinations in urine of patients with bladder carcinoma. Cancer 46:1802-1809, 1980.
72. Goldstein I, Selikowitz SM, Olsson CA, Krane RJ: A proposed tumor marker for urachal carcinoma. Abstr 434, 76. Annual meeting AUA, Boston, Massachusetts, 1981.
73. Kawamura J, Machida S, Yoshida I, Oseho F, Imura H, Hatori M: Bladder carcinoma associated with ectopic production of HCG. Cancer 42:2773-2780, 1978.

21

IMMUNOCHEMISTRY OF SOFT TISSUE TUMORS

AZORIDES R. MORALES, M.D., EDWIN W. GOULD, M.D. AND MEHRDAD NADJI, M.D.

I. INTRODUCTION

In the diagnostic evaluation of soft tissue tumors, more than in any other group of neoplasms, a large number of special diagnostic procedures are often performed. The application of these diagnostic tools underlines the difficulties in distinguishing undifferentiated carcinoma from sarcomas and one histogenetic type of sarcoma from another. In fact, the various histogenetic types of sarcomas have overlapping morphologic features, which is understandable since these mesenchymal neoplasms have a common cellular ancestor, the primitive mesenchymal neoplasms have a common cellular ancestor, the primitive mesenchymal cell undergoes proliferation and cellular differentiation which replicates the stages of development of its non-neoplastic counterpart. According to the cellular line of differentiation, during these various stages of development, a variety of different cytoplasmic products are elaborated. It follows therefore, that demonstration of these various cytoplasmic products could lead to histogenetic diagnosis. Consequently, the value of any one given "special stain" will depend on whether or not it demonstrates the characteristic cytoplasmic materials associated with these tumors.

Unquestionably, careful study of hematoxylin and eosin stained sections frequently permits histogenetic identification of a large number of sarcomas and demonstrates their infiltrative pattern, degree of pleomorphism, mitotic rate, grouping of tumor cells and other important criteria which are helpful in establishing whether a tumor is benign or malignant. However, a large number of histogenetic diagnoses would not be possible if this were the only stain available. Unfortunately, other commonly employed procedures such as stains for reticulin, collagen, mucopolysaccharides, glycogen, fat, and others are usually of little or no value in the histogenetic assessment of sarcomas. Likewise, enzyme histochemistry has failed to fulfill its expected diagnostic

---

The opinions or assertions contained herein are the private views of authors and are not to be construed as official or as reflecting the views of the Department of the Army or the Department of Defense.

value and tissue culture yields hardly any diagnostic information in spite of careful handling of the tissue and the employment of a specialized laboratory and trained personnel.

Ultrastructural evaluation of sarcomas has expanded our knowledge of mesenchymal tumors and permits the establishment of histogenetic diagnosis in a number of them by demonstrating cytoplasmic organelles that are beyond the resolution of light microscopy (1). Electron microscopy has been particularly helpful in the study of suspected cases of 1) rhabdomyosarcoma via identifications of small aggregates of sarcomere material not visible by light microscopy, 2) smooth muscle tumors in which there are intracytoplasmic masses of actin fibers, dense cell membrane plaques on the internal surface of the cell membrane, pinocytic vesicles and a basement membrane interposed between the cell membrane and the adjacent collagenous stroma 3) liposarcoma by way of demonstration of the spectrum of lipoblastic differentiation in various tumor cells 4) neurogenic sarcomas, because of their rather characteristic branching cytoplasmic processes which contain neurofilaments and microtubules, 5) malignant fibrous histocytoma, by the demonstration of primitive mesenchymal cells with predominantly fibroblastic features together with other neoplastic cells which resemble histiocytes in that they contain lysosomes and exhibit phagocytosis, 6) other more uncommon sarcomas such as hemangiopericytoma, Ewing's sarcoma, mesenchymal chondrosarcoma, etc. with less well defined ultrastructural features. Notwithstanding the fact that most of the technical difficulties associated with ultrastructural studies have been resolved electron microscopy continues to be a very time consuming procedure, for the technician. Moreover, its expense and its requirements for proper handling of tissue and specialized instrumentation raise serious questions about its routine applicability in the realm of tumor pathology.

While initially immunochemical procedures using fluorescent labeled antibodies to myosin and other substances were rather discouraging, it is now clear that no other special procedure can be as useful or as accurate as immunohistochemical techniques in determining the histogenesis of a number of tumors. The immunoperoxidase techniques, and particularly peroxidase antiperoxidase procedure, provides a simple, highly sensitive stain applicable to fresh frozen tissues and, more importantly, to formalin-fixed, paraffin embedded material. In fact, the one significant disadvantage of this technique is the lack of availability of antibodies to some tumors, such as liposarcoma.

On the other hand, with the rapid expansion of the field of immunohistochemistry, it is anticipated that in the very near future polyclonal, monoclonal or both types of antibodies will be developed to supplement those already used in the differential diagnosis of neoplasms including sarcomas. The purpose of this review is to summarize briefly the most common antibodies currently in use and their principal applications in the pathologic assessment of tumors suspected of having mesenchymal origin.

2. EPITHELIAL ANTIGENS

In this regard, the primary value of this group of antigens lies in the fact that demonstration of any or all of them distinguishes undifferentiated carcinoma from lymphoma and sarcoma. Carcinoembryonic antigen (CEA), keratin, epithelial basement membrane antigen, blood group isoantigens and milk fat globules membrane antigen are substances that, with rare exceptions, are found exclusively in epithelia and tumors derived from them. We find the first two antigens particularly helpful since their respective antibodies are readily available and there already exists a rather large body of information concerning their distribution in normal and neoplastic tissues. With the possible exception of granular cell tumors, reported by Shousha and Lyssiotis as staining positively for CEA (2), (a finding we have been unable to confirm), benign and malignant mesenchymal tumors as well as lymphomas are negative for CEA. Thus, positive staining of a poorly differentiated tumor with CEA antisera establishes the epithelial nature of the neoplasm. On the other hand, since CEA is not present in all types of carcinoma (3), a negative reaction does not exclude the possibility of an epithelial origin.

The identification of five major subgroups of intermediate filaments and the use of antibodies raised against them has greatly enhanced our capability to distinguish between epithelial and mesenchymal neoplasms and to establish the histogenesis of a number of sarcomas (4,56,7,9). Of these filaments cytokeratin is present only in epithelial cells; it is absent from mesenchymal cells. Conversely, vimentin and desmin are mesenchymal markers. The former is found in a variety of different mesenchymal cells whereas the latter is expressed only by muscle cells whether smooth, cardiac or skeletal. The remaining two intermediate filaments, glial fibrillary acid protein and neurofilaments are localized in glial cells and neurons respectively. The principal advantage of using cytokeratin antisera in the differential diagnosis of soft tissue tumors relates to the fact that its demonstration in a poorly differentiated tumor establishes its epithelial nature (9); it is particularly helpful in distinguishing spindle cell squamous carcinomas from sarcoma (Fig. 1). The demonstration of immunoreactivity for keratin in synovial sarcoma particularly in the epithelial (Fig. 2) but also in the spindle cell component as well as in a number of epithelioid sarcomas (9,10,11,12) not only permit distinction of these tumors from other sarcomas, but raise some question concerning the alleged mesenchymal lineage of these neoplasms.

3. MUSCLE ANTIGENS

Of the various antigens - actin, myosin, isoenzymes BB and MM of creatinine kinase, desmin and myoglobin, found in either or both smooth and striated muscle, only desmin and myoglobin are muscle specific and hence, are the most valuable in distinguishing muscle tumors from other soft tissue neoplasms.

The intermediate filament desmin is expressed by smooth skeletal and cardiac muscle (13). It has been demonstrated in leiomyoma (Figs. 3,4) (5,14) as well as leiomyosarcoma (Fig.5) (14) and rhabdomyosarcoma (5,14), but not in other histologic types of soft tissue tumors with the exception of an alveolar soft part sarcoma (7) a fibrosarcoma (5) and a malignant fibrous histiocytoma (5). These three reported instances of desmin immunoreactivity in non-myogenous tumors raise some doubts concerning either the specificity of desmin as a muscle marker or the accuracy of the criteria employed in classifying these three tumors. Alternatively, one can also speculate about the possibility that the primitive mesenchymal cell from which these tumors derived followed a bidirectional line of differentiation including that of smooth muscle.

It is becoming increasingly apparent that immunohistochemical staining for myoglobin is the most sensitive and practical procedure for the histologic diagnosis of rhabdomyosarcoma (Figs. 6,7). Myoglobin is found exclusively in skeletal and cardiac muscle (15) and has not been reported in any mesenchymal tumor cells, except the rhabdomyoblasts of rhabdomyosarcoma (15,16,17,18,19,20), mixed Mullerian tumor (18,21), "triton" tumor (18) and testicular teratoma (18). Recently Brooks (18) and Eusebi et al (22) have

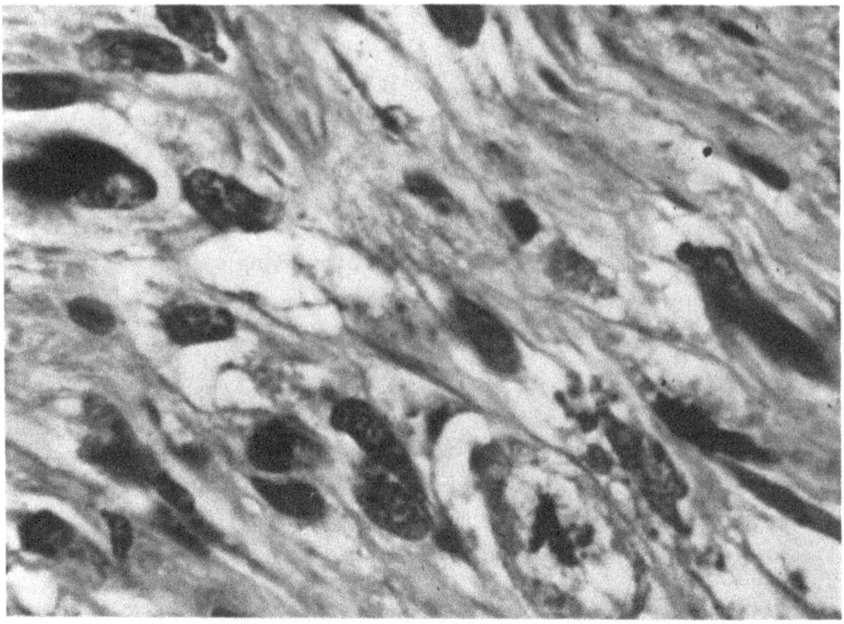

Figure 1. Spindle cell carcinoma. Intracellular keratin is readily detectable in a few tumor cells using the peroxidase antiperoxidase technique.

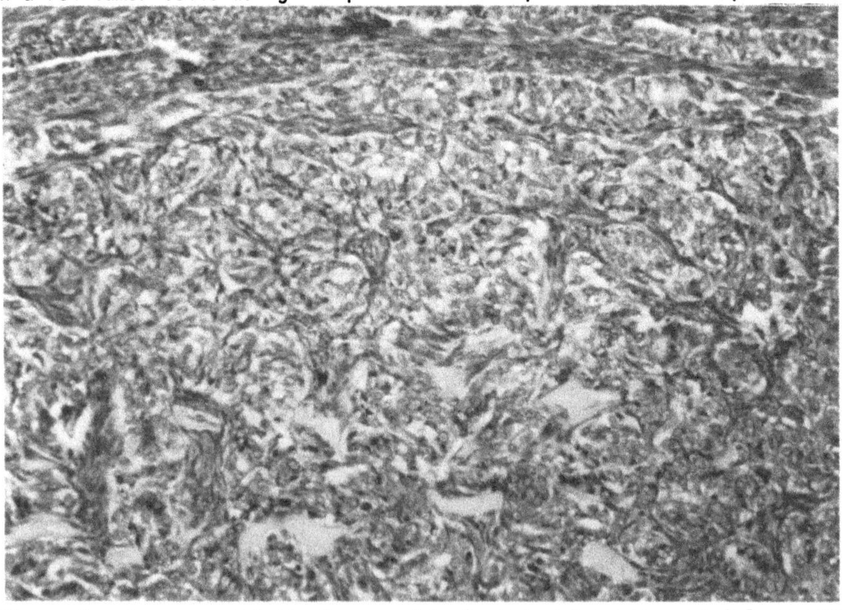

Figure 2. Immunoreactivity for keratin in this biphasic synovial sarcoma is apparent in epithelial component.

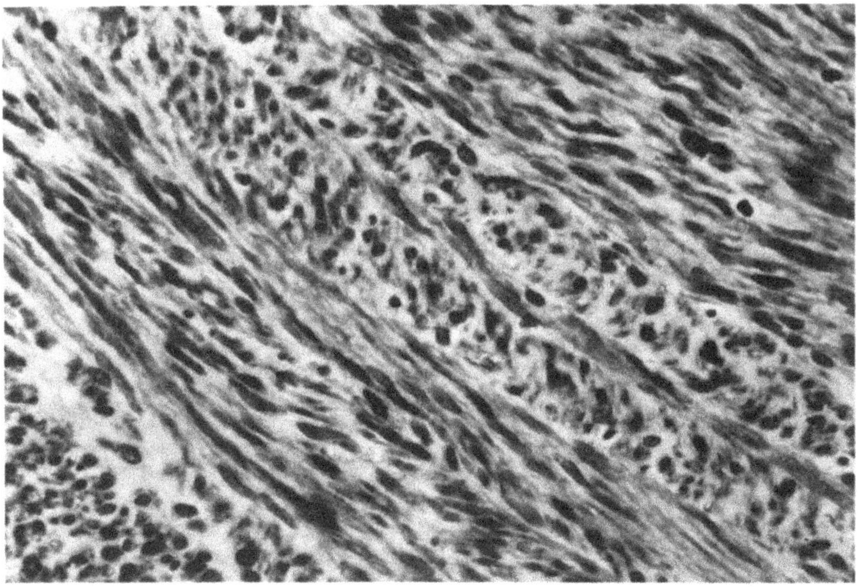

Figure 3. Universal intracytoplasmic immunostaining of desmin is demonstrated in this section of leiomyoma of uterus.

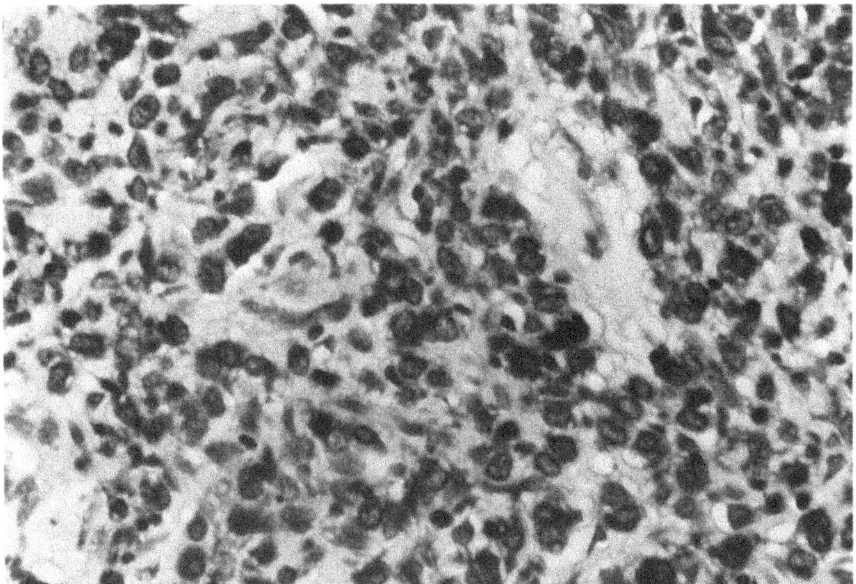

Figure 4. Leiomyoblastoma of the stomach. Note strong cytoplasmic staining indicating the presence of desmin.

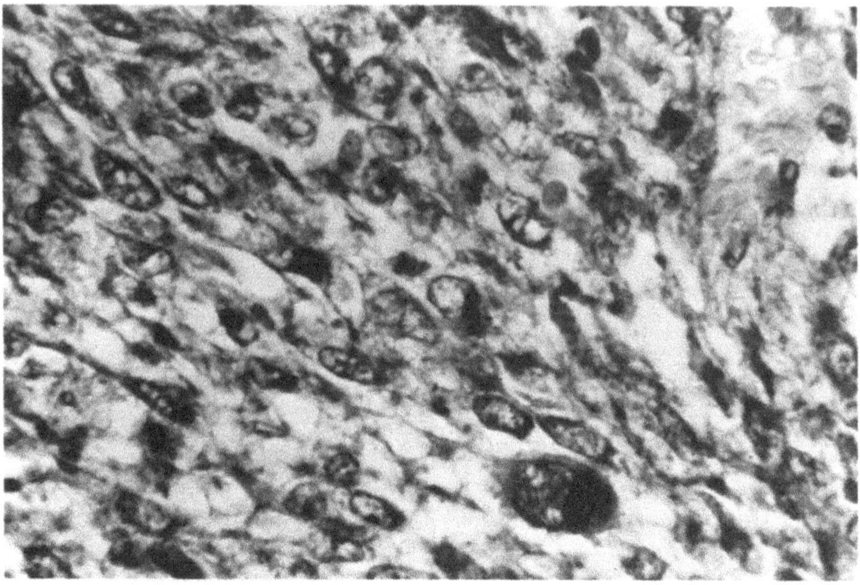

Figure 5. Leiomyosarcoma. The muscular nature of this poorly differentiated tumor was established by the demonstration of desmin in a number of tumor cells.

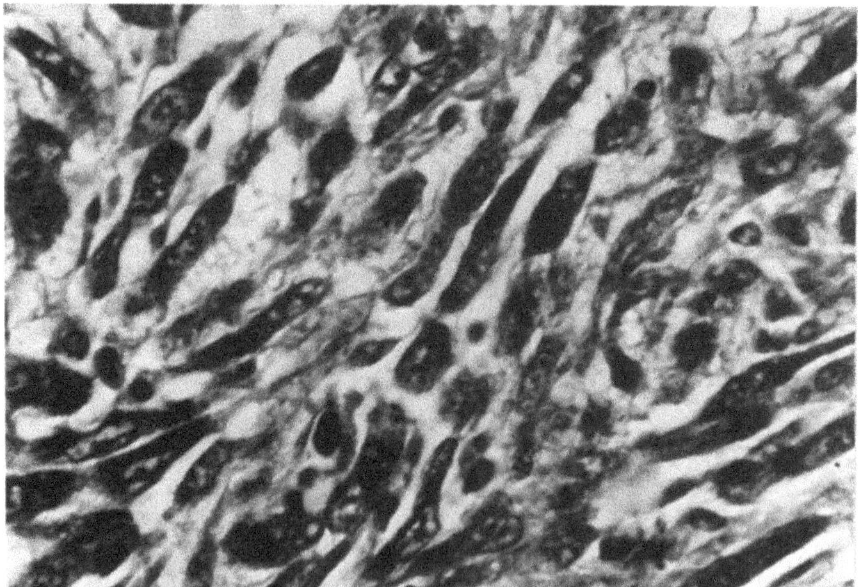

Figure 6. The intracytoplasmic immunoreactivity for myoglobin conclusively established the rhabdomyoblastic nature of this poorly differentiated spindle cell neoplasm.

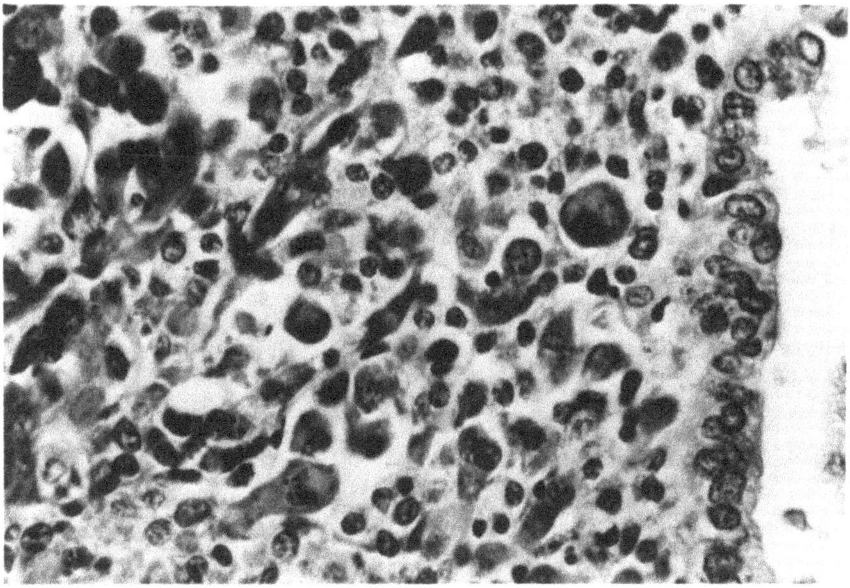

Figure 7. Mixed mullerian tumor. The rhabdomyoblastic elements of this tumor are highlighted by their immunostaining for myoglobin. Note the negative reaction of neoplastic glandular epithelium.

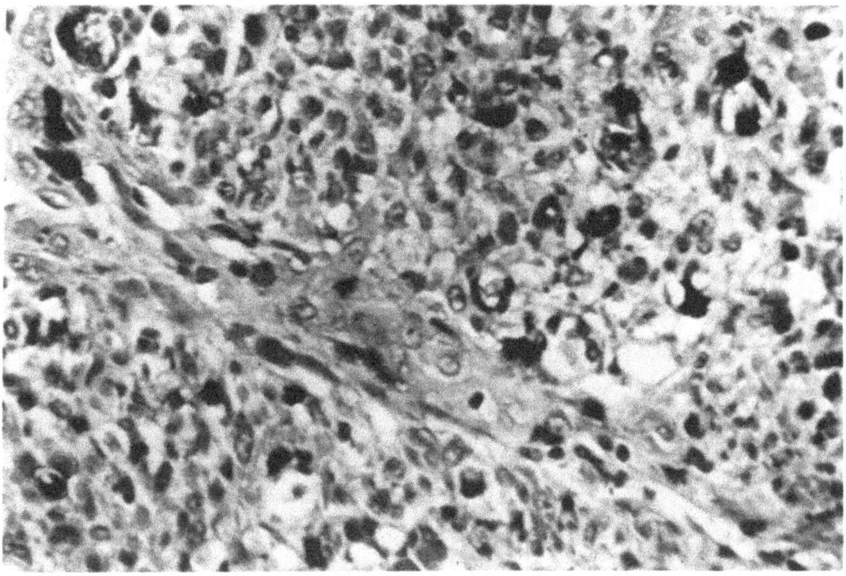

Figure 8. Malignant schwannoma. Myelin basic protein stained section showing irregular aggregates of this antigen throughout this neurogenic sarcoma.

pointed out the rare and unexpected occurrence of non-muscle cells exhibiting myoglobin immunoreactivity. They surmise that the myoglobin is probably released from muscle and phagocytized by inflammatory cells near areas of necrotic muscle (18) or by carcinoma cells in some instances of invasion of muscle by tumor (22).

The value of myoglobin staining in the diagnosis of rhabdomyosarcoma is underscored by its high positivity rate, from 76 to 100% of rhabdomyosarcomas in different series. This frequency can be explained by the fact that, contrary to desmin, myoglobin is expressed in the earliest stages of embryogenesis of skeletal muscle predating the formation of muscular striations.

4. NEURAL TISSUE ANTIGENS

Myelin basic protein and S100 protein are neural tissue antigens which have practical value in the differential diagnosis of soft tissue tumors. Myelin basic protein has been demonstrated in peripheral nerve (23) and is found in neurofibroma, schwannoma and their malignant counterparts (Fig. 8) whereas other spindle cell neoplasms do not stain for this substance (24). Its presence in granular cell tumors seems to support the concept of Schwann cell derivation of these lesions (Fig. 9) (25).

Although S100 protein is not specific for neural tissue, immunohistochemical assays for this substance assist in establishing the neurogenic nature of some poorly differentiated sarcomas (26,27). But, most importantly when used as a melanocytic marker, demonstration of this antigen permits to distinguish amelanotic malignant melanomas (Figs. 10,11) from some sarcomas which it often mimics such as rhabdomyosarcoma, alveolar soft part sarcoma, epithelioid sarcoma and malignant fibrous histiocytoma (9). In those instances in which differentiation between neurogenic sarcoma and malignant melanoma is uncertain, staining for both myelin basic protein and S100 protein may be helpful since S100 protein stains both and myelin basic protein does not stain melanocytes (24).

Although S100 protein is also present in chondrocytes and mature fat cells, staining of chondrosarcomas and liposarcomas yields rather inconsistent results; the procedure may not help in the evaluation of these lesions.

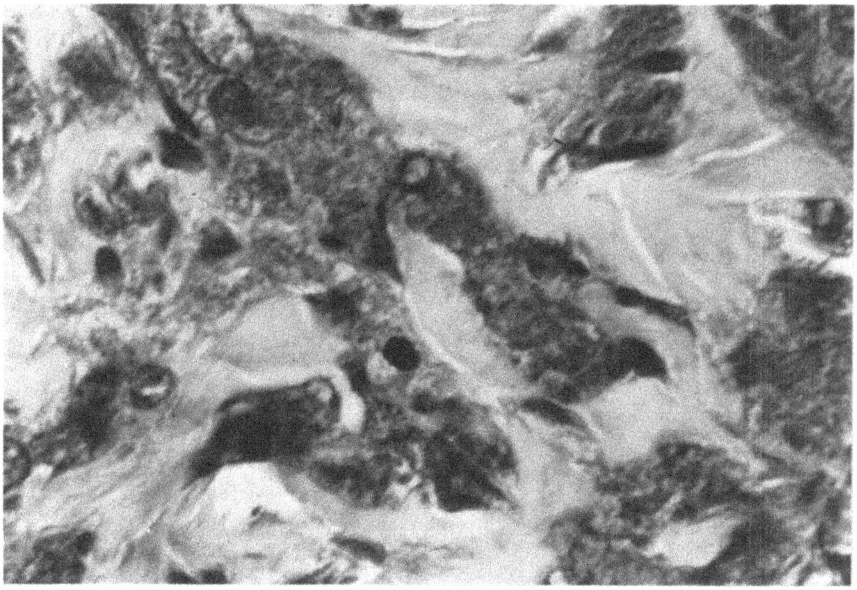

Figure 9. Granular cell tumor showing positive immunostaining with antibody against myelin basic protein.

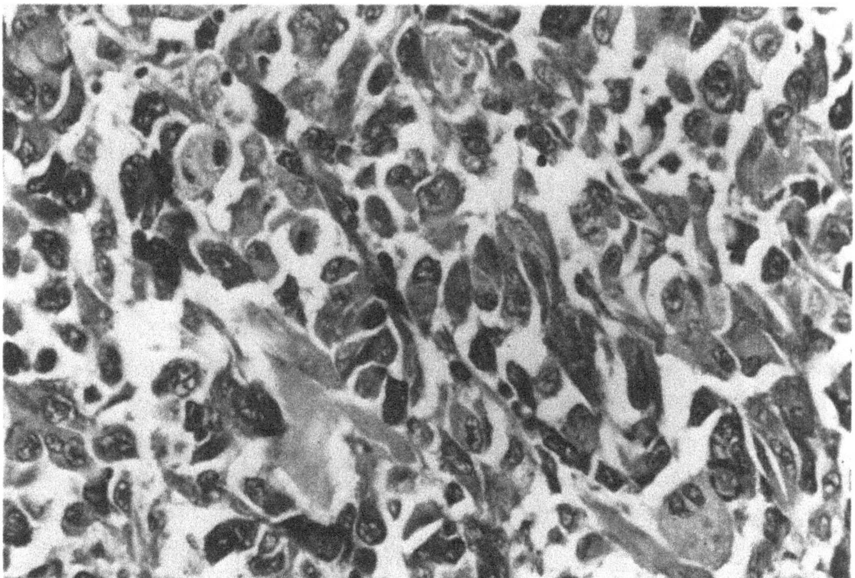

Figure 10. Staining for S100 protein help to distinguish malignant melanoma from sarcoma and fibromatosis as shown in this illustration of anaplastic malignant melanoma.

5. HISTIOCYTIC MARKERS

Muramidase, alpha-1 antitrypsin and alpha-1 antichymotrypsin, although present in a variety of different tissues including some epithelia, are usually regarded as lysosomal antigens and can usually be demonstrated in histiocytes. Attempts to demonstrate them in fibrous histiocytic tumors have shown that staining for muramidase is almost always negative, whereas only some cells in a few fibrous histiocytomas stain for alpha-1 antichymotrypsin or alpha-1 antitrypsin (24). It is becoming increasingly apparent that the malignant fibrous histiocytoma represents a tumor of very primitive mesenchymal cells with predominantly fibroblastic features which have a secondary differentiating line resembling histiocytes rather than representing a tumor of histiocytes with fibroblastic differentiation. It would seem, logical therefore, to assume that only those cells bearing lysosomes in their cytoplasm would stain for either alpha-1-antichymotrypsin or alpha-1-antitrypsin (Fig. 12).

6. ENDOTHELIAL CELL ANTIGENS

Actin, myosin, vimentin and blood group antigens have been demonstrated in endothelial cells and vascular tumors but they are not specific for endothelial cells. On the other hand, fact VIII related antigen is elaborated exclusively by megakaryocytes and endothelial cells (28); it has become one of the best available immunohistochemical markers for assessing whether or not reactive, hyperplastic and benign and malignant neoplastic type, express immunoreactivity for factor VIII related antigen. The reaction for this antigen in cystic lymphangiomas and lymphangiomatosis is weaker and fewer of their cells stain positively than do the cells of hemangiomas (30).

Factor VIII related antigen can usually be demonstrated in epithelioid hemangioendothelioma (Fig.13) and angiosarcoma (Figs. 14,15) but the intensity of the reaction varies from one vase to another and in some instances the immunoreactivity is confined to a few cells contrasting with an intense staining display by the adjacent non-neoplastic capillaries (29,30).

Immunoperoxidase staining for factor VIII related antigen has been helpful in establishing or confirming the endothelial nature of tumors of disputed histogenesis. Studies by Nadji et al (31) and Guarda et al (32) recently confirmed by Mukai and Rosai (30) have shown that, in addition to the cells

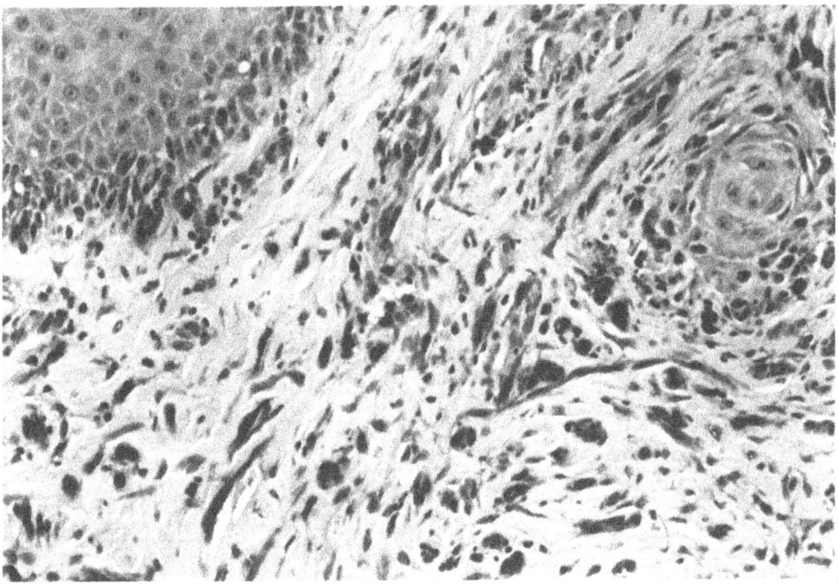

Figure 11. Staining for S100 protein helps to distinguish malignant melanoma from sarcoma and fibromatosis as shown in this illustration of desmoplastic malignant melanoma.

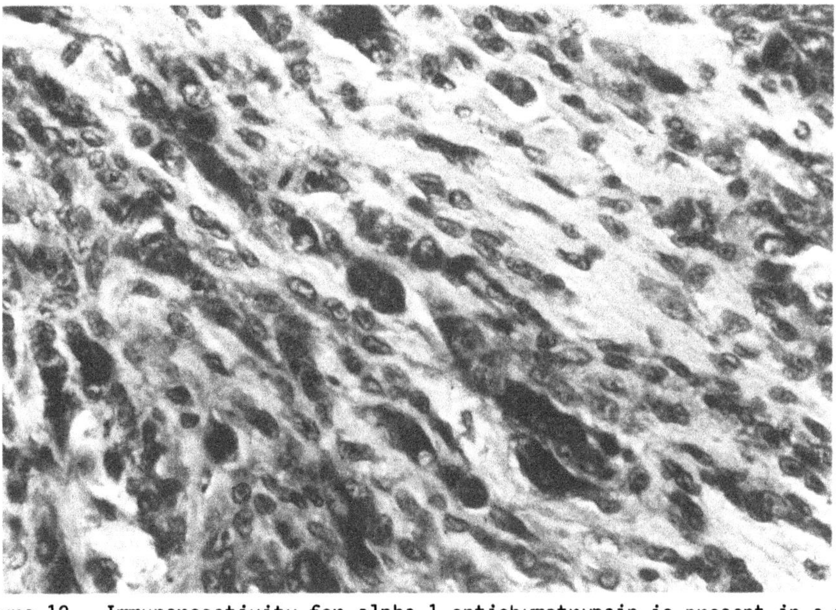

Figure 12. Immunoreactivity for alpha-1-antichymotrypsin is present in a few tumor cells of this malignant fibrous histiocytoma.

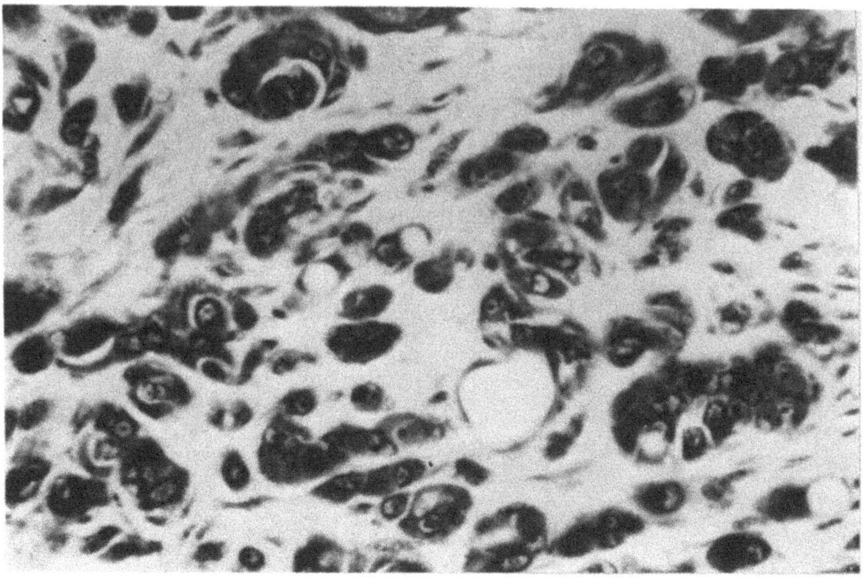

Figure 13. Epithelioid hemangioendothelioma. This tumor of the chest wall was initially interpreted as a metastatic carcinoma. Factor VIII related-antigen is universally present in the cytoplasm of tumor cells. Note a few cytoplasmic vacuoles indicative of vasoformative differentiation.

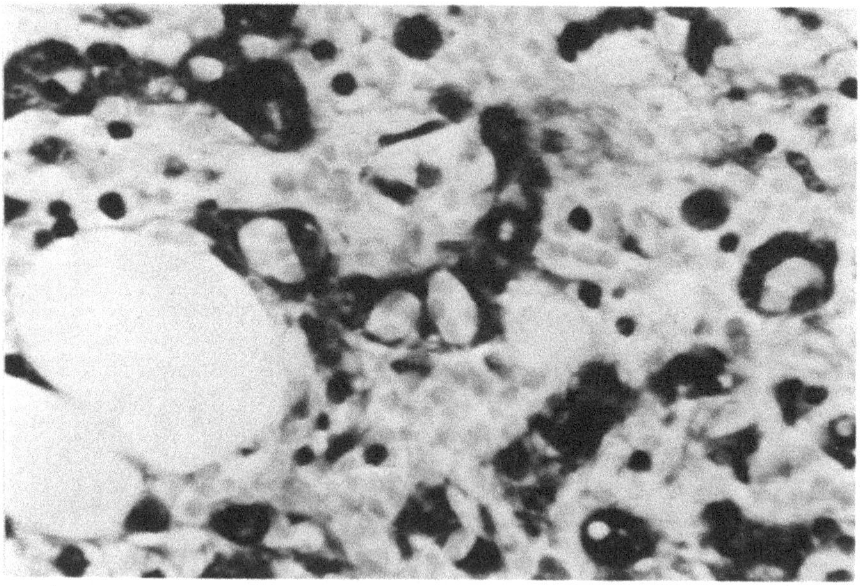

Figure 14. The endothelial nature of this tumor is confirmed by the strong reaction for factor VIII related-antigen.

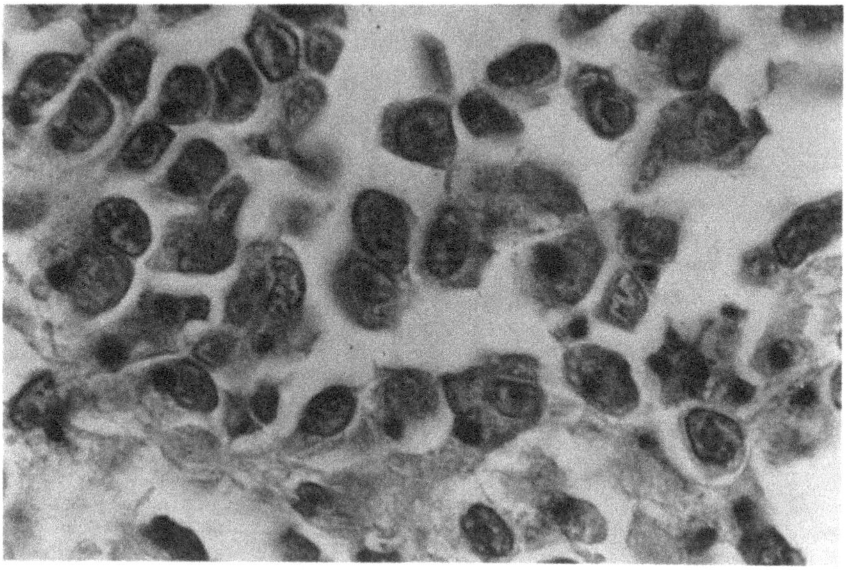

Figure 15. This poorly differentiated angiosarcoma contains paranuclear aggregates of factor VIII related-antigen.

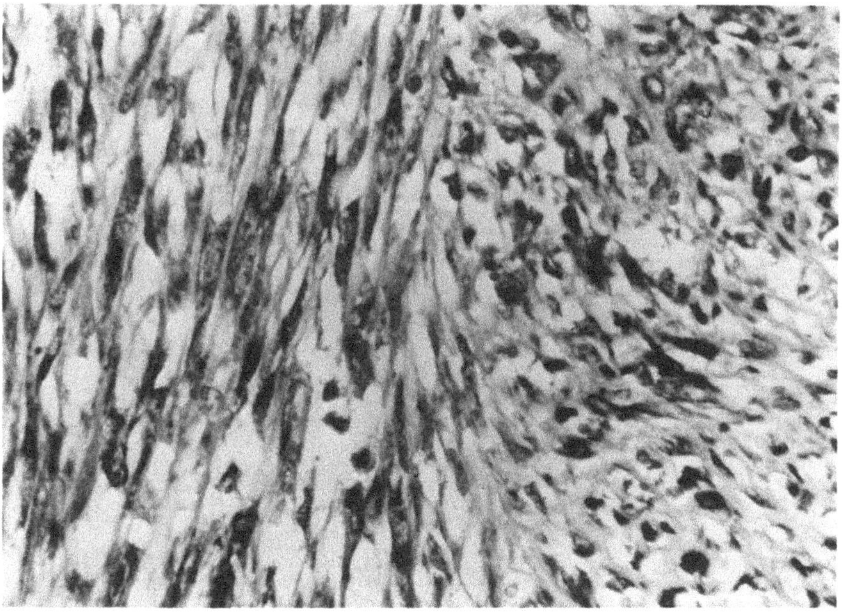

Figure 16. Immunostaining for factor VIII related-antigen in the spindle cells of Kaposi's sarcoma is clearly shown in this illustration.

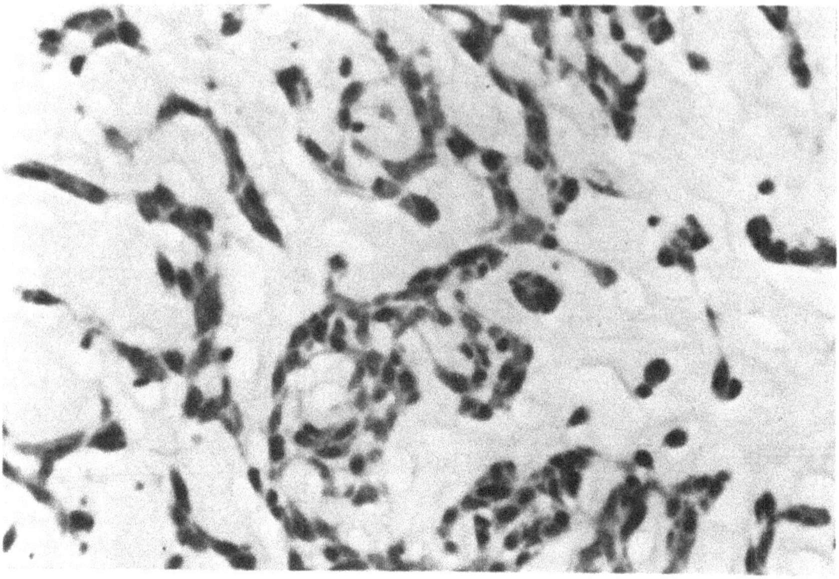

Figure 17. Cardiac myxoma. Anastomosing cords of tumor cells stain positively for factor VIII related-antigen. Note the lack of demonstrable antigen in the myxoid stroma.

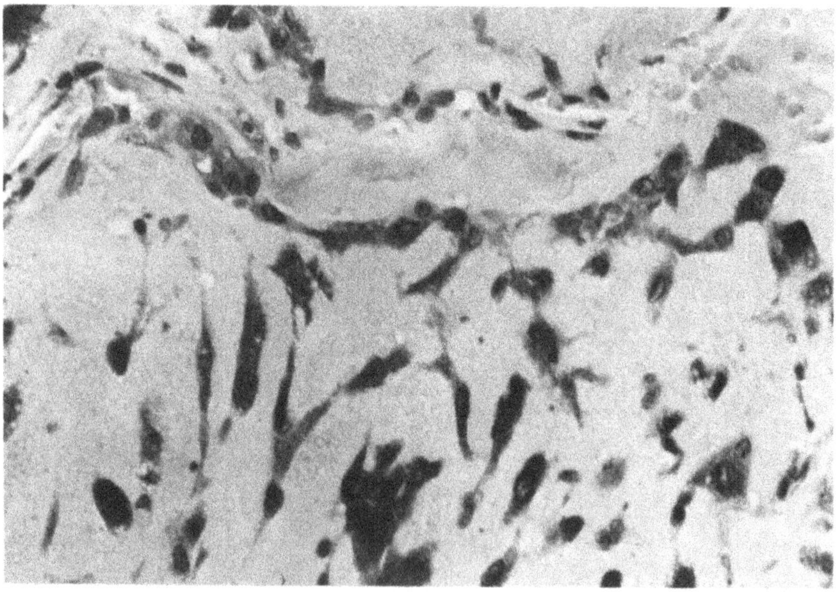

Figure 18. Intravascular bronchio-alveolar tumor. The endothelial nature of this tumor is demonstrated with immunoperoxidase staining for factor VIII related-antigen.

lining vascular spaces and slits, the characteristic spindle cells of Kaposi's sarcoma are also positive for factor VIII related antigen (Fig. 16). Although Morales et al (33) found universal staining of neoplastic cells in cardiac myxomas by factor VIII related antigens (Fig. 17), others have not been able to confirm that observation (30,34). The studies of Bhagavan et al (35) and Weldon-Linne et al (36) seem to indicate that the intravascular bronchial alveolar tumor, an uncommon pulmonary malignancy is of endothelial origin, an observation that we have confirmed in two of our cases (Fig.18). We have also found reactivity for factor VIII related antigen in the neoplastic elements of the rare malignant intraluminal tumors of large vessels (24).

In summary, factor VIII related antigen is helpful in the differential diagnosis of endothelial tumors allowing their differentiation from other neoplasms with which they are often confused such as sclerosing hemangioma, hemangiopericytoma, glomangiomas and, in particular, some primary and metastatic carcinomas.

REFERENCES

1. Morales AR: Electron microscopy of human tumors. Progr Surg Pathol 1:51-70, 1980.
2. Shousha S. Lyssiotis T: Granular cell myoblastoma: Positive staining for carcinoembryonic antigen. J Clin Pathol 32:219-224, 1979.
3. Primus FJ, Clark CA, Goldenberg DM: Immunohistochemical detection of carcinoembryonic antigen. In Diagnostic Immunohistochemistry. RA DeLellis, Ed., Masson Publishing, USA, New York, 1981, pp 263-276.
4. Gown AM, Gabbiani G: Intermediate sized (10 nm) filaments in human tumors. In Advances in Immunohistochemistry, RA DeLellis, Ed., Masson Publishing, USA, New York, 1984, pp 89-110.
5. Miettinen M, Lehto V-P, Virtanen J: Expression of intermediate filaments in soft tissue sarcomas. Int J Cancer 30:541-546, 1982.
6. Osborn M, Weber K: Biology of disease. Tumor diagnosis by intermediate filament typing. A novel tool for surgical pathology. Lab Invest 48:372-394,1983.
7. Denk H, Krepler R, Artlieb V, Gabbiani G, Rungger-Brandle E, Leoncini P, Franke WW: Proteins of intermediate filaments. An immunohistochemical and biochemical approach to the classification of soft tissue tumors. Am J Pathol 80:677-681, 1983.
8. Erlandson RA: Diagnostic immunohistochemistry of human tumors. Am J Surg Pathol 8:624, 1984.
9. Battifora H: Recent progress in the immunohistochemistry of solid tumors. Semin Diagn Pathol 1:251-271, 1984.

10. Miettinem M, Lehto V-P, Virtanen I: Keratin in the epithelial-like cells of classical biphasic synovial sarcoma. Virchows Arch (Cell Pathol) 40:151-157, 1982.
11. Miettinen M, Lehto V-P, Virtanen I: Monophasic synovial sarcoma of spindle cell type: Epithelial differentiation as revealed by ultrastructural features, content of prekeratin and binding of peanut agglutinin. Virchows Arch (Cell Pathol) 44:187-199, 1983.
12. Chase D, Ensinger F, Weiss SW, Langloss DVM: Keratin in epithelioid sarcoma. An immunohistochemical study. Am J Surg Pathol 8:435-441, 1984.
13. Lazarides E. Balzer DR Jr: Specificity of desmin to avian and mammalian muscle cells. Cells 14:429-438, 1978.
14. Gabbiani G, Kapanci Y, Barazzone P, Franke WW: Immunochemical identification of intermediate-sized filaments in human neoplastic cells: A diagnostic aid for the surgical pathologist. Am J Pathol 104:206-216, 1981.
15. Mukai, K, Rosai J, Hallaway BE: Localization of myoglobin in normal and neoplastic human skeletal muscle cells using an immunoperoxidase method. Am J Surg Pathol 3:373-376, 1979.
16. Miettinen M, Lehto V-P, Badley RA, Virtanen I: Alveolar rhabdomyosarcoma - demonstration of the muscle-type of intermediate filament protein, desmin, as a diagnostic aid. Am J Pathol 108:246-251, 1982.
17. Brooks JJ: Immunohistochemistry of soft tissue tumors. Myoglobin as a tumor marker for rhabdomyosarcoma. Cancer 50:1757-1763, 1982.
18. Brooks JJ: Immunohistochemistry of myoglobin. In Advances in Immunohistochemistry. RA DeLellis, Ed., Masson Publishing, USA, New York, 1984, pp 343-358.
19. Corson JM, Pinkus GS: Intracellular myoglobin - A specific marker for skeletal muscle differentiation in soft tissue sarcomas. An immunoperoxidase study. Am J Pathol 103:384-389, 1981.
20. Kindblom L, Eidal T, Karlsson K: Immunohistochemical localization of myoglobin in human muscle tissue and embryonal and alveolar rhabdomyosarcoma. Acta Path Microbiol Scand (Sect A) 90:167-174, 1982.
21. Mukai K, Varela-Duran J, Nochomontz LE: The rhabdomyoblast in mixed Mullerian tumors of the uterus and ovary: An immunohistochemical study of myoglobin in 25 cases. Am J Clin Pathol 74:101-104, 1980.
22. Eusebi V, Bondi A, Rosai J: Immunohistochemical localization of myoglobin in non-muscular cells. Am J Surg Pathol 8:51-56, 1984.
23. Uyemura RK, Susuki M, Kitamusa K: Studies on myelin proteins in human peripherhal nerve. Adv Exp Med Biol 100:95-115, 1977.
24. Nadji M, Morales AR: Unpublished data.
25. Penneys NS, Adachi K, Ziegels-Weissman J: Granular cell tumors of the skin contain myelin basic protein. Arch Pathol Lab Med 107:302-303, 1983.
26. Stefansson K, Wollmann R, Jerkovic M: S100 protein in soft-tissue tumors derived from Schwann cells and melanocytes. Am J Pathol 106:261-268, 1982.
27. Weiss SW, Langloss JM, Enzinger FM: The value of S100 protein in the diagnosis of soft tissue tumors with particular reference to benign and malignant Schwann cell tumors. Lab Invest 49:299-308, 1983.
28. Jaffe EA: Endothelial cells and the biology of factor VIII. N Engl J Med 296:377-383, 1977.
29. Nadji M, Gonzalez MS, Castro A, Morales AR: Factor VIII-related antigen. An endothelial cell marker. Lab Invest 42:139, 1980.
30. Mukai K, Rosai J: Factor VIII-related antigen. An endothelial marker, In Advances in Immunohistochemistry, RA DeLellis, Ed., Masson Publishing, USA, New York 1984, 253-261.

31. Nadji M, Morales AR, Ziegels-Weissman J, Penneys NS: Kaposi's Sarcoma. Immunohistologic evidence for an endothelial origin. Arch Pathol Lab Med 105:274-275, 1981.
32. Guarda LG, Ordonez EG, Nelson G, Smith LJ: Factor VIII in Kaposi's sarcoma. Am J Clin Pathol 76:197-200, 1981.
33. Morales AR, Nadji M, Castro A, Fine G: Cardiac myxoma (endocardioma). An immunocytochemical assessment of histogenesis. Human Pathol 12:896-899, 1981.
34. McComb RD: Heterogenous expression of factor VIII/von Willebrand factor by cardiac myxoma cells. Am J Surg Pathol 8:539-544, 1984.
35. Bhagavan BS, Dorfman HD, Murthy MSN, Eggleston SC: Intravascular bronchio-alveolar tumor. A low-grade sclerosing epithelioid angiosarcoma of lung. Am J Surg Pathol 6:41-52, 1982.
36. Weldon-Linne CM, Victor TA, Christ ML: Immunohistochemical identification of factor VIII-related antigen in the intravascular bronchio-alveolar tumor of the lung. Arch Pathol Lab Med 105:628-629, 1981.

22

A REVIEW OF DNA FLOW CYTOMETRIC PREPARATORY AND ANALYTICAL METHODS

JERRY T. THORNTHWAITE, RICHARD A. THOMAS, JOSE RUSSO, HELEN OWNBY, GEORGE I. MALININ, FRANCIS HORNICEK, THOMAS W. WOOLLEY, JIM FREDERICK. THEODORE I. MALININ, D. ANTONIO VAZQUEZ, DANIEL SECKINGER

The detection of cell surface antigens is the most familiar application of flow cytometry in clinical immunology. Rapid advances in immunocytochemical applications of monoclonal antibodies, which may now be regarded as "true" reagents in the clinical laboratory, have made possible the immunological characterization of various tumors (1-3) and the classification of cells of the immune system (4-6). This extensive immunological characterization was virtually unattainable a few years earlier.

The characterization of cells by their DNA content antedates the development of fluorescent antibody methods. In spite of this, DNA measurements, as opposed to fluorescent antibody measurements, have not been widely used for the characterization of cells. Even though the DNA measurements for the detection of cancerous cells was one of the first applications of flow cytometers in the late 1960s (7), this methodology, which has promise as a prognostic indicator (8,9), was unjustly neglected and is just beginning to gain acceptance in the clinical laboratory. We discuss three reasons why this application has been slow in developing as a valuable clinical and research tool. First of all, flow cytometers have not had the resolution (10-14) to measure DNA with coefficients of variation in the 1 - 2% range. Secondly, the standardization of materials and methods for preparing cells and tissues for DNA flow cytometery (15) with the use of appropriate DNA standards (16) have only recently been standardized. Lastly, the prognostic significance of DNA measurements has not been fully appreciated until recently (8,9,17,18).

In this chapter we present criteria for flow cytometric analysis of DNA in cells, some of which were isolated from tissues and the rest obtained from cell cultures. These criteria are as follows:

1. Isolation of nuclei

2. Specific fluorescent staining of DNA and the determination of DNA content

3. Stability of DNA in refrigerated and frozen tissues and cells

4. Adequate sampling

5. DNA standard

6. High resolution measurements

7. Some clinical applications of DNA flow cytometry

Without proper nuclear isolation procedures, judicious selection of DNA specific stain, adequate sampling, the use of a stable DNA standard, and sharp resolution of measurements, DNA flow cytometric analysis is a wasted effort.

This chapter briefly reviews our experience in flow cytometric measurements of DNA. For didactic reasons, these methodologies are illustrated by appropriate experimental evidence and are what we feel are "state-of-the-art" for the measurement of DNA.

1. Isolation of nuclei

The usefulness of flow cytometry in studies of cell proliferation and carcinogenesis to a large extent is predicated on the availability of a consistent and rapid method for the isolation of cells or nuclei from tissues. Although much analytical work has been performed with ascites tumor cells (19,20), cell cultures (21) and hemopoetic cells (22), none of these require special preparatory procedures. Cytometric analysis of these cells may be accomplished readily after staining DNA while avoiding cell clumping. However, sample preparation of solid tumors or tissues for flow cytometric analysis becomes more difficult when the cells must be completely separated from each other to obviate increased DNA values generated by the adherence of two or more cells to one another.

Several preparative methods have been employed for the isolation of cells from tissues. The most widely used procedures have relied on the enzymatic dissociation of cells. For example, trypsin was used to dissociate mouse squamous-cell carcinoma (23), pepsin for metastatic human tumors (24), and the combinations of trypsin-collagenase for a variety of tissues (25). The nonenzymatic, chemical (26,27), or physical (28,29) procedures were also used to recover isolated cells for flow cytometric studies. In general, these preparative methods are multi-step processes, specially adapted to each type of tissue to insure maximum dissociation and cell yields. Unfortunately, the reproducibility of these techniques has not been firmly established, particularly since cell dissociation is not always complete, thus rendering interpretations of flow cytometric DNA histograms suspect on account of elevated DNA values generated by the cellular aggregates.

The standard procedures for nuclear isolation from tissues usually require homogenization and centrifugation (30,31) which may lead to incomplete cell dissociation, release of DNA from the fragmented nuclei, and nuclear clumping. These procedures are therefore unacceptable for flow cytometric measurements. Hypotonic solutions (32) which may be supplemented by the nonionic surfactant, nonidet P 40 (NP 40) (33,34), have often been used to isolate nuclei from dispersed cells for the subsequent flow cytometric analysis of propidium iodide stained nuclei. A hypertonic saline solution supplemented with NP 40 has also been utilized to obtain nuclei from solid tumor cells (34).

In view of the diversity of existing techniques for isolation of nuclei, one of our initial objectives was the development of a dependable, rapid method for isolation of fluorochrome stained nuclei from normal and cancerous tissues. This one-step procedure, which combines nuclear isolation and the concomitant DNA staining with 4',6-diamidino-2-phenylindole (DAPI), does not require centrifugation, thus eliminating a main cause of nuclear clumping (15).

Nuclear Isolation Medium (NIM): The composition of NIM was fully described elsewhere (15) and therefore will not be reiterated here. The main advantages of NIM are rapid isolation of stained nuclei with less than 2% clumping. Practical implementation of nuclear isolation with NIM is depicted in Fig. 1. Tissues are teased in fluorochrome containing NIM, syringed and filtered. The syringing step is optional since most tissue preparations result in monodispersed nuclei without it.

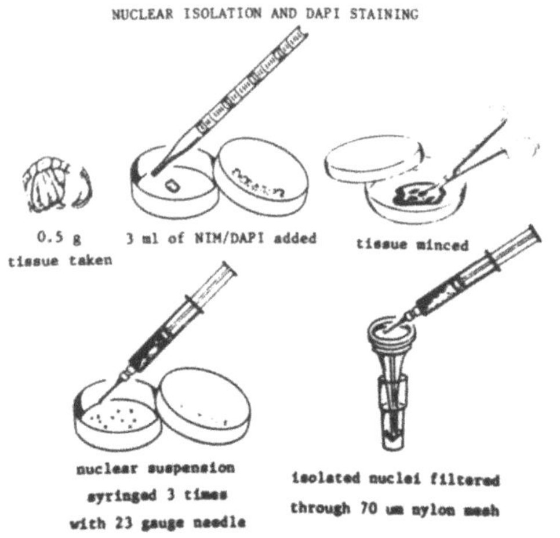

Figure 1. Isolation of nuclei with nuclear isolation medium (NIM) (15) and simultaneous staining of DNA with DAPI. The syringing step is optional. The entire procedure, performed at room temperature, requires only 5 minutes.

While the nuclei can be isolated in solutions with low (3-10 mM) (20,34) and high (550 mM) NaCl concentrations (34), we have found (35) tonicity of the nuclear isolation media to be a very important determinant for the retention of nuclear volume within normal range. Nonetheless, it is possible to isolate nuclei by resorting to the non-ionic extraction fluids. For example, the nonionic surfactant, NP40, was successfully used by us to isolate nuclei from a variety of tissues. Generally speaking, a 0.6% NP40 concentration proved to be the optimum for most of the tissues, although 1-2% concentrations have been utilized without impairment of nuclear integrity. Still higher NP40 concentrations may be useful in isolation nuclei if the tissue in question is hard to dissociate. On the other hand, nuclear isolation may likewise be attained by very low NP40 concentrations, such as 0.025% in the case with human mammary and prostatic tissues.

2. Specific fluorescent staining of DNA and the determination of DNA content

In recent years, a number of antibiotic drugs which bind to nucleic acids (36-44) have been characterized as fluorochromes. Key factors in their usefulness for DNA determinations are the enhancement of their fluorescence that occurs on binding of the fluorochromes to DNA, and minimal cross-reactivity of these reagents with other substances. For instance, DNA intercalating dyes, such a propidium iodide and ethidium bromide, show enhanced fluorescence on binding to DNA, but they also react with RNA, thus necessitating treatment of tissue with ribonuclease.

Fluorescent non-intercalating DNA-specific dyes have been used for the rapid quantitative determinations of DNA. These include the guanine-cytosine binding mithramycin (38), and adenine-thymine binding dyes, Hoechst 33258 (36,37,44) and 4',6-diamidino-2-phenylindole (DAPI) (39,45). Unlike intercalating fluorochromes, these compounds can be added directly to tissue homogenates without interference from RNA. Although cytometric assays with fluorochromes are very sensitive, they are equally affected by cell ploidy, DNA containing cell fragments, and inaccuracies in cell counting.

A very suitable fluorochrome for measuring DNA in cells by flow cytometry is DAPI. This dye has a very high quantum yield and is reasonably resistant to photodegradation. Under appropriate conditions, DAPI will pass through the nuclear envelope to bind stoichiometrically to the adenine-thymine rich regions of the DNA molecule (40). The DNA-DAPI complex is maximally excited at 365 nm and emits maximum fluorescence at 465 nm. There is a 20-fold increase in fluoresence yield when

DAPI binds to DNA as compared to DAPI alone (42,43). Degradation of RNA with RNase has no effect on DAPI-DNA fluorescence (39,41) and therefore is not necessary.

If one wishes to employ the channel ratio method for calculating the amount of DNA in a sample, the following relationship may be used:

$$C_x = \frac{\text{peak channel number}_x}{\text{peak channel number}_{st}} C_{st}$$

where the peak channel number $_x$ refers to the sample; peak channel number $_{st}$ refers to the standard; C_{st} is the DNA content per nucleus, in picograms, of the standard; and C_x is the DNA content per nucleus, in picograms, of the sample.

It is clear from the above that for the determination of DNA in a sample, a stable DNA standard is required. Moreover, DNA values over the calibration range must show linear relationship to the channel number. Figure 2, a flow histogram of CFI mouse liver cells with four ploidy peaks at 2C, 4C, 8C and 16C DNA levels, demonstrates the linearity of the DNA values in the 7 to 112 pg range. The ordinate represents the number of nuclei. The 1000 channels on the abscissa represent fluorescence intensity of the nuclear DAPI-DNA complex. The correlation coefficient squared of the DNA content and channel number was $r^2 = 0.999$.

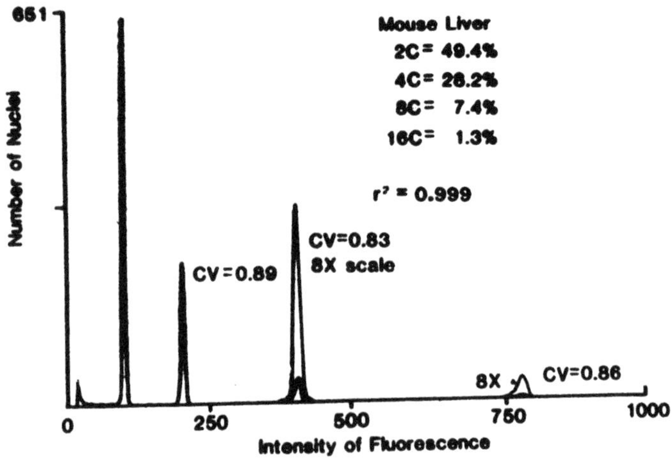

Figure 2. Distribution of DNA content in mouse liver nuclei isolated with NIM and stained with DAPI shows a consistently linear correlation of ploidy levels with the fluorescence intensity. C represents the haploid DNA content of the nuclei. The heights of the 8C and 16C nuclei peaks have been magnified eight times. The correlation coefficient squared is $r^2 = 0.999$. (Anal. Biochem 137:221, 1984)

3. Stability of DNA in refrigerated and frozen tissues

The processing of tissues for the subsequent flow cytometry may be time consuming particularly if one has to deal with a large number of specimens. Consequently, the storage of tissues for various periods becomes a practical necessity.

From the vantage point of flow cytometry, the one overriding question is how the tissue storage conditions affect stability and detectability of DNA. Generally speaking, the tissues may be refrigerated for short-term and frozen for long-term storage. Storage of refrigerated tissues may be readily attained at temperatures of 4°C and below in any commercial refrigerator. However, one should bear in mind that tissues are poor heat conductors, and therefore they must be cut or minced into small pieces to ensure rapid and uniform cooling of the specimens. The second factor to be borne in mind is the fact that low temperatures only inhibit, but by no means abolish, enzymatic reactions. Thus, essential degradation of DNA in the refrigerated tissue specimens is inevitable. In practical terms, as is shown in Figure 3, tissue specimens may be stored for at least 3 weeks without any apparent effect on their DNA content.

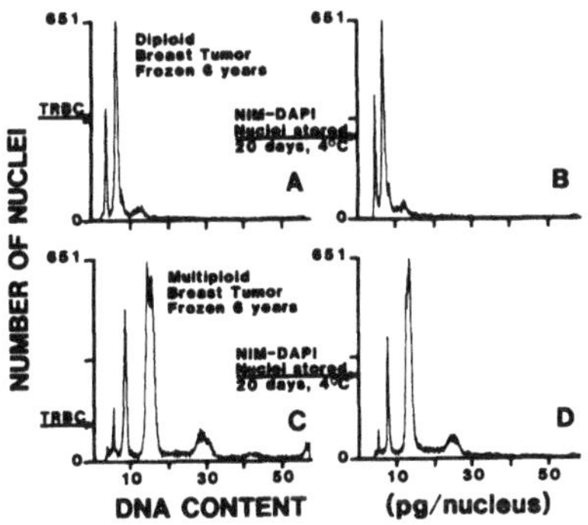

Figure 3. The DNA histograms of a (A) essentially diploid and (C) multiploid carcinomas of the breast stored for 6 years at - 70°C. The NIM nuclei were additionally refrigerated for 20 days at 4°C and their DNA content was then determined (B,D). Note that the DNA content of the respective samples was unaffected by 20 days storage at 4°C. The reference standard, in this case trout red blood cells, were stored under the same conditions as pointed out on the histograms.

Data presented here indicate that tissue samples may be refrigerated for over approximately 20 days without any detectable decline of their DNA content.

Whereas the loss of DNA by the refrigerated tissues will eventually be apparent, this is not the case with tissues frozen to -70°C and below. As was shown in Fig. 3, tissues may be stored indefinitely at -70°C.

Moreover, the freeze-thaw cycle (Table 1) likewise has no effect on the DNA levels detected by flow cytometry.

TABLE 1 - DNA ANALYSIS OF RAT TISSUE TYPE (pg/NUCLEUS)

	CEREBELLUM		LIVER		TESTIS		
Fresh	6.35±0.1	12.6±0.2	6.25±0.1	12.6±0.2	3.1±0.1	6.25±0.1	12.6±0.2
Frozen	6.25±0.1	12.5±0.1	6.45±0.1	13.2±0.1	3.2±0.1	6.35±0.0	12.4±0.1

± SD (n = 4 - 10)

This demonstrable stability of DNA in refrigerated and frozen tissues should not be misconstrued to imply that other macromolecules, which may be detected by flow cytometry, will remain equally unaffected by refrigeration and by the freeze-thaw cycle.

4. Adequate Sampling

One of the major practical determinants of quantitative cytometry is the acquisition of representative cell samples (46,47). For example, in the analysis of malignant tissues, there is always a posibility that a "pocket" of atypical cells, obtained during sampling procedure, may be considered to represent the predominant cell mass comprising a given tumor. In order to minimize such an unwanted possibility, multiple parts of the tissue should be analyzed. For example, Figure 4 is a schematic across-section of a human sarcoma of the leg. In this case, multiple parts of this tumor were analyzed for their DNA content.

Whereas the percentages of S-phase nuclei increased from the peripheral (6.68 ± 0.33 SD) to the intermediate (10.5 ± 1.14) parts of the tumor, the degree of aneuploidy varied only slightly in these samples. Two to three samples (1-3 mm^3), in our opinion, are sufficient to characterize the nuclear DNA distribution in the malignant breast tissue. Figure 5 shows an example of DNA histograms obtained from one $3mm^3$ primary breast tumor sections. The data are equivalent.

5. DNA standard

Criteria for selecting a DNA standard were accessilibity and storage stability, constancy of DNA content, CV in the 1 to 2% range, and absence of hyperdiploid nuclei which would overlap the DNA distribution of the sample so that minor fluctuations in instrumentation or staining would be evident in the channel shifts of the standard. Nucleated erythrocytes serve as the best DNA standards by the above criteria. For instance, trout (TRBC) (8,16,48) and chicken (CRBC) (16,38,41,48-53) erythrocytes have been used as DNA standards. For determinations of DNA levels in mammalian cells, the TRBC are prefered by us, since their DNA content is close to that of mammalian cells 2C peak (Fig. 6). TRBC do not show sex determined variations in DNA content as do cells derived from the chicken (48). The DNA peak of TRBC has a CV of 1% and the cells can be stored for several weeks at 4°C or frozen at -70°C for long

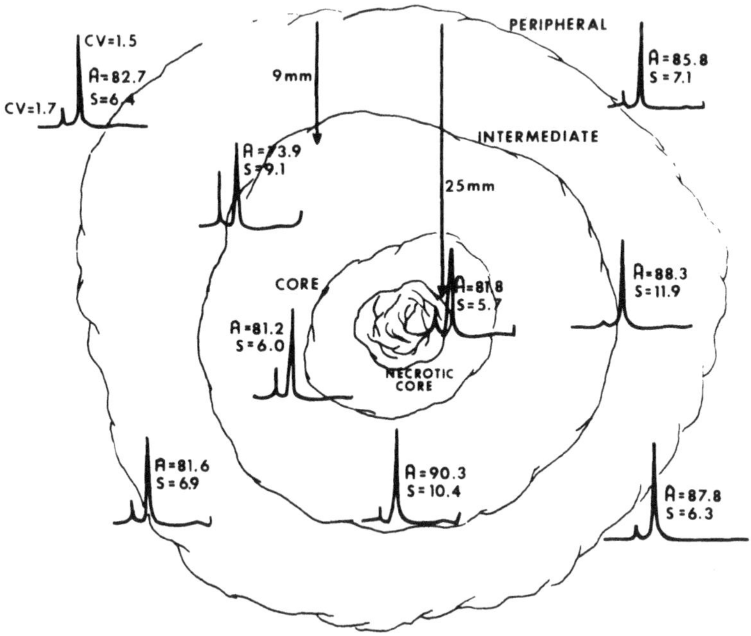

Figure 4. Equal masses of tissue were obtained from the tumor periphery, its intermediate part (9mm) and its core. Here S = percentage of hyperdiploid nuclei in the hyperdiploid S region. A = percentage of aneuploid nuclei (% of hyperdiploid nuclei out of the total nuclei analyzed). (Cytometry 1:229, 1980)

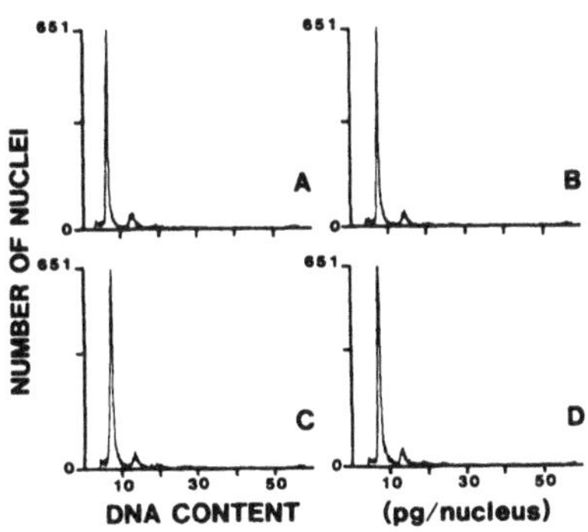

Figure 5. Four DNA histograms obtained from four $3mm^3$ tissues of a 5 year old MCF. Frozen, primary breast cancer tissue

periods of time (16,48) with no detectable change in DNA content. Evident superiority of TRBC as compared to CRBC is illustrated in Fig. 6.

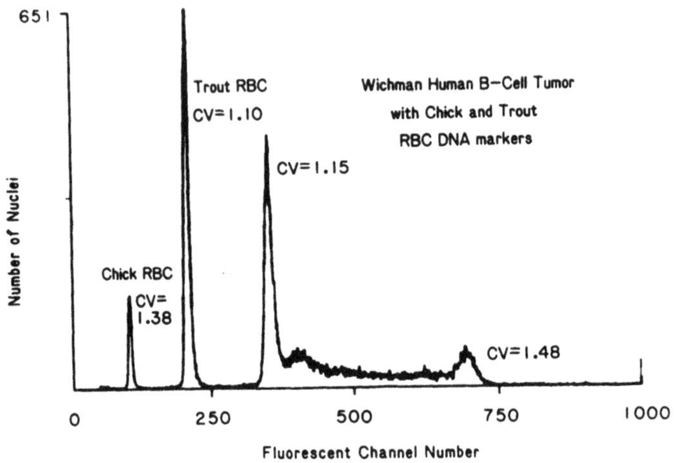

Figure 6. Comparison of chicken (CRBC) and trout (TRBC) red blood cell DNA standards with human Wichman B-cell line (courtesy of Dr. R. Braylan) nuclei. This graph demonstrates the clear separation of the sample peaks from those of the standards when CRBC and TRBC are added directly to the sample.

If possible, an additional internal standard should be analyzed in parallel with the tumor sample. It is defined as a part of control tissue of the same histologic type and hopefully obtained from the same donor. This, however, is not always possible, and thus the TRBC marker is always used. Cells isolated from many normal mammalian tissues (e.g. pancreas, liver, muscle, bone marrow, breast, pleural effusions) have been found to be diploid (or polyploid) (8-10,12,15), whereas prostatic epithelial cell populations contain cells with aneuploid DNA content. All cells isolated from fetal prostates were diploid as compared to cells derived from multiple samples of histologically normal young adults (18-28 yr old) (Fig. 7). Aneuploid cell populations were detected in the 23 normal human prostates obtained from accidental death victims. Table 2, using the TRBC marker, summarizes the multiple sampling data obtained from one of these normal prostate subjects. These data show the importance of determining the DNA distribution of cells obtained from normal tissue before measuring the DNA content of cells derived from diseased tissue.

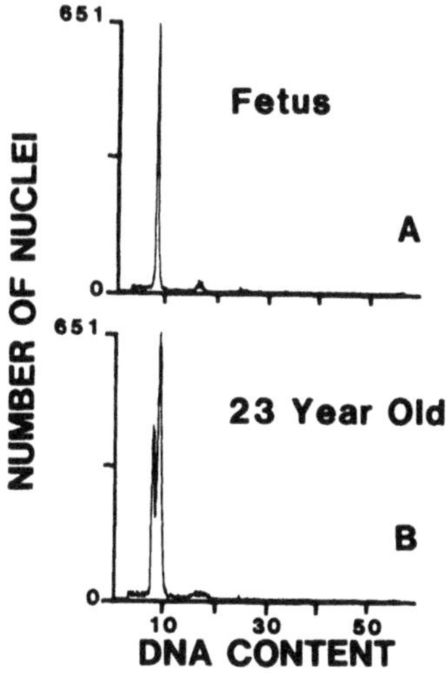

Figure 7. DNA flow cytometric histograms of prostatic epithelial cells obtained from (A) a fetus and a (B) 23 year old.

Table 2 reveals DNA flow cytometric data obtained from 5 sections of a normal prostate from the 28 year old. TRBC were used as the DNA standard (5.2 pg/nucleus). The percentage of aneuploid prostate nuclei was calculated by dividing the number of prostate nuclei, which were not contained in the 2C distribution, by the total number of prostate nuclei enumerated, and multiplying by 100%.

Table 2: DNA Flow Cytometric Data from 5 Sections of Prostate Tissue from a 28 yr old.

Section #	1	2	3	4	5	Mean ± SD[c]
Peak #1[a]	8.3	8.0	8.5	ND	8.2	8.3 ± 0.2
Peak #2[a]	10.9	9.4	10.3	9.7	10.8	10.2 ± 0.7
% Aneuploidy[b]	55	54	33	79	56	55 ± 16

[a] Data shown is in pg/nucleus as determined with TRBC standard (5.2 pg/nucleus).
[b] % of non-diploid nuclei
[c] Mean ± standard deviation (n = 5).
ND-Not clearly distinguishable

6. High Resolution Measurements

The resolution of DNA histograms may be defined as an unambiguous separation of two or more closely spaced DNA distributions. The resolution of these populations is inversely proportional to the coefficient of variations (CV) between, at least two, DNA histogram curves. The CV is derived through a relationship:

$$CV = \frac{\text{width of the curve at } 1/2 \text{ height}}{\text{Peak channel number x 2.35}} \times 100$$

We have obtained consistently high resolution CVs in the 0.8 to 2.0% range for most of the cells also analyzed elsewhere (8-10,12,55). The reasons for this consistency are of interest and therefore appear to merit a few remarks.

It is important to use standardized nuclear isolation and staining techniques (in this case NIM-DAPI procedures) to minimize variations between the samples. In addition, the flow cytometer we use is equipped with a mercury arc lamp which is ideally suited for the excitation of DNA-DAPI complex at 365 nm. The maximum fluorescence is emitted at 465 nm which is the optimum sensitivity range of S 20 photomutiplier tubes. In contrast, the conventional argon laser of commercially available flow cytometers fails to excite the DNA-DAPI complex (54). Moreover, epi illumination used in our instrument allows optimal focusing of excitation light, while making it possible by means of high aperature optics to capture most of the emitted light. This is not possible with the conventional flow cytometers (14-18) since they are capable of exciting only parts of large nuclei (D = 7um) with slit-scan cylindrical optics system, and register only a small quantity of fluorescence emission at 90° to the incident beam. The importance of high resolution measurements to generate DNA histograms is illustrated in the following figures. Figure 8A, DNA histogram of human blood leukocytes, shows them to be diploid cells with an excellent CV of 0.75. Conversely, the DNA histogram of pleural effusions (Fig. 8B) reveals that 57.6% of the nuclei are aneuploid. Without the high resolution, pleural effusion in this case could have easily have been interpreted as consisting of diploid cells with a low resolution measurement above CV = 3%. We have found high resoluton to be very important in differentiating diploid from near diploid primary breast cancers (8,9). Without the low CV = 1-2%, some cell populations can be falsely identified as having diploid DNA content. Example are shown in Figure 9.

The final example of the importance of resolution is shown in Figure 10. All but one of the primary breast tumors, characterized by cells with diploid DNA content, were from patients who survived more than five years. In Figure 10F, this patient only survived six months after tumor removal. Since two resolvable DNA populations were not found, this sample was classified as diploid. However, the CV was 5% compared to CV of less than 2% for the others.

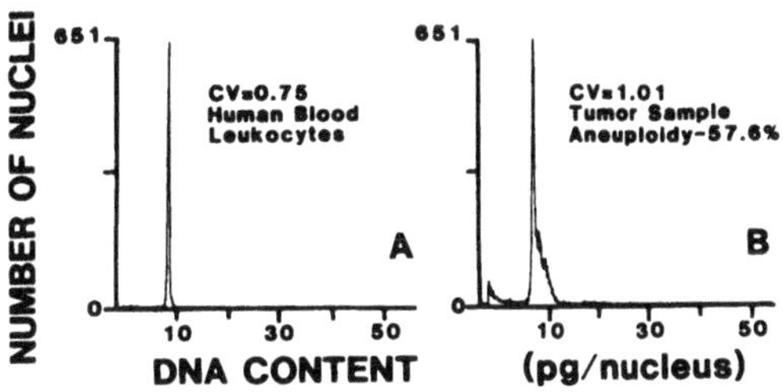

Figure 8. DNA histograms of a patient's (A) blood leukocytes and (B) pleural effusion.

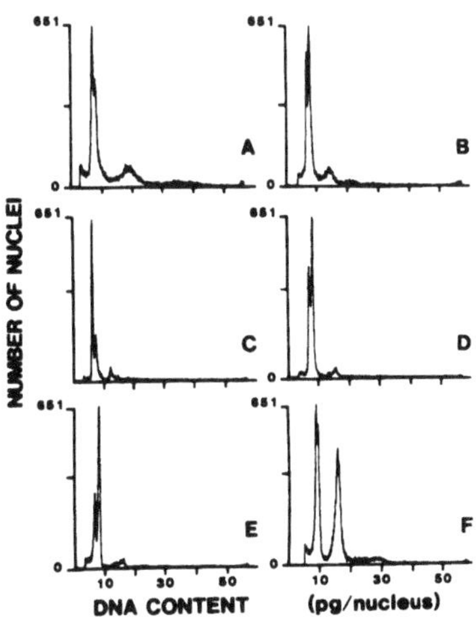

Figure 9. Examples of DNA histograms from (A-E) near-diploid MCF primary breast cancer tumors. The CVs were less than 2%.
(F) multiploid tumor with near-diploid cell population.

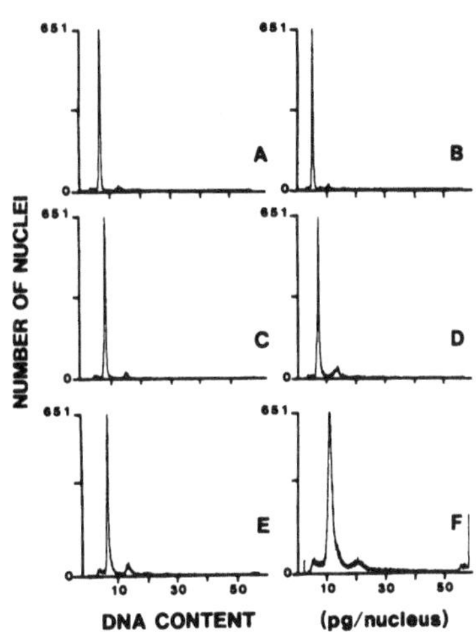

Figure 10. Examples of DNA histograms from MCF primary breast cancer tumors. (A-E) diploid tumors, surviving at 5 years, CV - 1-2%
(F) diploid tumor, death at six months, CV = 5%.

7. Some clinical applications of DNA flow cytometry

Space will not permit a detailed discussion of all clinical applications of DNA flow cytometry. The reader is therefore referred to two recent, excellent review articles on this subject (55,56). However, one important aspect will be reviewed briefly, namely, the correlation between DNA histogram parameters and survival of primary breast cancer patients (8,9). Figure 11 shows a DNA histogram of cells derived from a tumor and gives the relevant parameters for analysis of the data.

Primary mammary carcinomas were evaluated for the biochemical presence of steroid cytosolic receptors and by flow cytometry (8). These parameters were compared with the histological staging and the patients' survival over a 36-month period. A total of 74 patients were evaluated. The tumors were classified into five DNA histogram types based on their DNA content. The results of this study showed that 21% of the tumors were diploid and thus indistinguishable from the diploid population of normal breast cells, 8% were hypodiploid, 11% were hypertetraploid, 8% were multiploid, and the remaining 52% were hyperdiploid. All the breast samples invariably demonstrated a peak population of diploid $G_{0/1}$ cells which contained 2C amounts of DNA.

Figure 12 shows the survival curves generated by the DNA type and surgical stage using the Kaplan-Meier method on data from the Tennessee study (8). It is evident that the DNA type is superior to staging in dividing these 74 cases into groups of similar risks ($p<.05$ and $p<.08$, respectively). Estrogen receptor (E_2R) status was also tested and found not to be significant.

Similar results were found in a preliminary study of MCF data reported in Table 3. The percentage of aneuploid cells was the most important single variable. The diploid type per se was not significant in this preliminary data set. For comparison, other commonly used prognostic indicators were also tested. Although the percent aneuploid (tumor load, Fig. 11) was correlated with E_2R status ($p<0.04$) (9), E_2R status was not significantly related to survival. Tumor-node-metastasis (TNM) stage may be a relevant factor, but the data do not demonstrate this as clearly as they show the importance of the percent aneuploid. There was no relation between the percent aneuploid and staging of the tumor ($p>0.5$).

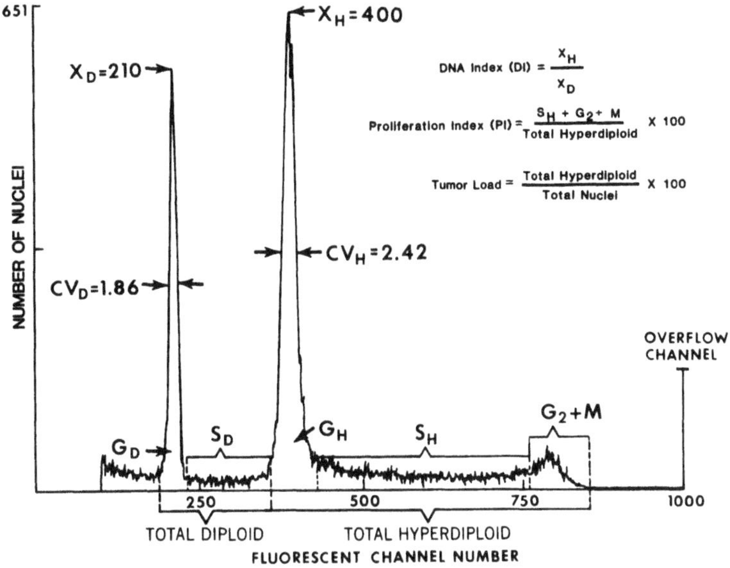

Figure 11. Data from an aneuploid FC histogram. CV of the diploid (CV_D), hyperdiploid (CV_H), peaks are shown with their normalized ratio(CV_N). The fluorescent peak channels of the diploid (X_D) and hyperdioloid (X_H) populations are shown with their normalized ratio, DNA index, DI. The areas under the curves show the diploid (G_D) and hyperdiploid (G_H) $G_1 + G_0$ populations, while only the hyperdiploid $G_D + S$ curve is shown since the diploid $G_2 + M$ component is overlapped by G_H. The S regions are defined as those areas of the curve not encompassed by G_D, G_H, and $G_2 + M$. They may or may not include only the diploid (S_D) or hyperdiploid (S_H) cells undergoing DNA synthesis. An increase in the S region has been interpreted as an increase in the proliferation of diploid and hyperdiploid populations of the tumor. The proliferation index of the aneuploid (hyperdiploid) population is defined in the Figure. The total hyperdiploid cells are equal to all of the cells in G_H, S_H and $G_2 + M$, while the total diploid cells are in the G_D and S_D regions. The % aneuploid (tumor load) is calculated as shown in the figure. The overflow channel (channel 1000) shows the number of nuclei with fluorescence greater than channel 999. (Cytometry 1:229, 1980)

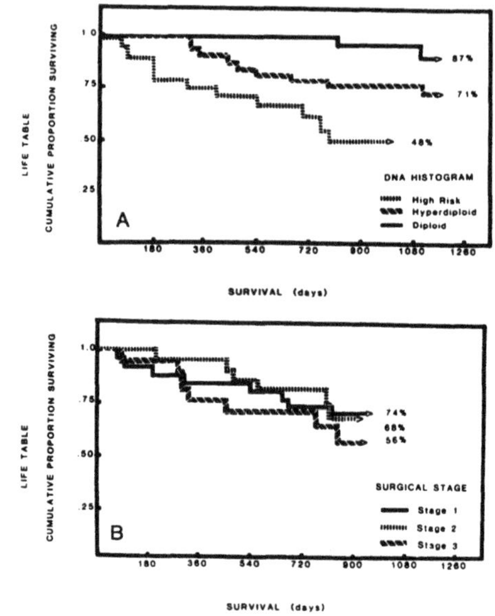

Figure 12. A, life expectancy table correlation of breast cancer patients with five DNA histogram types (n = 74). The 36 month survival of diploid tumor patients was 87%. Reference: Kaplan Meier product-limit estimate of survivorship (57,58). Survival = days from receptor assay (breast surgery) to death. B, life expectancy table of breast cancer patients in relation to surgical stage groups (n = 60). The 36-month survival for Stage 1 patients was 74%; for Stage 2 patients it was 68%, and for Stage 3 patients, it was 56%. Cancer Res. 44:4187, 1984.

Table 3. Statistical Analysis of the Preliminary Data from MCF Breast Tumors

	MCF Data					
	30-mo survival (n = 33)			60-mo Survival (n = 28)		
	X^2	df	P value	X^2	df	P-value
% Aneuploid ≤49	8.17	2	0.017	5.41	2	0.067
% Aneuploid ≤49 and PIa ≤17	9.46	4	0.050	9.69	4	0.046
Diploid Type	3.60	4	0.463	3.97	4	0.410
TNM Stage	11.51	6	0.074	7.45	6	0.281
E_2R Status	0.32	2	0.85	1.34	2	0.512

Note: Since the cases used in this study were selected on the basis of their recurrence status, survival was tested in conjunction with recurrence. This is reflected in the degrees of freedom. (df)

While more data are needed, the importance of the DNA measurements as prognostic indicators is apparent in the two studies. With the small sample size used in these studies, the DNA variables are significant when commonly accepted indicators are marginally significant at best.

REFERENCES

1. Knowles DM II, Dodson LD, Raab R, Mittler RS, Talle MA, Goldstein G: The application of monoclonal antibodies to the characterization and diagnosis of lymphoid neoplasms: a review of recent studies. Diag Immuno (1):142-149, 1983.
2. Janossy G, Thomas JA, Pizzolo G, Granger SM, McLaughlin J, Habeshaw JA, Stansfeld AG, Sloane J: Immuno-histological diagnosis of lymphoproliferative diseases by selected combinations of antisera and monoclonal antibodies. Br J Cancer (42):224, 1980.
3. Knowles DM II: Non-Hodgkin's lymphomas. Current immunologic concepts. In: Fenoglio CM, Wolff M, (eds) Progress in surgical pathology, Vol 2, New York, Masson Publishing, pp 107-143, 1980.
4. Bach MA, Bach J-F: The use of monoclonal anti-T cell antibodies to study T cell imbalances in human diseases. Clin Exp Immunol (45):449-456, 1981.
5. Engleman EG, Warnke R, Fox RI, Dilley J, Benike CJ, Levy R: Studies of a human T lymphocyte antigen recognized by a monoclonal antibody. Proc Natl Acad Sci USA (78):1791-1795, 1981.
6. Fairbanks TR: Current status of lymphocyte subpopulation testing in humans.

Am J Med Technol (46):471-475, 1980.
7. Kamentsky LA, Melamed MR, Derman H: Spectrophotometer: a new instrument for ultrarapid cell analysis. Science 150, 1965.
8. Coulson PB, Thornthwaite JT, Woolley TW, Sugarbaker EV, Seckinger D: Prognostic indicators including DNA histogram type, receptor content, and staging related to human breast cancer patient survival. Cancer Res (44):4187-4196, 1984.
9. Russo J, Thornthwaite JT, Thomas RA, Woolley TW, Ownby H, Frederick J, Sapereto S, Seckinger D: Relationship of DNA flow cytometric analysis to survival in human primary breast cancer. Proceedings of the International Academy of Pathology
10. Collins J, Bagwell CB, Block NL, Claflin AJ, Irvin G III, Pollack A, Stover B: Flow cytometric monitoring of R 3327 rat prostate carcinoma. Invest. Urol. (19):8-13, 1981.
11. White RV, Deitch AD, Olsson CA: Limitations of DNA histogram analysis by flow cytometry as a method of predicting chemosensitivity in a rat renal cancer model. Cancer Res (43):604-610, 1983.
12. Goldberg ID, Rosen EM, Shapiro HM, Zoller LC, Myrick K, Levenson SE: Isolation and culture of a tetraploid subpopulation of smooth muscle cells from the normal rat aorta. Science (226):559-561, 1984.
13. Shapiro HM: Multistation multiparameter flow cytometry: a critical review and rationale. Cytometry (3):227, 1983.
14. Loken MR, Herzenberg LA: Analysis of cell populations with a fluorescence-activated cell sorter. Ann NY Acad Sci (254):163, 1975.
15 Thornthwaite JT, Rasch EM: Picogram per cell determination of DNA by flow cytometry. Anal Biochem (137):221-226, 1984.
16. Lee GL, Thornthwaite JT, Rasch EM: Picogram per cell determination of DNA by flow cytometry. Anal Biochem (137):221-226, 1984.
17. Wolley RC, Schreiber K, Koss LG, Karas M, Sherman A: DNA distribution in human colon carcinomas and its relationship to cinical behavior. J Natl Cancer Inst (69):15-22, 1982.
18. Evans D, Thornthwaite JT, Sugarbaker EV, Ng ABP: DNA flow cytometry of human pleural effusions: comparison with pathology for the diagnosis of malignancy. Quant Anal Cytol (5):19-27, 1983.
19. Schumann J: Die wirkung von bleomycin auf die DNA von tumorzellen in vivo und in vitro. In: Wust G (ed.) Aktuelle probleme der therapie malinger tumoren, Stutgart, pp 85-95, 1973.
20. Zante J, Schumann J, Barlogie B, Gohde W, Buchner TH: New preparating and staining procedures for specific and rapid analysis of DNA distributions. In: Gohde W, Schumann J, Buchner T (eds) Second international symposium on pulse cytophotometry, European Press, Medikon, Ghent, pp 97-106, 1976.
21. Dosik GM, Barlogie B, Johnston DA, Murphy WK, Drewinko B: Lethal and cytokinetic effects of anguidine on a human colon cancer cell line. Cancer Res (38):3304, 1978.
22. Barlogie B, Hittelman W, Spitzer G, Trujillo JM, Hart JS, Smallwood L, Drewinko B: Correlation of DNA distribution abnormalities with cytogenetic findings in human adult leukemia and lymphoma. Cancer Res (37):44000, 1977.
23 Horan PK, Romero A, Steinkamp JA, Petersen DF: Detection of heteroploid tumor cells. J Natl Cancer Inst (52):843, 1974.
24. Barlogie B, Gohde W, Johnston A, Smallwood L, Schumann J, Drewinko B, Freireich DJ: Determination of ploidy and proliferative characteristics of human solid tumors by pulse cytophotometry. Cancer Res (38):3333, 1978.
25. Noel JS, Zucker RM, Wu NC, Demaray SY: The dissociation of transplantable tumors. J. Histochem Cytochem (25): 544, 1977.
26. Escobar GJ, Todd P, Sattilaro RF: The dispersal of cells from human gyneologic

specimens: chemical agents. J Histochem Cytochem (25):513, 1977.
27. Leif RC, Nordquist G, Clay S, Cayer M, Ingram D, Cameron BF, Bobbit D, Gaddis R, Leif SB, Cabanas A: A procedure for dissociating ayre scrape samples. J Histochem Cytochem (25):525,1977.
28. Goerttler K, Balmain A, Sauerborn R: Comparison of various cell dispersal techniques applied to the model of the mouse skin. In: Second International Symposium on Pulse Cytophotometry, Gohde W, Schumann J, Buchner T (eds.) European Press, Medikon, Ghent, 1976, p. 156-161
29. Waymouth C: To disaggregate or not to disaggregate. Injury and cell disaggregation, transient or permanent? In Vitro (10):97, 1974.
30. Blobel G, Potter VR: Nuclei from rat liver: isolation method that combines purity with high yeild. Science (154):1662, 1966.
31. Horvat A: Insulin binding sites on rat liver nuclear membranes: biochemical and immunofluorescent studies. J Cell Physiol (97):37, 1978.
32. Krishan A: Rapid flow cytofluorometric analysis of mammalian cell cycle by propidium iodide staining. J Cell Biol (66):188, 1975.
33. Krishan A, Ganapathi RN, Israel M: Effect of adriamycin and analogs on the nuclear fluorescence of propidium iodide-stained cells. Cancer Res (38):3656, 1978.
34. Vindelov LL: Flow microfluorometric analysis of nuclear DNA in cells from solid tumors and cell suspensions. Virchows Arch (Cell Pathol) (24):227, 1977.
35. Thornthwaite JT, Thomas RA, Leif SB, Yopp TA, Cameron BF, Leif RC: The use of electronic cell volume analysis with the AMAC II to determine the optimum glutaraldehyde fixative concentration for nucleated mammalian cells. In Scaning Electron Microscopy, Vol II SEM INC, AMF O'Hare, Illinois, 1978, p 1123-1130.
36. Cesarone CF, Bolognesi C, Santi L: Improved microfluorometric DNA determination in biological material using 33258 Hoechst. Anal Biochem (100):188-197, 1979.
37. Labarca C, Paigen K: A simple, rapid, and sensitive DNA assay procedure. Anal Biochem (102):344-352, 1980.
38. Williams SK, Sasaki AW, Matthews MA, Wagner RC: Quantitative determination of deoxyribonucleic acid from cells collected on filters. Anal Biochem (107):17-20, 1980.
39 Coleman AW, Maguire MJ, Coleman JR: Mitharmycin and 4',6-diamidino-2-phenylindole (DAPI) DNA staining for fluorescence microspectrophotometric measurements of DNA in nuclei, plastids, and virus particles. J Histochem Cytochem (29):959-968, 1981.
40. Russel WC, Newman C, Williamson DH: A simple cytochemical technique for demonstration of DNA cells infected with mycoplasmas and viruses. Nature (253):461-462, 1975.
41. Taylor IW, Milthrope BK: An evaluation of DNA fluorochromes, staining techniques, and analysis for flow cytometry. J Histochem Cytochem (28):1224-1232, 1980.
42. Dann O, Bergen G, Demant E, Volz G: Trypanocide diamidine des 2-phenyl-indols. Justus Liebigs Ann Chem (748):68-79, 1971.
43 Lin MS, Comings DI, Alfi OS: Optical studies of the interaction of 4'-6-diamidino-2-phenylindole with DNA and metaphase chromosomes. Chromosoma (Berlin) (60):15-25, 1977.
44. Latt SA; Fluorometric detection of deoxyribonucleic acid synthesis; possibilities for interfacing bromodeoxyuridine dye techniques with flow cytometry. J Histochem Cytochem (25):913-926, 1977.
45. James TW, Jope C: Visualization of fluorescence of chloroplast DNA in higher plants by means of the DNA specific probe 4'6'-diamidino-2-phenylindole. J Cell Biol (79):623-628, 1978.
46. Leif RC, Easter, HN Jr, Warters RL, Thomas RA, Dunlap LA, Austin MF:

Centrifugal cytology. I. A quantitative technique for the preparation of glutaraldehyde-fixed cells for the light and scanning electron microscope. J Histo and Cyto (19)No 4:203-215, 1971.
47. Thornthwaite JT, Leif RC: The plaque cytogram assay. I. Light and scanning electron microscopy of immunocompetent cells. J Immuno (113)No 6:1897-1908, 1974.
48. Vindelov LL, Christensen IJ, Keiding N, Spang-Thomsen M, Nissen NI: Long term storage of samples for flow cytometric DNA analysis. Cytometry (3):317-327, 1983.
49. Pogany GC, Corzett M, Weston S, Balhorn R: DNA and protein content of mouse sperm. Implications regarding sperm chromatin structure. Exp Cell Res (136):127-136, 1981.
50. Noguchi PD, Browne WC: The use of chicken erythrocyte nuclei as a biological standard four flow microfluorometry. J. Histochem Cytochem (26):761-762, 1978.
51. Tannenbaum E, Cassidy M, Alabaster O, Herman C: Measurement of cellular DNA mass by flow microfluorometry with use of a biological internal standard. J. Histochem Cytochem (26):145-148, 1978.
52. Rasch EM, Prehn LM, Rasch RW: Cytogenic studies of Poecilia (Pisces) II triploidy and DNA levels in maturally occurring populations associated with the gynogenetic teleost, Poecilia Formosa (Girard). Chromosoma (31):18-40, 1970.
53. Sugarbaker EV, Thornthwaite JT, Temple WT, Ketcham AS: Flow cytometry: general principles and applications to selected studies in tumor biology. Int Adv Surg Oncol (2):125-153, 1979.
54. Peters DC: A comparison of mercury arc lamp and laser illumination for flow cytometers. J Histochem Cytochem 27:241, 1979.
55. Lovett EJ III, Schnitzer B, Keren DF, Flint A, Hudson JL, McClatchey KD: Application of flow cytometry to diagnostic pathology. Lab Invest (50):115-140, 1984.
56. Friedlander M, Hedley DW, Taylor IW: Clinical and biological significance of aneuploidy in human tumors. J Clin Pathol (37):961-974, 1984.
57. Kaplan EL, Meier P: Nonparametric estimation from incomplete observations. J Am Stat Assoc (53):357-381, 1958.
58. Lee ET: Statistical methods for survival data analysis. Belmont, CA: Lifetime Learning Publications, 1980.

Acknowledgements

We thank Mrs. Buchanan for typing the manuscript, and Mrs. Bradley, Ms. Lee and the Medical Media Department of Cedars Medical Center for preparation of the figures. We also thank the publishers of Analytical Biochemistry, Cytometry and Cancer Research for the modified reproduction of Figures 2, 4, 11 and 12, respectively. We thank Dr. B. Buck for the fetal prostate tissue, and Mrs. Castiglione for freezing tissues and obtaining patient data.

INDEX

A

ABC immunoperoxidase technique,4,12,14,36,40,45,84,87,91,151,184,215,236,271
Acid phosphatase (AP), 84,99,102,103
Acromegaly, 186
ACTH, 175,186,187,188,191,192,194,298,350
Actin, 6,25,27,73,207,208,300,363,372
Activated cells 7
Acquired immunodeficiency (AID), 155
Acute lymphoblastic leukemia, 141,142,156
Acute lymphocytic lymphoma, 120,155
Acute monocytic leukemia, 100
Adenocarcinoma, 5,22,23,24,25,34,44,337
Adenoma, salivary gland, 42
Adrenocorticotrophin, 6
Adrenaline, 190
Adult T cell leukemia/lymphoma, 104
Adult tissue, 282
AE1, 32,36,37,38,40,45,46,49,51
AE3,32
Aldosterone, 205
Alkaline phosphatase (ALP) 6,84,85,107
Allergic encephalitis, 16
Alpha-1-anti-chymotrypsin, 372
Alpha-1-Antitrypsin, 5,106,108,121,129,297,302,372
Alpha fetoprotein, 6,25,26,207,297,302,303,322,323,324, 325,326,327,329,330, 331,335
Alpha lactalbumin, 5,208,213,214
Alpha naphtyl acetate esterase (AEST), 84, 104, 107
Alpha naphtyl butyrate esterase (B-EST) 84,105,107
Alpha subunit (hCG),187
Algorithms, 21
Alveolar soft sarcoma, 370
Alzheimer's disease, 12, 18
Amelanotic melanoma, 35,40,42,50
Amino ethyl carbazole (AEC), 79, 152
Aneuploid, 388, 391
Angiocentric immunoproliferative lesions, 104
Angiocentric lymphomas, 104
Angiosarcomas 25, 27,76,372
Anti basal lamina, 31
Antibodies (Ab) 281,282,285,287,288
Antibodies against:
    Breast tissue, 208
    BA1, 154
    B4, 120,121,125,126
    B1:1, 120,121,124,129,131,141,161
    B6:2, 215, 218, 219
    B7, 129
    B72:3, 215,217,218,219,224
    Casein, 208, 214
    Collagen IV, 208, 214

T29/33 31,40,41,49,52
T200, 31,40,41,49,52
Elastin, 208,214,215
Epithelial membrane, 208
Fat globule membrane 208, 224
human mammary epithelial cells, 233, 243
kappa light chain, 154
keratin, 22,23,25, 208, 209, 219, 356
lactoferrin, 208, 214
lambda light chain 154
laminin, 208,214
lung cancer, 22,26
mu chain 154
myosin, 208
perikaryonal neurofibrillar antibody, 17
synapse associated complex, 17
Tac, 87
Uro1, 283,284,285
Uro2, 283,284,285,286
Uro3, 283,284,285,286
Uro4, 283,285,286
Uro5, 283,284,285,290
Uro7, 286
Uro9, 286,288
Uro10, 286,288
Antidiuretic hormone (ADH), 194
Arachis hipogaea, 352
Argyrofil stain, 293
Ascitis tumor cells, 2
ASD - Chloroacetate esterase (ASD-CL), 84, 85,107
Astrocytoma, 287
Atrial myocardium, 202, 204,205
Atypical carcinoids, 174
Atypical fibrous histiocytoma, 52
Autoimune diseases, 155

B

Basement membrane 47,48, 345
Basset granules, 105
B Cells, 7,120,142,148,149
B cell lymphoma, 7, 25,27,83,85
Beta endorphin, 191
B 5-fixative, 27,144,150,160,216
Biotin-Avidin 116,119
Bladder, 5,283
Cancer, 283, 286, 287, 288
Papillomas, 287
Blood brain barrier, 16
Blood group antigens, 351
Blood group isoantigen, 5
B lymphocytes 7
Bombesin, 175,179
Bone marrow, 35,142,143,158

Bouin's fixative, 118,152,176
Breast, 25,26,46,47,48,75,207,265,266,272,385
Breast carcinoma, 5,35,233,274,287
Breast epithelium, 210
Bronchi, 75
Bronchogenic carcinoma, 289
Bronchopulmonary tract, 174
Buffered formalin, 151,161
Burkitt's lymphoma, 97,118

C

Calcitonin, 6,25,26,125,189, 190, 191, 192, 304
Calcium Chloride, 10
CALLA, 93,95,97,98,121,125,126,150,154,158,159
Capping, 148,149
Carbodiimide, 203
Carcinoembryonic antigen (CEA) 5,8,22,23,44,45,46,52,161,207,215, 218,219,220,223,224,323,353,355,364
Carcinoid, 5,35,174,183
Carcinoma of pancreas,297
Carcinoma of prostate, 342
Carcinoma of stomach, 297
Cardionatrins, 202,203,204
Casein, 5,214
C cells, 189,190
C cell hyperplasia 6
Cell lines, 269, 276
Cell suspension, 116,118,146,148,152
Cell types, 131,184
Cell viability, 142
Cerebellum, 14,17,386
Cerebral spinal fluid, 141,144,159,160
Cervical Intraepithelial neoplasia, 63
Cervix, 5,24
Channel ratio method, 384
Chondroblast, 75
Chondroma, 39
Chondrosarcoma 39,43, 370
Chordoid sarcoma, 34
Chordoma,34,39,42,187
Choriocarcinoma, 25,26,322, 332
Chorionic gonadotropin, 6,295,296,301
Chromagranin, 193, 304,308
Chromosomal analysis, 353
Chromosomal translocation, 97,98
Chronic lymphocytic leukemia (CLL),93,94
Chronic lymphocytic lymphoma, 126
Chronic lymphocytic lymphoma B cell type, 155
" " " Non B-Non T cell type, 155,156,159
" " " T cell type, 156
Clinical application, 381
Clinical imaging, 282
Clonal excess value, 162,163
Clonal expansion, 124

Coefficient variation, 389,390
Collagenase, 381
Collagen type IV, 47,48,49,50,301
Collecting duct, 285
Colloidal gold, 203,205
Colon, 5,24,46,287,294
Common acute lymphoma leukemia antigen (CALLA) 285
Common epithelial membrane antigen (CEMA), 151,161,170
Common leukocyte antigen (CLA, T200), 25,27,85,98,151,161
Concanavalin, 236,241,254
Congenital Immunodeficiency, 155
Corneocyte, 59
Coronary bypass, 203
Corpus Pineale, 185,189
Corticoliberin, 186, 192
Corticotrophs, 187
Craniopharyngiomas, 188
C_3b, 129
C_3d, 9,95,96,97,98,99
C_3 receptors, 105,124,153
Cutaneous T cell lymphoma, 120
Cyst, 207
Cystosarcoma phylloides, 209
Cytosol, 264
Cytospin, 142,146,147,148
Cytotoxic T lymphocytes, 7

D

DAB (Diaminobenzidine), 151
DAPI (4'-6'-diamino-2-phenylindole)-, 382,383, 384
DAPI-DNA complex, 384,390
Defatted human milk, 210
Dendritic reticulum cells, 105,106
Desmin, 6,25,32,72,73,74,75,76,77,299,302, 365, 370
Desmoplakin, 176,177
Diaminobenzidine, 79
Differentiation antigen, 281
Diffuse aggressive lymphoma, 96
Diffuse neuroendocrine system, 6
Di George syndrome, 155
Diploid, 385,391,393,
Distal Tubule, 205
DMSO (Dimethylsulfoxide),88,123
DNA content 353
DNA histogram 386, 389, 392, 394
DNA Index, 393
DNA intercalating dyes, 383
DNA measurements, 380
DNA stability, 381, 385
DNA standard, 380, 381,384,386,388
Down syndrome, 18
Ductal carcinoma, 208, 209, 213
Duodenum, 295

Dysgerminoma, 303
Dysplasia, 63

E

EAC,84,107
Early thymocytes,120
Eccrine ducts, 62
Ectopic, 184,192
EMA (epithelial membrane antigen), 210,212
Embryonal carcinoma, 38, 322, 324, 325, 327, 328, 335
Endocervix, 301
Endocrine cells, 202
Endocrine glands, 183
Endocrine tumors, 183
Endodermal sinus tumor, 302
Endogenous peroxidase, 10,151,152
Endometrial carcinoma, 299, 298, 299, 300, 305, 309
Endometrium, 272, 301
Enzymatic disociation, 381
Ependymomas, 25, 305, 306
Epidermis, 33, 75
Epidermoid, 59, 60, 63
Epinephrine, 191
Epithelial antigen, 364
Epithelial cells, 43, 72, 207, 208
Epithelial mesothelioma, 34, 74
Epithelial tumors, 299
Epithelioid sarcoma, 34, 39, 365, 370
Epithelioid schwanoma, 40
E Rosettes, 84,99,142,149,153,154,159
Estradiol,193,270,306
Estrogen, 268
Estrogen receptor (E2R), 223,224,225,237, 238, 239, 240,241,242, 264, 266, 268 270, 273, 301, 392
Estrogen regulated protein, 268
Estrone, 193
Estrophilin, 264
Ethidium bromide, 4
Eutopic, 184
Ewing's sarcoma, 178, 363
Exocrine pancreas, 214

F

Fab fragment, 10
Fab_e fragment, 18,148
Factor VIII, 5,25,27,372,377
Fat globule membrane monoclonal Ab-(MC5), 5
FC receptor, 105,148
Ferritin, 303
Fetal tissue, 282
Fibroadenoma, 209
Fibroblasts, 75
Fibrocystic disease, 213, 216

Fibromatosis, 43
Fibronectin, 323
Fibrosarcoma, 76
Fibrous histiocytoma, 38
Ficoll, 118
Ficoll-hypaque, 143,145
Fillagrin, 59,65,66,67
Flow cytometry, 84,90,114,117,353, 380, 385
Fluorescein, 47
Fluorescence, 284
Fluorochromes, 146,147,380,382,383
Follicular center cell tumor, 25
Follicular lymphoma 94,131
Follicular small cleaved lymphoma, 120,132
Follicle stimulating hormone, 6, 187, 195
Fresh tissue, 117,386,
Frozen sections, 2,3,41,84,116,118,142,151,184,264,283
Frozen tissue, 142,151,385

G

Gamma glutamyl transptidase, 323
Gangliocytomas, 186
Gastric lymphomas, 141
Gastrin, 5, 175, 192, 298, 304
Gastrointestinal tract, 75
Germ cell tumors, 6, 25, 26, 34, 37, 301, 322
Glial fibrillary acidic protein, 5, 72, 73, 74,75, 78, 80, 186, 305, 306, 364
Glial fibrillary antigen, 25, 27
Glial filaments, 32
Gliomas, 5, 3, 7, 76
Glomangiomas, 377
Glomerulus, 285
Glucagon,5,192,298,304,305
Glucose oxidase, 152
Glutaraldehyde, 203
Glycoproteins, 283
Glycoprotein GP52, 216
Glycosaminoglycans, 52
Glycosyltransferase, 351
Golgi complex, 202, 205
Gonadoblastoma, 303
Gonadoliberin, 185
Granules, 205
Granular cell tumor, 370
Granulosa cells, 321
Granulosa cell tumor 42, 296, 321
Granulocytes, 7
Granulocytic sarcoma, 25, 27
Growth hormone,6,185,186

H

Hairy cell leukemia, 88
Hassal's corpuscles, 33
Hamartoma, 185
Hanks balanced salt solution (HBSS), 172
Helper, 7,101,120,121,126
Helper/inducer T cells, 150
Hemangiomas, 5
Hemangioendothelioma, 372
Hemangiopericytoma, 377, 363
Hemangiosarcomas, 5
Hematopoietic stem cell, 7
Hemocyanin, 203
Henle's loop, 285
Hepatitis, 34
Hepatitis B antigen, 5
Hepatocellular carcinoma, 5, 34, 297
Hepatoid yolk sac tumor, 302
Hepatoma, 25, 26
Hepatosplenomegaly, 104
Histaminase, 6
Histidine rich protein, 65
Histiocytic cells, 105
Histiocytic proliferation, 27, 106
Histiocytosis X, 108
Histochemical markers, 207
Histoplasma capsulatum, 156
Hodgkin's disease 109,117,133,155,156,169,171
Hoechtst, 33, 258, 383
Hormone Precursors, 185, 195
Hormone receptors, 185, 194, 195, 350
Human chorionic gonadotropin (hCG), 25, 26, 189, 219, 221, 222, 224, 277, 323, 325, 327, 332, 333, 335, 346
Human mammary glycoprotein, 216
Human milk, 43
Human placental lactogen, 297, 302, 323, 325, 334
Hyaline bodies, 302
Hyaluronic acid, 52
Hybridomas, 269
Hydrogen peroxide, 10
Hypercalcemia, 104, 194
Hyperdiploid, 8,14
Hypergammaglobulinemia, 102
Hyperplasia, 208, 213, 340,341
Hypogammaglobulinemia, 94,101
Hypothalamic gangliocytoma, 189
Hypothalamus, 184, 185, 186

I

Ia antigen 120,125,126,127
Idiotypic sites, 13
Immature B cells, 120
Immature cortical thymocytes, 120
Immature teratoma, 322, 330

Immunoanatomy, 283
Immunoblastic lymphoma, 132
Immunoblotting tests, 282
Immunodeficiency syndromes,143,156
Immunoferritin, 4
Immunofluorescence, 2,3,77,146,184,287,288
Immunogen, 283,286
Immunoglobulins,
  IgA 7,89
  IgD, 89
  IgE 90
  IgG, 88,89
  IgJ, 7
  IgM, 7,89,131,148
Immunohistogenesis, 281, 282
Immunoperoxidase, 3,79,150,184,287
Immunoprecipitation, 282
Immunotherapy, 282
Inducer, 120,121,126
Inducer T lymphocytes, 7
Infiltrating ductal carcinoma, 236, 237, 253
Insulin, 192, 304, 305
Interdigitating reticulum cells,105,106
Intermediate B type cell, 155,163,164,166
Intermediate filaments, 32, 72, 73, 79, 81, 208, 299, 369
Intestine associated antigens, 295
Intracellular bridges, 21
Intracytoplasmic lamina, 245, 246, 247, 249, 255, 260
Intraductal carcinoma, 212
Intravascular bronchiolo alveolar tumor, 377
Inventory, 9
Involucrin, 60,61,62,63,64,300
Isoantigen A 351
  B 351
  O 351
  H 351
Isoantigens, 349

J

J5, 80,98,120,121,125,126

K

Kaposi, 25,27,377
Kappa chain, 7,25,27, 94,125,126,130,132,135,136,147,161
Keratin, 5,8,31,32,36,59,60,68,73,161,229,303,307,349,364
Keratinocyte, 60
Keratoacanthomas, 62
Keratohyalin, 65
Keratolinin, 68
Kidney, 34,46,75,283
Krukemberg tumor, 296

L

Laboratory equipment, 3
Laboratory organization, 1,2
Lactalbumin, 24, 25
Lactic acid dehidrogenase, 323
Lactotrophs,186
Lacunar cells,117
Lambda chain, 7,25,27,94,125,126,130,135,136,147,161
Laminin, 47, 48, 301
Langerhans cells, 42, 105,109
Langerhans islets, 192
Large cell undifferentiated carcinoma, 65
Large cell lymphoma, 42, 49, 163,164,167
Large cell non cleaved lymphoma, 121, 125, 129,130
Large granular lymphocyte, 128
Larynx, 51
Lectin, 233, 241, 242, 253, 254, 349
Leiomyosarcoma, 76
Leukocytes 40,75
Leukocyte common antigen (T200), 31,40,41,49,52
Leukoenkephalin, 175,179
Leukoplakias, 62, 63,64,68
Leydig cells, 277, 321
Leydig cell tumor, 6
Lichen planus, 62
Light chain Ig,118
Lipoma, 43
Liposarcomas, 25,43,76,363,370
Liquid nitrogen, 8
Liver, 75, 386
Lobular carcinoma, 208, 213
Lobular carcinoma in situ, 208
Lung, 24,26,46,47,63,75
Lung carcinoma, 207,287
Luteinizing hormones, 6
Lymphangiomas, 372
Lymph node, 35,141,144,161
Lymph node status, 222, 224,225
Lymphoblasts, 88
Lymphoblastic lymphoma, 97,120,132
Lymphocytic differentiation antigen (LDA),126
Lymphocytic lymphoma, 95
Lymphomas, 25, 27, 35, 37, 116,118,178,282,287
Lymphopenia, 155
Lymphoproliferative diseases 116,118
Lymphoreticular proliferation, 141,141
Lysosomal enzymes, 83,108
Lysozyme, 5, 25,27,295

M

Malignant fibrous histiocytoma 76, 363, 365, 370
Malignant histiocytosis, 106
Malignant lymphomas, 83, 188
Malignant melanoma, 35, 40, 42
Malignant mesothelial tumor, 297, 300
Malignant schwanoma, 43
Malignant transformation, 72
Mallory alcoholic hyaline bodies, 34
Mammary epithelial membrane antigen 349, 357
Mature teratoma, 322, 329
Mature thymocyte, 120
McCoy medium, 145
MC-5 (Fat globule membrane monoclonal Ab) 5, 210, 211, 212, 213, 219, 223, 224
MCF-7 cells, 216, 264, 265, 268, 269, 391, 392, 395
Medullary carcinoma, 48
Medullary carcinoma of thyroid 6, 25, 26, 184, 189, 190,
Melanin, 22
Melanin stimulating hormone, 175
Melanocytes, 75, 288, 289
Melanoma, 22, 25,26, 76, 281, 282, 287, 288, 308
Melanoma associated antigens, 289
Meningioma, 35, 188
Merkel cells, 181
Merkel cell tumors, 40
Mercury lamp, 390
Mesenchymal cell, 72
Mesenchymal chondrosarcoma, 363
Mesodermal cells, 72
Mesothelial cells, 43, 44
Mesothelial cells, reactive, 47
Mesothelial tumors, 24
Mesothelioma, 5,46,47,53
Metaplasia, 63
Metastatic carcinoma, 188
Methyl green, 87
Microfilaments, 73, 74, 75, 78
Micropapillary carcinoma, 236
Microspectrum analyzes, 237
Microtubules, 363
Milk fat globule antigen 25, 31, 43, 45, 46, 210, 217, 234, 244, 308
Mithramycin, 383
Mitotic Index 224, 225
Mitochondria, 204
Mixed (Large cell and small cleaved cell/B cell lymphoma),163
Mixed mesothelioma, 34
Monoclonal antibodies, 3, 12, 31, 207, 264, 300
    BA1,86,94,95,96,97,98
    BA2, 86,95
    BA3,86
    B1, 86,93,94,95,96,97,98
    B1:1,215, 218, 219, 220,223

B2 - 86,98
B4 - 86,97,
D547, 264
D58, 264
Fatty acid synthetase - 236, 237, 289, 240, 241, 242
HLADR (OKlal), 7,86,94,97,107
H222, 264
H226, 264
Ia, 85,97
J5, 85,92,119,120,124,125
LCA (Leukocytic Common Antigen) 31, 40, 41
Leu 1, 85,102
Leu 2,120,121,124,125,126,127,131
Leu 3, 85,120,124,125,126,127
Leu 4, 85,119,120,126,131
Leu 5, 120,124,125,127,131
Leu 7, 121,129
Leu 9, 124,126
Leu 10,129,131
Leu 11,121,129
Leu 15,121,129
Leu M3,120,129
Li, 120
LICR-LON-M8, 210, 212
LICR-LON M18, 209, 210, 212
LN-1, 25, 27, 129
LN-2, 22, 25, 27, 121,125,126,129
LN-3, 27,121,129,131
LyT, 83,84
MBr1 (Monoclonal Ab against breast), 308
M OV2(Monoclonal Ab against ovary), 308
MC1, 236, 237, 238, 239, 240, 241, 243, 244, 245, 251, 258, 260
MC5, 236, 237, 238, 239, 240, 241, 243, 244, 245, 251, 258, 260
OC-125, 300
OKB2, 7
OKB7, 7
OK1a1 (anti HLA DR), 7, 154
OKM1, 7
OKM5, 7
OKT1 (anti Leu1),7
OKT3, 7, 86,102,150,151,154,161
OKT4, 85,103,150,151,154,161
OKT5, 102
OKT6, 86,102
OKT8 (Leu 2),102,150,151,154,169
OKT9, 7, 86,120,121,125,127
OKT10, 7,85,99,120,121,125,127
OKT11,150,154,157,161
PCA1, 83,99
T101, 85
Monocytes, 7
Monocytic leukemia, 5
Mononuclear phagocytes (MP) 84,85,106
Mortality, 224
Mouse liver cells, 384

Mucin, 293
Mucinous cystoadenoma, 298
Mucinous ovarian carcinoma, 207
Mucinous prostatic carcinoma, 344
Mu chains, 147
Mucocutaneous candidiasis, 155
Multiple myeloma,99
Multiploid, 6
Muscle antigens, 365
Muscle cells, 6, 202
Muraminidase, 372
Mycosis fungoides,126,133
Myeloma, 25
Myeloid cells, 84,85
Myoepithelial cells,6,207,208
Myofibrils, 204
Myogenic cells, 73
Myoglobin, 6,300,365,380
Myosarcomas, 25, 27
Myosin, 6, 25, 27, 73, 207, 300, 363, 372

N

N-acethylgalactosamine, 351
Naphtol acetate,79
Natural killer cells,121,129
Neoplasia, 59, 60,63
Neural crest,40,284
Neural tissue antigens, 370
Neurilemomas, 25
Neuroblastoma, 178
Neuroectodermal cells, 72
Neuroendocrine carcinomas, 174
    Intermediate cell type, 174,176
    Small cell type, 174,176
    Well differentiated, 174,175,176,178
Neuroendocrine neoplasms, 174
Neuroendocrine tumors, 23,26
Neuroendoencrine skin carcinomas, 178
    Intermediate cell type 178,179
    Small cell type 178,180
    Trabecular type, 177, 178
Neurofilaments, 32, 73, 76,77,180,181,363
Neurogenic sarcoma, 363
Neuron, 75
Neuron specific enolase, 6, 26,175,177,180,191,192,304,308
Neurosecretory granules, 175,179
Neurotensin, 298
Non Hodgkin's lymphoma,88,129,162
Non Hodgkin's lymphoma t cell type,167,168
Non enzymatic dissociation, 381
Non oncocytic, 188
Non specific binding, 10
Non specific cancer antigen (NCA), 24

Non specific sterase, 106
Noradrenaline 191
Norepinephrine, 191
Normal tissues, 271
Normal values, 153
Nuclear grade, 345
Nuclear isolation medium, 383
Nucleated erythrocytes, 386
Nuclei isolation, 380
Nucleolus, 265
Null cells, 7,156
Null cell adenoma, 187
Null cell lymphoma, 129

O

Oat cell carcinoma, 34, 35
Odland bodies, 59
Oncocytic changes, 187
Oncogenes, 281
Osteoblasts, 75
Osteoclast activating factor, 103
Ovarian teratoma, 305
Ovarian tumors, 293, 294, 296, 298, 300
Ovary, 46, 47, 193, 295, 300
Oxytocin, 186

P

PAP complex, 13, 15
PAP method, 12
PAP monoclonal Ab, 10, 12, 17, 19
PAP technique, 175,177,180
Paget's disease, 5, 236,242,258,261
Pancreas, 24,75
Pancreatic islets, 184,198, 192
Pancreatic polypeptide, 298, 304
Paneth cells, 295
Pan T cells, 7
Pan T markers, 119
Papain, 151
Papillary bladder tumor, 288
Papillary carcinoma, 344, 346
Paraffin embedded, 151
Paraganglioma, 35
Parathyroid, 25, 185,191
Paratohormone, 25, 26
PAS reaction, 22
Patch work configuration, 208, 211, 216
Peanut agglutinin, 236, 341, 254
Peanut lectins, 349, 350
Peptide hormones, 298

Peripheral blood, 141,142,143,154
Peripheral T cells, 7,119,120,126,150
Peripheral T cell lymphomas, 103
Peroxidase, 84,85,107
Phagocytic assay, 84
Phenotype, 124
Pheochromocytoma, 190, 191, 308
Phorbol ester (TPA), 95
Phosphatase, 17, 18, 19
Phosphorylation, 12, 14, 18
Pituitary adenomas, 184
Pituitary anterior 185, 186
Pituitary oncocytoma, 187
Pituitary posterior, 185, 186
Placenta, 272
Placental antigens, 295
Placental lactogen, 5,6
Placental like alkaline phosphatase, 297, 303
Placental, proteins, 5
Plasma cells, 120
Plasmocytoid lymphoma,130
Plasmocytomas, 41
Platelets, 7
Pleural effusion, 141,143,153,159,160,391
Pneumocystic cariini pneumonia, 156
Pokeweed mitogen (PWM),172
Polar body, 251, 252, 253
Polyembryoma, 322
Polypeptide hormones, 202
Poorly differentiated lymphoma B type, 155,156,160,163,164
Poutrier microabscesses, 104
Pre B acute lymphocytic leukemia,120,125
Pre B cell acute lymphoblastic leukemia,92,93
Pre Pre-B-leukemia,120,121,125
5regnancy specific globulin (SP1) 323, 325
Preneoplasia, 59, 60
Prepropeptide, 202
Prostate, 193
Prostate specific antigen 6, 8, 339, 341, 342, 343, 344, 345, 346, 347, 348, 349
Pseudolumina, 248, 250
Progesterone, 193, 306
Progesterone receptor, 270, 301
Prolactin, 6, 187
Proliferating cells, 7
Proliferation index, 393
Propidium iodide, 383
Propiomelanocortin, 187, 188, 191
Prostate, 25, 26, 46, 75, 337, 350, 389
Prostate acid phosphatase, 6, 8, 337, 341, 342, 343, 344, 345, 346, 347, 348, 349
Prostatic carcinoma, 6
Prostatic specific acid phosphatase, 24, 25, 26
Prostate specific antigen, 24, 25, 26
Protein A gold method, 4

Protein S100, 31,41, 50,51
Proximal Tubules, 285
Pulmonary Carcinoma, 300
Pylorus, 295

Q

Quality control, 9

R

Receptor poor, 265, 266
Receptor Rich, 265, 266
Records, 9
Recurrence, 224, 225
Recurrent herpes genitalis, 155
Reed Sternberg cells, 109,133,137
Renal Carcinoma, 34, 283, 286, 287
Renin Release, 205
Repeated infections, 155
Reticulum cells, 105
Reticulin stain, 293
Rhabdomyosarcoma, 21, 28, 39, 42, 75, 79, 363, 365, 370
Rhodamine, 147
Ribonuclease, 383, 384
RNA, 353, 383, 384
Rosettes, 119
Roswell Park Memorial Institute (R.P.M.I),172
Rough endoplasmic reticulum,202
Russel bodies, 136

S

Sarcomas, 5, 22, 282
Schwann cells, 370
Schwanomas, 25,42,76
Schwartz-Bartter syndrome, 207, 208, 213
Sclerosing adenosis, 207, 208, 213
Sclerosing hemangioma, 377
Seborrheic keratosis, 62
Second antibodies, 13
Secretin, 288, 304
Secretory granules, 187
Seminomas, 34, 35, 37, 38, 322, 331, 333
Sensitivity, 13, 14
Serotonin, 128,175,
Serous carcinoma of ovary, 309
Serous ovarian neoplastic amylase (SONA), 297
Serous Papillary cystoadenoma, 300
Sertoli cells, 321
Sertoli cell tumor, 6
Sertoli-leydig cell tumors, 294, 295, 308
17, B Estradiol, 64
Sex cord stromal tumor, 245, 306, 321

Sexual precocity, 302
Sezary syndrome 102,103
Sheep red blood cell receptor (lyt 3),85
Sheep erythrocytes, 119
Sinus macraphages, 121
Skeletal muscle, 75
Skin, 33, 51, 61, 63, 175,177,214,272
Small cell carcinoma of lung, 193
Small cell non cleaved lymphomas,121
Small lymphocytic leukemia, 94,95
Small lymphocytic lymphoma 120,130
Small lymphocytic T cell type, 169
Smooth muscle, 75
Snap-freezing, 41
Sodium hydroxide, 10
Soft tissue tumors,362
Solid tissues, 281
Somatoliberin, 186, 192, 194
Somatostatin, 5, 184, 191, 192, 195, 298, 304, 305
Somatotrophs, 187
S100 protein, 6, 25,187,308,370
SP1 glycoprotein, 5, 219, 221, 222, 223, 224
Specific red blood cell adherence, 352
Specimen collection, 142
Spermatocytic seminoma, 322
Spindle cell carcinoma, 38
Spindle cell melanoma, 51, 52
Spinous layer, 62
Squamous cell carcinoma, 21, 22, 23, 25, 34, 62, 64
Squamous differentiation, 300
Stem cells, 176
Steroid producing endocrine tissues, 185, 193
Stomach, 24, 46
Strumal carcinoid, 304
Suppresor T cells, 7,107
Suppressor cytotoxic T cells, 150
Surface immunoglobulins, 84,93,94,95,96,102,132,147,152
Survival, 392, 395
Synciotrophoblast, 303, 346
Synovial sarcoma, 34, 38, 39, 365

T

T antigens, 120, 352
T cells, 21,120,121
T cell chronic lymphocytic leukemia, 100,142
T cell growth factor (TCGF), 98
T cell leukemia, 41,99
TdT (terminal deoxynucleotidil transferase),82,93,97,99,103,125,
146,150,157,161
2 methyl butane, 88
27K protein, 276
28K protein, 268, 269, 272, 273, 274, 276
Tartrate resistant acid phosphatase (TRAP) 84,85,98
Teratocarcinoma, 287, 324

Teratoma, 303, 322, 324
Testosterone, 6
Testicular tumors, 321
Testis, 193
Theca cells, 321
Teca cell tumors, 6
Thecomas, 306
Thomson-Friedenreich, 352
Thymic carcinoids, 193
Thymocytes, 7,150
Thymoma, 33, 37, 120
Thymus, 33, 191
Thyroglobulin, 6, 25, 26, 189, 190, 304, 305
Thyroid, 25, 26, 75, 185, 189, 305
Thyroid adenoma, 6
Thyroid follicular cells, 189
Thyroid stimulating hormone 6
Thyroliberin,192
Thyrotrophs, 187
Thyroxine, 191
Tissue sections,116,118
Tonofilaments, 59
Transitional cell carcinoma, 26, 26, 281, 286, 287, 288, 299, 244
Transferrin, 303
Transglutaminase, 60
Triiodothyronine, 191
Triton tumor, 365
Trypsin, 10, 17, 18, 19, 151
Trypsinization, 24
Tuberculosis, 155
Tubulin, 73
Tumor associated antigens, 207, 216, 281

U

Ultrastructural immunocytochemistry, 4
Undifferentiated non lymphoid tumors, 169
Undifferentiated carcinomas, 344
Unlabeled immunoperoxidase, 116
Urachal adenocarcinoma, 354
Ureter, 75
Urinary bladder, 75, 285
Urothelium, 285
Uterus human, 265
Uterus rabbit, 265

V

Vagina, 64, 272
Vasoactive agents, 202, 205
Vasointestinal polypeptide, 5, 175, 191
Vasopressin, 186, 194
Verrucous carcinoma, 68
Viability 142,144
Vimentin, 32, 72, 73, 74, 75, 76, 77, 80, 176, 299, 303, 307

Virilization, 302

W

Waldenstrom's macroglubulinemia, 94
Well-differentiated lymphocytic lymphoma, 147
Well-differentiated B cell lymphomas, 163,164,165
Wright-Giemsa, 87,101,117,143,145

Y

Yolk sac elements, 302, 303
Yolk sac tumors, 322, 324, 325, 328, 331, 335

Z

Zenker's fixative, 66, 151
Zollinger Ellison syndrone,192, 299

www.ingramcontent.com/pod-product-compliance
Ingram Content Group UK Ltd.
Pitfield, Milton Keynes, MK11 3LW, UK
UKHW020237160926
475610UK00001B/27
9781461296362